Radiographic Pathology
for Technologists

W9-CCA-192

Radiographic Pathology for Technologists

James D. Mace, MBA, RT (R)
Senior Director—Professional Services
Riverside Methodist Hospitals
Columbus, Ohio

Nina Kowalczyk, MS, RT (R)
Associate Director—Radiology
The Ohio State University Hospitals
Columbus, Ohio

Third Edition

with 496 *illustrations*

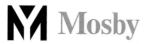

St. Louis   Baltimore   Boston   Chicago   Naples   New York   Philadelphia   Portland   London
Madrid   Mexico City   Singapore   Sydney   Tokyo   Toronto   Wiesbaden

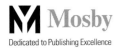

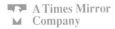

Publisher: Don E. Ladig
Senior Editor: Jeanne Rowland
Senior Developmental Editors: Lisa Potts, Carolyn Kruse
Project Manager: Mark Spann
Production Editor: Julie Eddy
Book Design Manager: Judi Lang
Manufacturing Manager: Betty Mueller

THIRD EDITION

Copyright 1998 by Mosby–Year Book, Inc.
A Mosby imprint of Mosby–Year Book, Inc.
Previous editions copyrighted 1988, 1994

Composition by Graphic World, Inc.
Printed by Maple-Vail Book Manufacturing Group
Printed in the United States of America

Mosby–Year Book, Inc.
11830 Westline Industrial Drive
St. Louis, Missouri 63146

Library of Congress Cataloging-in-Publication Data
Mace, James D.
    Radiographic pathology for technologists / James D. Mace,   Nina
    Kowalczyk.—3rd ed.
        p.   cm.
    Rev. ed. of: Radiographic pathology for technologists, 2nd ed.,
c1994.
    Includes bibliographical references and index.
    ISBN 0-8151-4568-3
    1. Diagnosis, Radioscopic.   2. Diagnostic imaging.   3. Pathology.
    4. Radiologic technologists.   I. Kowalczyk, Nina.   II. Mace, James
    D.   Radiologic pathology for technologists.   III. Title.
    [DNLM: 1. Pathology—methods.   2. Radiography—methods.   QZ 4
    M141r   1997]
    RC78.M185   1997
    616.07'57—dc21
    DNLM/DLC   97-23176
    for Library of Congress   CIP

98 99 00 01 02 / 9 8 7 6 5 4 3 2 1

Dedicated to David W. Mace,
a good man fallen far before his time.

Preface

It is our sincere hope that radiography instructors and students found the first two editions of this textbook helpful in enhancing their appreciation of radiography as an art as much as a science. We believe the revision and expansion of this, our third edition, furthers that goal. With each edition, this enhancement becomes a bit more difficult. Certainly there are new treatments, new modalities to visualize disease, and improved results—these are all covered inside. The trickiness is to continually improve, yet not disturb, a format our readers like; additions and changes were needed and add more than just extra pages.

We think you'll like the changes in the third edition. Our intention was to improve the quality of the product while making it simpler to use. We have expanded the text to augment and clarify information, as well as added a number of new illustrations to more comprehensively represent the pathologies discussed. Additionally, key terms for each chapter have been highlighted in advance so readers can focus on the main ideas as they move through the material. Open-ended questions have been added to the multiple-choice questions so that more critical-thinking skills can be applied. Finally, traumatic conditions have been consolidated into a chapter of their own to allow a better appreciation of the multisystem impact of trauma. We believe this approach and the revisions contained within this edition will meet with your satisfaction.

Certainly, instructors have a variety of choices for how to approach a course in radiographic pathology. They are aided by textbooks of varying levels of complexity, directed to a wide variety of audiences. Some use their own teaching files of actual radiographs or those purchased commercially—perhaps on CD ROM. Course length varies from a few weeks to several months. Some programs teach pathology at the beginning, some weave it throughout the course, and others present it toward the end of the students' experience. It is clear that no one methodology to teach this subject matter is applied universally.

Because of that, educators have preferences. Thankfully, there are a lot of options to satisfy those preferences, including our textbook. And, of course, we have our own ideas about the place of radiographic pathology in a student's education. We believe this text best serves the radiography student who has had previous anatomy and physiology experience. Because of the need for so much up-front technical knowledge, this course is often deferred to the latter part of a student's program. That may be for the best, anyway, as students' on-the-floor experiences begin to transform their sheer concentration on not making a mistake to more critical thinking about *why* they're doing their job.

That's where we want our students' attention focused. Thinking about why they're doing what they are will help them become better technologists. All modalities now offer more latitude than ever in determining how the image is represented for interpretation. The continued evolution of computer technology and its entrance in all parts of imaging open a wide variety of possibilities. Having some sense of what disease looks like, how it might have originated, and what prognosis the patient has can only help the technologist portray the given condition in an optimal fashion. This, in turn, elevates the ability of the technologist in detection, prevention, and treatment of disease—a goal in which we all believe strongly. It is our sincere hope that you'll find our textbook useful in this endeavor.

James D. Mace
Nina Kowalczyk

Acknowledgments

Each year we seem to get busier, making it more difficult for us to do projects like this. As with the prior two editions, we could not have completed the book without a great team of people around us who wanted this text to be successful and accomplish its primary mission. First and foremost, we thank our spouses, Cheryl and Doug, for going on without us at the most inopportune moments as a deadline from our publisher was coming. Their support is, in large part, why we succeeded. Also, a huge thanks goes to Mosby as well, for their unending patience, and particularly to Lisa Potts, who coaxed and cajoled us through this effort despite our protestations about how busy we were. We clearly couldn't have done it without her.

Our sincere gratitude is extended to our physician reviewers: Rebecca Gibbons, M.D., and Greg Gibbons, M.D. Their thorough reviews have once again helped improve the quality of the text—particularly its accuracy. As former educators, we both know how important accuracy is. The assistance of both Becky and Greg was invaluable, and we appreciate, too, their willingness to fit us in with their family obligations and busy medical practices. As with the previous two editions, other physicians were helpful as well. These include Phil Shaffer, M.D., Bill Wiand, D.O., Geoff Wiot, M.D., Mark Alfonso, M.D., Bill Briggs, M.D., and Peter Pema, M.D. We thank them for their help in procuring images as well as in lending guidance to text development.

As with the last edition, our images come from a variety of fine organizations who are to be thanked for graciously allowing us to use their material. They include the American College of Radiology, as well as Riverside Methodist Hospitals, Grant Medical Center, The Ohio State University Hospitals, and Children's Hospital—all located in Columbus, Ohio. Much credit, too, goes to our photographer, Grant Arthur of Riverside Methodist Hospitals. The artistry of his photography will hopefully show up in improved image quality throughout this new edition.

Also, there were a number of technologists, sonographers, and others who contributed images to this text; they include Jeff Bradley, RDMS, Shelley

Wheeler, RDMS, Cindy Burns, R.T., Meg Reis, R.N., Karla Rusk, R.N., and Scott Rossmiller, R.T. If we've left anyone out, forgive us. Thanks to all. One technologist, in particular, deserves special recognition for his efforts. Ken Goodwin, editorial research consultant, went to great lengths to produce the best example of a given condition as well as ran errands ad nauseam, and all with a smile on his face! We simply couldn't have done this text without his significant help.

As in the prior edition, it simply wouldn't be fair not to give credit to those who inspired us many years ago to take on difficult tasks like this, not for personal gain but for the betterment of our profession. Bill Finney and Phil Ballinger (retired) of the School of Allied Medical Professions at The Ohio State University have been friends of ours for a long time and really great role models for us both. We are truly grateful for their ongoing encouragement and support.

Finally, our own students from years past have served as a source of inspiration who helped get this project going initially. All of those from our prior lives as teachers of radiologic technology at Providence Hospital in Sandusky, Ohio; Riverside Methodist Hospitals in Columbus, Ohio; and The Ohio State University in Columbus, Ohio have played at least some small role in this production and its predecessors. Hopefully, texts such as ours contribute to their development and play a role in appreciating the art, as well as science, of radiography. Thanks to all!

James D. Mace
Nina Kowalczyk

Reviewers

M. Elia Flores, MEd, RT (R)
Program Director
Radiologic Technology Program
Blinn College
Bryan, Texas

Diane Gronefeld, MEd, RT (R)
Associate Professor
Radiologic Technology Program
Northern Kentucky University
Highland Heights, Kentucky

Steven G. Hayes, Jr., RT (R)
Radiologic Technology Instructor
USAF
Sheppard Air Force Base
Wichita Falls, Texas

Steven G. Hayes, Sr., BSRT, MEd, RT (R)
Formerly Assistant Professor
Department of Radiologic Technology
Midwestern State University
Wichita Falls, Texas

Edna Jones-Holmes, RT (R), ARRT
Director
Radiologic Technology Program
Lake Michigan College
Benton Harbor, Michigan

Bette Schans, MS, RT (R)
Program Director
Assistant Professor
Radiologic Technology Program
Mesa State College
Grand Junction, Colorado

Contents

1 Introduction to Pathology   1

Pathologic Terms   2
Disease Classifications   6

2 The Skeletal System   12

Anatomy and Physiology Review   13
Imaging Considerations   16
Congenital and Hereditary Diseases   17
Inflammatory Disease   22
Metabolic Disease   30
Vertebral Column   34
Neoplastic Disease   35

3 The Respiratory System   45

Anatomy and Physiology Review   46
Imaging Considerations   46
Chest Tubes, Vascular Access Lines, and Catheters   57
Congenital and Hereditary Diseases   60
Inflammatory Diseases   61
Neoplastic Diseases   74

4 The Abdomen and Gastrointestinal System   78

Anatomy and Physiology Review   79
Imaging Considerations   82
Congenital and Hereditary Anomalies   91
Inflammatory Diseases   94
Esophageal Varices   102
Degenerative Diseases   104
Bowel Obstructions   107

Neurogenic Diseases   110
Diverticular Diseases   111
Neoplastic Diseases   114

5   The Hepatobiliary System   120

Anatomy and Physiology Review   121
Imaging Considerations   123
Inflammatory Diseases   128
Metabolic Diseases   133
Neoplastic Diseases   133

6   The Urinary System   138

Anatomy and Physiology Review   139
Imaging Considerations   140
Congenital and Hereditary Diseases   146
Inflammatory Diseases   152
Degenerative and Metabolic Disease   155
Neoplastic Diseases   159

7   The Reproductive System   166

The Female Reproductive System   167
The Male Reproductive System   182

8   The Cardiovascular System   189

Anatomy and Physiology Review   190
Imaging Considerations   193
Congenital and Hereditary Diseases   203
Valvular Disease   206
Congestive Heart Failure   207
Degenerative Diseases   208
Aneurysms   213
Venous Thrombosis   214

9   The Hemopoietic System   217

Anatomy and Physiology Review   218
Imaging Considerations   220
Acquired Immune Deficiency Syndrome   222
Neoplastic Disease   223

10   The Central Nervous System   227

Anatomy and Physiology Review   228
Imaging Considerations   231
Congenital and Hereditary Diseases   235
Inflammatory Diseases   238
Degenerative Diseases   240

11   Traumatic Disease   255

Introduction   256
Trauma of the Vertebral Column and Head   258
Skeletal Trauma   266
Trauma of the Chest and Thorax   283
Abdominal Trauma   287

Answer Key   290
Glossary   292
Bibliography   311
Index   313

Introduction to Pathology

Pathologic Terms
    Monitoring disease trends
    Health care resources
Disease Classifications
    Congenital and hereditary disease
    Inflammatory disease

Degenerative disease
Metabolic disease
Traumatic disease
Neoplastic disease
    The staging of cancer
Conclusion

Upon completion of Chapter 1, the reader should be able to:

- Define common terminology associated with the study of disease.

- Differentiate between signs and symptoms.

- Distinguish between a disease diagnosis and its prognosis.

- Describe the different types of disease classifications.

- Cite characteristics that distinguish benign from malignant neoplasms.

- Describe the system used to stage malignant tumors.

- Identify the difference in origin for carcinoma and sarcoma.

KEY TERMS

Disease	Acute	Hereditary
Pathogenesis	Chronic	Inflammatory
Symptom	Diagnosis	Degenerative
Sign	Prognosis	Metabolism
Syndrome	Epidemiology	Traumatic
Etiology	Mortality rate	Neoplastic
Nosocomial	Morbidity rate	Benign neoplasm
Iatrogenic	Congenital	Malignant neoplasm

Pathology is basically the study of disease. Many types of disease exist, and, in general, many conditions can be readily demonstrated radiographically. The radiography student who wants to better understand specific pathologic conditions must first have a working knowledge of common pathologic terms. This chapter serves as a brief introduction to terms associated with pathology.

PATHOLOGIC TERMS

Any abnormal disturbance of the function or structure of the human body as a result of some type of injury is called a **disease.** After injury, **pathogenesis** occurs. This refers to the sequence of events producing cellular changes that ultimately lead to observable changes known as *manifestations*. These manifestations can display in a variety of fashions. A **symptom** refers to the patient's perception of the disease. Symptoms are subjective, and only the patient can identify these manifestations. For example, a headache is considered a symptom. A **sign** is an objective manifestation that can be detected by the physician during examination. Fever, swelling, and skin rash are all considered signs. A group of signs and symptoms that character-

izes a specific abnormal disturbance is a **syndrome.** However, some disease processes, especially in the early stages, do not produce symptoms and are termed *asymptomatic*.

Etiology is the study of the cause of a disease. In addition to the normal agents that can cause disease (e.g., viruses, bacteria, trauma, heat), a number of other causes are known. Proper infection control practices are important in a health care environment to prevent **nosocomial** disease. Staph infection following hip replacement surgery is an example of a nosocomial disease, that is, one acquired from the environment. The etiology of the disease in this case could be poor infection-control practices. **Iatrogenic** reactions are those adverse responses that occur from medical treatment itself (e.g., a collapsed lung that occurs in response to a complication that arises in arterial line placement). If no causative factor can be identified, the disease is termed *idiopathic*.

The length of time over which the disease is displayed may vary. **Acute** diseases usually have a quick onset and last a short period of time, whereas a **chronic** disease may present more slowly and last a very long time. An example of an acute disease is pneumonia, whereas multiple sclerosis is considered a chronic condition.

Two additional terms refer to the identification and outcome of a disease. A **diagnosis** is the name of a disease an individual is believed to have, and the prediction of the course and outcome of the disease is called a **prognosis.**

Government agencies compile statistics annually regarding the incidence, or rate of occurrence, of disease (Table 1-1). **Epidemiology** is the investigation of disease in large groups. The *prevalence* of a given disease refers to the number of cases found in a given population. The *incidence* of disease refers to the number of new cases found in a given time period. Diseases of high prevalence in an area where a given causative organism is commonly found are said to be *endemic* to that area. For example, histoplasmosis is a fungal disease of the respiratory system endemic to the Ohio and Mississippi River valleys. It is not uncommon to see a relatively high prevalence of it in these areas. Its appearance in great numbers in the far west, however, could represent an epidemic.

Monitoring Disease Trends

The **mortality rate** is the number of deaths caused by a particular disease averaged over a population. One common mortality rate monitored by governmental health agencies is the infant mortality rate. In 1992, the infant mortality rate was 8.5 deaths per 1000 live births. In addition, the U.S. Department of Health and Human Services monitors and reports mortality rates in terms of leading causes of death, according to sex, race, age, and specific causes of death such as heart disease or breast cancer. Trends in these mortality patterns are identified and tracked to help identify necessary interventions. For instance, the age-adjusted death rate for heart disease (the leading cause of death in both sexes in the United States) has demonstrated a downward trend since the 1970s and declined 29% between 1980 and 1992. This decline is due

in part to health education and changes in lifestyle behaviors.

The incidence of sickness sufficient to interfere with an individual's normal daily routine is referred to as the **morbidity rate.** One agency responsible for trending morbidity rates is the Center for Disease Control (CDC). It is fairly easy to obtain accurate data concerning the mortality rate of a specific population, but somewhat more difficult to obtain accurate data about the morbidity rate. This information comes primarily from physicians and other health care workers reporting morbidity statistics and information to the various governmental and private agencies.

Health Care Resources

Over the past decade, there have been major changes in the delivery of health care. Since the early 1990s, the use of ambulatory care centers has greatly increased, especially among the elderly. The type of ambulatory care center varies from hospital outpatient and emergency departments to physicians' offices. In response to this shift, emphasis has been placed on increasing the numbers of physician generalists including family practitioners, internal medicine physicians, and pediatricians. Inpatient services and hospital length of stay have continued to decline, averaging less than 5.9 days.

The cost associated with health care in the United States is staggering. In 1992, U.S. health spending accounted for a larger share of gross domestic product (GDP) than in any other major industrialized country. In 1993, U.S. health care expenditures totaled $884.2 billion and comprised 18.6% of total federal government expenditures. This equates to approximately $3,299 per U.S. citizen. Emphasis on wellness and disease prevention must continue to help reduce these costs. Studies have shown it is much more cost-effective to provide preventive care than to wait until a disease has progressed. One good example of this trend is the emphasis placed on mammography in the

Table 1–1   Deaths, Death Rates, and Percent of Total Deaths for the 10 Leading Causes of Death, 1993

Age and Rank Order	Cause of Death	Deaths
	1993	
Under 1 Year		
	All causes	33,466
1	Congenital anomalies	7,129
2	Sudden infant death syndrome	4,669
3	Disorders relating to short gestation and unspecified low birthweight	4,310
4	Respiratory distress syndrome	1,815
5	Newborn affected by maternal complications of pregnancy	1,343
6	Newborn affected by complications of placenta, cord, and membranes	994
7	Unintentional injuries	898
8	Infections specific to the perinatal period	772
9	Intrauterine hypoxia and birth asphyxia	549
10	Pneumonia and influenza	530
1-4 years		
	All causes	7,066
1	Unintentional injuries	2,590
2	Congenital anomalies	804
3	Malignant neoplasms	522
4	Homicide and legal intervention	464
5	Diseases of heart	296
6	Human immunodeficiency virus infection	204
7	Pneumonia and influenza	182
8	Certain conditions originating in the perinatal period	100
9	Septicemia	96
10	Benign neoplasms	77
5-14 years		
	All causes	8,658
1	Unintentional injuries	3,466
2	Malignant neoplasms	1,089
3	Homicide and legal intervention	656
4	Congenital anomalies	485
5	Suicide	321
6	Diseases of heart	303
7	Human immunodeficiency virus infection	155
8	Chronic obstructive pulmonary diseases	138
9	Pneumonia and influenza	135
10	Cerebrovascular diseases	79

NOTES: For data years shown, the code numbers for cause of death are based on the *International Classification of Diseases, Ninth Revision,* described in Appendix II, Table V. Categories for the coding and classification of human immunodeficiency virus infection were introduced in the United States beginning with mortality data for 1987.

Table 1–1 Deaths, Death Rates, and Percent of Total Deaths for the 10 Leading Causes of Death, 1993—cont'd

Age and Rank Order	1993	
	Cause of Death	Deaths
15-24 years		
	All causes	.35,483
1	Unintentional injuries	.13,966
2	Homicide and legal intervention	.8,424
3	Suicide	.4,849
4	Malignant neoplasms	.1,738
5	Diseases of heart	.981
6	Human immunodeficiency virus infection	.609
7	Congenital anomalies	.472
8	Pneumonia and influenza	.251
9	Cerebrovascular diseases	.208
10	Chronic obstructive pulmonary diseases	.206
25-44 years		
	All causes	.155,683
1	Unintentional injuries	.27,277
2	Human immunodeficiency virus infection	.27,228
3	Malignant neoplasms	.21,834
4	Diseases of heart	.16,660
5	Suicide	.12,477
6	Homicide and legal intervention	.11,815
7	Chronic liver disease and cirrhosis	.4,477
8	Cerebrovascular diseases	.3,316
9	Diabetes mellitus	.2,299
10	Pneumonia and influenza	.2,275
45-64 years		
	All causes	.373,396
1	Malignant neoplasms	.133,057
2	Diseases of heart	.104,722
3	Cerebrovascular diseases	.14,682
4	Unintentional injuries	.14,434
5	Chronic obstructive pulmonary diseases	.13,165
6	Diabetes mellitus	.10,927
7	Chronic liver disease and cirrhosis	.10,316
8	Human immunodeficiency virus infection	.8,330
9	Suicide	.7,229
10	Pneumonia and influenza	.5,583

SOURCES: Centers for Disease Control and Prevention, National Center for Health Statistics: Vital Statistics of the United States, Vol. II, Mortality, Part A, for data years 1980 and 1992. Public Health Service. Washington. U.S. Government Printing Office; Data computed by the Division of Health and Utilization Analysis from data compiled by the Division of Vital Statistics.

National Center for Health Statistics, Health, United States, 1994, 1995, Hyattsville, Maryland, Public Health Service.

Continued

Table 1–1 Deaths, Death Rates, and Percent of Total Deaths for the 10 Leading Causes of Death, 1993—cont'd

	1993	
Age and Rank Order	Cause of Death	Deaths
65 years and over		
	All causes	1,654,294
1	Diseases of heart	619,755
2	Malignant neoplasms	371,549
3	Cerebrovascular diseases	131,551
4	Chronic obstructive pulmonary diseases	86,425
5	Pneumonia and influenza	73,853
6	Diabetes mellitus	40,502
7	Unintentional injuries	27,784
8	Nephritis, nephrotic syndrome, and nephrosis	19,743
9	Septicemia	16,846
10	Atherosclerosis	16,460

management of breast disease. The percentage of women 50 years of age or older having routine mammograms more than doubled between 1987 and 1993, again in part because of aggressive health education programs.

DISEASE CLASSIFICATIONS

Diseases can be grouped into several broad categories. Those in the same category may not necessarily be closely related, but groupings such as those discussed in the following tend to produce lesions that are similar in *morphology,* that is, their form and structure. Pathologies discussed in this text are generally grouped into classifications of

1. Congenital and hereditary
2. Inflammatory
3. Degenerative
4. Metabolic
5. Traumatic
6. Neoplastic

Congenital and Hereditary Disease

Diseases that are present at birth and result from genetic or environmental factors are termed **congenital.** It is estimated that 2% to 3% of all live births show one or more congenital abnormalities, although some of these may not be visible until a year or so after birth. A major category of congenital diseases is due to abnormalities in the number and distribution of chromosomes. In somatic cells (those other than germ cells), chromosomes exist in the nucleus of each cell in pairs, with one member from the male parent and the other from the female parent. In humans, chromosomes are normally composed of 22 pairs of autosomes (those other than the sex chromosomes) and 1 pair of sex chromosomes. Down syndrome is a congenital condition caused by an autosomal mitosis error, leading to an extra twenty-first chromosome so that the affected individual has 47 chromosomes rather than the normal 46.

Hereditary diseases are caused by developmental disorders genetically transmitted from either parent to child through abnormalities of individual genes in chromosomes and are derived from ancestors. For example, hemophilia is a well-known hereditary disease in which proper blood clotting is absent. A genetic abnormality present on the sex chromosome is a sex-linked inheritance; those on one of the other 22 chromosomes is an autosomal inheritance. The inherited disease may be dominant (transmitted by a single gene from either parent) or recessive (transmitted by both parents to an offspring). Amniocentesis, typically guided by ultrasound, is a standard procedure used prenatally to assess the presence of certain hereditary disorders.

A congenital defect is not necessarily hereditary, because it may have been acquired in utero. Intrauterine injury during a critical point in development can occur from maternal infections, radiation, or drugs. Abnormalities of this type occur sporadically and cannot generally be recognized before birth. However, their likelihood is greatly lessened by following proper precautions against infection, avoiding radiation (particularly during the early term of pregnancy), and avoiding of drugs or agents not specifically recognized by a physician as safe.

Inflammatory Disease

An **inflammatory** disease results from the body's reaction to a localized injurious agent. Types of inflammatory diseases include infective diseases, which result from invasion by microorganisms such as viruses, bacteria, or fungi; toxic diseases, which result from poisoning by biologic substances; and allergic diseases, which are an overreaction of the body's own defenses. Pneumonia is a type of inflammatory disease.

Some diseases in this classification are considered *autoimmune disorders.* Under normal conditions, antibodies are formed in response to foreign antigens. In certain diseases, however, they form against and injure the patient's own tissues. These are known as autoantibodies, and diseases associated with them are autoimmune disorders. Rheumatoid arthritis is an example of an autoimmune disorder.

An inflammatory reaction (i.e., inflammation) is a generalized pathologic process that is nonspecific to the agent causing the injury. The body's purpose in creating an inflammatory

reaction is to localize the injurious agent and prepare for subsequent repair and healing of the injured tissues. Substances released from the damaged tissues can cause both local and systemic effects (Fig. 1-1). Those effects seen local to the injury include capillary dilatation to allow fluids and leukocytes, specifically, to infiltrate into the area of damage. Cellular *necrosis* (death) is common to acute inflammation, and the leukocytes serve to remove the dead material through phagocytosis. The characteristics of such acute inflammation include heat, redness of skin, swelling, pain, and some loss of function as the body tends to protect the injured part. If the inflammatory process is significant, system effects such as an elevation of body temperature become evident.

Chronic inflammation differs from that of the acute stage in that damage caused by an injurious agent may not necessarily result in tissue death. In fact, necrosis is relatively uncommon in cases of chronic inflammation. It differs also in the duration of the inflammation, with chronic conditions lasting for long periods. Certain conditions discussed in this text evidence chronic inflammation (e.g., pulmonary emphysema as described in Chapter 3).

The repair of tissues damaged from an inflammatory process attempts to return the body to normal. Tissue regeneration is the process in which damaged tissues are replaced by new tissues that are essentially identical to those replaced. While this is the most desirable type of repair, tissues vary in their ability to replace themselves. Damaged nerve cells, for example, are not likely to readily regenerate. Fibrous connective tissue repair is the alternative to regeneration, but it is less desirable because it leads to scarring and fibrosis. Damaged tissues are replaced by a scar and lack the structure and function of the original tissue.

Debridement (removal of dead cells and materials) is an essential component of the healing process. It may be accomplished at both the cellular level and through human intervention, as in the case of burns or removal of foreign objects such as glass. The repair process begins with the migration of adjacent cells into the injured area and replication of the cells via mitosis to fill the void in the tissue. This new growth includes capillaries, fibroblasts, collagen, and elastic fibers. Remodeling of the new tissue, the last phase in the healing process, occurs in response to normal use of the tissue. For instance, remodeling of the bone following a skeletal fracture may take months, but the results often return the injured bone to its original contour.

Infection refers to an inflammatory process caused by a disease-causing organism. Under favorable conditions, the invading pathogenic agent multiplies and causes injurious effects. Generally, localized infection is usually accompanied by inflammation, but inflammation can occur without infection. *Virulence* refers to the ease with which an organism can overcome body defenses. An organism with high virulence is likely to produce progressive disease in susceptible persons; one of low virulence can pro-

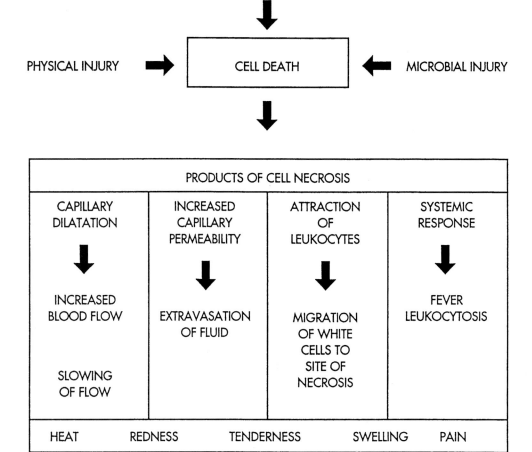

Fig. **1-1** Local and systemic effects of cell necrosis induced by various agents. (From Crowley LV: *Introductory concepts in pathology,* Chicago, 1972, Mosby.)

duce disease only in highly susceptible persons under favorable conditions.

Degenerative Disease

Degenerative diseases are caused by a deterioration of the body. Although they are usually associated with the aging process, some degenerative conditions may exist in younger patients. For instance, an individual may develop a degenerative disease following a traumatic injury, regardless of age.

The process of aging results from the gradual maturation of physiologic processes that reach a peak, then gradually fade (i.e., degenerate) to a point where the body can no longer survive. Heredity, diet, and environmental factors are known to affect the rate of aging. Over time, the functional abilities of tissues decrease because either their cell numbers are reduced or the function of each individual cell declines, with both typically participating in pathologies resulting from aging. Atherosclerosis, osteoporosis, and osteoarthritis are three diseases commonly associated with the aging process. Each is discussed later in this text.

Metabolic Disease

Metabolism is the sum of all physical and chemical processes in the body. Diseases caused by a disturbance of the normal physiologic function of the body are classified as metabolic diseases. These include endocrine disorders (e.g., diabetes and hyperparathyroidism) and disturbances of fluid and electrolyte balance.

Endocrine glands secrete their product (hormones) into the bloodstream to regulate various metabolic functions. The major endocrine glands include the pituitary, thyroid, parathyroids, adrenal glands, pancreatic islets, ovaries, and testes. An endocrine disorder may consist of hypersecretion, causing an overactivity of the target organ, or insufficient secretion, resulting in underactivity. The clinical effects of endocrine disturbance depend on the degree of dysfunction and the age and sex of the individual.

Dehydration is the most common disturbance of fluid balance. It is due to insufficient intake of water or excessive loss of it. Electrolytes are mineral salts (most commonly sodium and potassium) dissolved in the body's water. Depletion of them may occur because of vomiting, diarrhea, or use of diuretics (substances that promote the excretion of salt and water). Disturbance of either the fluid or electrolyte balances upset homeostasis, the body's normal internal resting state.

Traumatic Disease

Another general classification of diseases is **traumatic.** These diseases may result from mechanical forces such as crushing or twisting of a body part or from the effects of ionizing radiation on the human body. In addition, disorders resulting from extreme hot or cold temperatures, such as burns and frostbite, are also classified as traumatic.

Trauma may injure a bone, resulting in fractures, which are covered extensively in Chapter 11. It may also injure soft tissues. A wound is an injury of soft parts associated with rupture of the skin. Traumatic injuries may injure soft tissues even if the skin is not broken. Bleeding into the tissue spaces as a result of capillary rupture is known as a bruise or contusion.

Neoplastic Disease

Neoplastic disease results in new, abnormal tissue growth. Normally, growing and maturing cells are subject to mechanisms that control their growth rate. When this control mechanism goes awry, an overgrowth of cells develops, resulting in a neoplasm. *Lesion* is a term used to describe the many types of cellular change that can occur in response to disease. Some lesions may be visible immediately (e.g., a burn); others may be detectable initially only through diagnostic means such as laboratory testing.

An abnormal growth of cells leads to the formation of both benign and malignant tumors, or neoplasms. A **benign neoplasm** remains localized and is generally noninvasive, as opposed to a **malignant neoplasm,** which continues to grow, spread, and invade other tissues. *Cancer* is a general term often used to denote various types of malignant neoplasms. The spread of cancer cells is termed *metastasis.* Certain types of cancer appear more often as metastases from other areas rather than originating in a given organ. More discussion of this topic occurs in subsequent chapters.

Note that the terms cancer and carcinoma are not synonymous. A *carcinoma* is one type of cancer and is derived from epithelial tissue. Another cancer is a *sarcoma,* which arises from connective tissue. Radiography plays a major role in the diagnosis of a variety of neoplastic diseases.

The treatment of cancer consumes enormous financial, emotional, and other resources in health care. While the state of the art is continually advancing, the primary treatment modalities are surgery, chemotherapy, and radiation therapy. The choice of which modality or combination of modalities depends on many factors, including the type of cancer, its location and stage, and the treating oncologist. The goal of treatment may be *curative,* allowing the patient to remain free of disease for 5 years or more, or *palliative,* which is designed to relieve pain when curing is not possible.

The Staging of Cancer

Decisions regarding the appropriate treatment of malignant tumors and in determining prognosis and end results are guided by classifications that "stage" the disease. Although several clinical classifications of cancer exist, the *TNM system* emerged in the 1950s and is now considered a recognized standard, as endorsed by the American Joint Committee on Cancer (AJCC). The AJCC is cosponsored by several prominent health organizations, including the American Cancer Society and the American College of Radiology.

The TNM system is based on the premise that cancers of similar histology or origin are similar in their patterns of growth or extension. The *T* refers to the size of the untreated primary cancer or tumor. As the size increases, lymph node involvement (i.e., *N*) occurs, eventually leading to distant metastases (i.e., *M*). The addition of numbers to these three letters indicates the extent of malignancy and the progressive increase in size or involvement of the tumor. For example, T0 indicates that no evidence of a primary tumor exists, while T1, T2, T3, and T4 indicate an increasing size or extension. Lack of regional lymph node metastasis is indicated by N0, while N1, N2, and N3 indicate increasing involvement of regional lymph nodes. Finally, M0 indicates no distant metastasis, while M1 indicates the presence of distant metastasis.

In addition, other descriptors are used to categorize a given tumor further according to its primary site, histopathologic type and grade, lymphatic or venous invasion, and residual tumor classification. Neoplastic cells are examined histologically, and these growths are categorized or "graded" according to their degree of differentiation. The degree of differentiation or grading is used to distinguish between degrees of malignancy, with grade 1 categorized as least malignant and grade 4 as most malignant. The combination of all of these allows the TNM system to serve as a shorthand notation for description of the clinical extent of a given malignant tumor. It facilitates treatment planning, provides an indication of prognosis, assists in evaluating treatment results, facilitates information exchange between treatment centers, and allows unambiguous categorization of malignancies to aid in the continuing investigation of cancer.

CONCLUSION

There is no doubt that technological advances in the field of radiology have done much to relieve human suffering, but radiography alone cannot provide a definitive diagnosis. Radiography must be used in conjunction with other diagnostic and therapeutic modalities to provide the best treatment for each specific disease process. The following chapters provide the student radiographer with a better understanding of the disease processes of the various physiologic systems. This information should help students to analyze and critique each radiograph to ensure that it provides optimal information to assist physicians in their diagnosis.

QUESTIONS

1. The prediction of the course and end of a disease and an outlook based on that prediction best define its:
   a. diagnosis
   c. prognosis
   b. etiology
   d. syndrome

2. A compression fracture of the lumbar spine that results from steroid treatments for pain reduction of arthritis would be an example of _____ disease.
   a. degenerative
   c. idiopathic
   b. iatrogenic
   d. traumatic

3. A disease such as Tay-Sachs syndrome that is transmitted genetically is termed:
   a. congenital
   c. metabolic
   b. hereditary
   d. neoplastic

4. Sickness sufficient to interefere with normal daily routines is termed:
   a. etiology
   c. mortality
   b. morbidity
   d. pathogenesis

5. Which of the following would be considered a symptom of a disease process?
   a. bloody stool
   c. skin rash
   b. nausea
   d. swelling

6. A disease that presents slowly and lasts over a long period of time is said to be:
   a. acute
   c. chronic
   b. asymptomatic
   d. congenital

7. Which of the following types of disease classifications is usually associated with the normal aging process?
   a. congenital
   c. inflammatory
   b. degenerative
   d. metabolic

8. If 4,000 cases of a given disease are found in the inhabitants of a given population, its is _____ defined.
   a. incidence
   c. metabolism
   b. morphology
   d. prevalence

9. The relative ease with which an organism can overcome normal bodily defenses against the organism refers to:
   a. infection
   c. pestulence
   b. necrosis
   d. virulence

10. A general term to describe the many types of cellular changes that occur in response to disease is:
   a. contusion
   c. metastasis
   b. lesion
   d. morphology

11. Specify two pathologies that are iatrogenic in origin and explain the probable cause of each pathology. Are any specific to the use of ionizing radiation?

12. What is the difference between mortality and morbidity rates? How is each important to the practice of medicine and to public health agencies?

13. Differentiate between an acute illness and a chronic illness. Give two examples of each type of disease.

14. Explain the concept of neoplastic disease. Are all neoplasms cancer?

15. Describe the TNM classification system and specify how it may be used by physicians in a health care setting.

Chapter 2

The Skeletal System

Anatomy and Physiology Review
Imaging Considerations
  Radiography
  Other studies
Congenital and Hereditary Diseases
  Osteogenesis imperfecta
  Achondroplasia
  Osteopetrosis
  Hand and foot malformations
  Congenital dislocation of the hip
  Vertebral anomalies
  Cranial anomalies
Inflammatory Disease
  Osteomyelitis
  Tuberculosis
  Arthritis
    Acute arthritis
    Rheumatoid arthritis
  Ankylosing spondylitis
  Osteoarthritis

Inflammation of associated joint structures
  Gouty arthritis
Metabolic Disease
  Osteoporosis
  Osteomalacia
  Paget's disease (osteitis deformans)
  Hyperparathyroidism
  Acromegaly
Vertebral Column
Neoplastic Disease
  Osteochondroma (exostosis)
  Osteoma
  Endochondroma
  Simple bone cyst
  Osteoid osteoma and osteoblastoma
  Osteoclastoma (giant cell tumor)
  Osteosarcoma (osteogenic sarcoma)
  Ewing's sarcoma
  Chondrosarcoma
  Metastases from other sites

Upon completion of Chapter 2, the reader should be able to:

- Describe the anatomic components of the skeletal system on a macroscopic and basic microscopic level.

- Identify and explain the criteria for assessing technical adequacy of skeletal radiographs.

- Characterize a given condition as congenital, inflammatory, arthritic, metabolic, traumatic, or neoplastic.

■ Specify the pathogenesis, signs and symptoms, and prognosis of the skeletal pathologies cited in this chapter.

■ Discuss the healing process involved with fractures and identify complications associated with skeletal trauma.

■ Describe and classify skeletal fractures according to the various classifications discussed in this chapter.

■ Explain the role of various imaging modalities in the diagnosis and treatment of skeletal pathologies.

KEY TERMS

Compact bone	Anencephaly	Paget's disease
Cancellous bone	Osteomyelitis	Hyperparathyroidism
Medullary canal	Sequestrum	Acromegaly
Trabeculae	Involucrum	Whiplash
Osteoblasts	Tuberculosis	Spondylolysis
Osteoclasts	Arthritis	Spondylolisthesis
Osteogenesis imperfecta	Pyogenic arthritis	Osteochondroma
Achondroplasia	Rheumatoid arthritis	Exostosis
Osteopetrosis	Juvenile rheumatoid arthritis	Osteoma
Albers-Schönberg disease	Ankylosing spondylitis	Hyperostosis frontalis interna
Craniotubular dysplasias	Osteoarthritis	Endochondroma
Syndactyly	Osteophytes	Simple bone cyst
Polydactyly	Tenosynovitis	Osteoid osteoma
Clubfoot	Ganglion	Osteoblastoma
Congenital hip dislocation	Bursitis	Osteoclastoma
Scoliosis	Gouty arthritis	Osteosarcoma
Transitional vertebra	Osteoporosis	Ewing's sarcoma
Spina bifida	Osteomalacia	Chondrosarcoma
Craniosynostoses	Rickets	

ANATOMY AND PHYSIOLOGY REVIEW

The skeletal system is comprised of 206 separate bones and is responsible for body support, pro-tection, movement, and blood cell production. It contains more than 98% of the body's total calcium and up to 75% of its total phosporus. The system is commonly divided into the axial

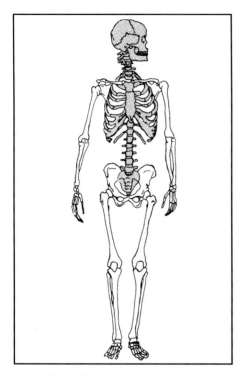

Fig. 2-1, left. Axial skeleton. (From Bontrager KL: *Textbook of radiographic positioning and related anatomy,* ed 3, St Louis, 1993, Mosby.)

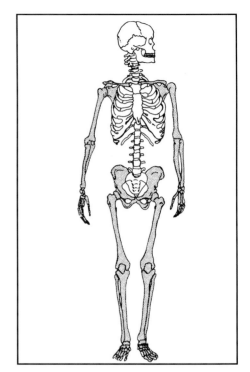

Fig. 2-2, right. Appendicular skeleton. (From Bontrager KL: *Textbook of radiographic positioning and related anatomy,* ed 3, St Louis, 1993, Mosby.)

skeleton (Fig. 2-1), which contains 80 bones, and the appendicular skeleton (Fig. 2-2), which contains 126 bones. Bone is a type of connective tissue, but it differs from other connective tissue because of its matrix of calcium phosphate. The construction of this matrix further classifies bone tissue as either **compact** (dense) or **cancellous** (spongy) (Fig. 2-3).

The outer portion of bone is composed of compact bone, and the inner portion, termed the **medullary canal,** is made up of cancellous bone. Bone marrow is located within the medullary canal and is interspersed between the **trabeculae.** This intricate, weblike bony structure is visible on a properly exposed radiograph of the skeletal system and is often referred to as the trabecular pattern. The term *diploë* is specific to the cancellous bone located within the skull.

The red bone marrow is responsible for the production of bone erythrocytes and leukocytes. Red bone marrow is found, in a normal adult, primarily in the bones of the trunk. At the approximate age of 20 years, the majority of the red bone marrow is replaced by yellow bone marrow composed mainly of fat.

Osteoblasts are the bone-forming cells that line the medullary canal and are interspersed throughout the periosteum. They are responsible for bone growth and thickening, ossification, and regeneration. **Osteoclasts** are specialized cells that break down bone to enlarge the medullary canal and allow for bone growth. This production and breakdown of bone play an important role in serum calcium and phosphorus equilibrium. Certain metabolic disease processes may alter the percentage of

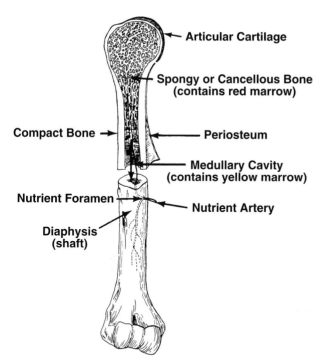

← Articular Cartilage

← Spongy or Cancellous Bone
(contains red marrow)

Compact Bone →

← Periosteum

← Medullary Cavity
(contains yellow marrow)

Nutrient Foramen →

← Nutrient Artery

Diaphysis
(shaft)

Fig. 2–3 Bone composition. (From Bontrager KL: *Textbook of radiographic positioning and related anatomy,* ed 3, St Louis, 1993, Mosby.)

calcium, resulting in either hypocalcemia or hypercalcemia.

The bones of the skeletal system may also be classified according to their shape to include long, short, flat, and irregular bones. The diaphysis of a long bone refers to the shaft portion, whereas the epiphysis refers to the expanded end portion (Fig. 2-4). The metaphysis refers to the growth zone between the epiphysis and diaphysis. It is the area of greatest metabolic activity in a bone. A cartilaginous growth plate is located between the metaphysis and the epiphysis in the bone of a growing child. Radiographically, these growth areas appear radiolucent. As the body matures, this cartilage calcifies and is no longer radiographically visible in the adult.

The periosteum is a fibrous membrane that encloses all of the bone except the joint surfaces

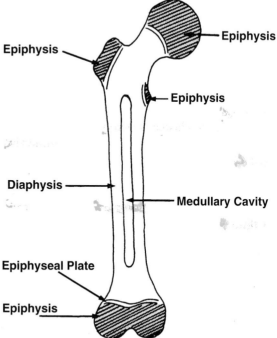

Epiphysis →

Epiphysis ←

← Epiphysis

Diaphysis →

← Medullary Cavity

Epiphyseal Plate →

Epiphysis →

Fig. 2–4 Endochondral ossification. (From Bontrager KL: *Textbook of radiographic positioning and related anatomy,* ed 3, St Louis, 1993, Mosby.)

and is crucial to supplying blood to the underlying bone. Osteoblasts located within the periosteum increase bone thickness relative to individual activities. The more physical stress a bone is under, the thicker the compact portion develops; therefore, it is common medical practice to allow patients with healing fractures of the hip or femur to bear weight on the injured bone, thus helping to reduce the healing period. Disuse atrophy occurs when a bone is not allowed to bear weight and results in significant decalcification and thinning of the bone.

The 206 bones of the body are connected to each other by one of three types of joints. Fibrous (synarthrodial) joints form firm, immovable joints, such as the sutures of the skull. Cartilaginous (amphiarthrodial) joints, such as those found between the vertebral bodies, are slightly movable. Synovial (diarthrodial) joints, such as the knee, are freely movable. The ends of the bones composing a synovial joint are lined with articular cartilage and are held together by ligaments. The joint capsules are lined by a synovial membrane responsible for the secretion of synovia, a lubricating fluid containing mucin, albumin, fat, and mineral salts.

IMAGING CONSIDERATIONS

Radiography

In examining a skeletal radiograph, it is important to begin by properly orienting the film and recognizing the radiographic projection. The radiographic exposure technique selected can be very important in achieving a proper diagnosis. Proper technique is achieved when the soft tissues and bony structures of interest are both visible. Any motion of the part in question impairs the visibility of the detail present.

Soft tissue areas often hold clues to the diagnosis and are examined by the interpreting physician. Any signs of muscle wasting, soft tissue swelling, calcifications, opaque foreign bodies, or the presence of gas may indicate disease. Analysis of the configuration of the bone and

its relationship to other bones serves to detect or exclude fractures, dislocations, congenital anomalies, or acquired deformities.

The interface between cortical (compact) bone and soft tissue is also important. Any periosteal new bone formation seen may be a response to trauma, tumors, or infection. Juxtaarticular erosions are often seen in cases of arthritis. Cortical reabsorption can be demonstrated as smudgy, irregular loss of the cortical margin. In addition, the internal bone structure is important and should be examined for abnormally altered texture, alterations in the amount of mineralization, or foci of destruction. Careful consideration of all areas mentioned assists the physician in achieving the correct diagnosis.

Other Studies

Magnetic resonance imaging (MRI) has assumed a larger role in imaging of skeletal pathology, particularly in providing soft tissue detail related to MRI's superior contrast resolution. It is considered the modality of choice for detection and staging of soft tissue tumors involving the extremities. It is also extremely useful in evaluation of joints, particularly the knee and shoulder. Enhanced by the emergence of kinematic studies of joints, especially the cervical spine, knee, wrist, shoulder, and temporomandibular joint (TMJ), the value of MRI should further increase with echoplanar imaging, offering the potential for "fluoroscopic" MRI. Bone marrow imaging done with MRI is superior to the older nuclear medicine bone scan, particularly for subtle abnormalities (e.g., edema). Also, MRI may play a larger role in trauma medicine, particularly with the refinement of open bore technology.

Computed tomography (CT) is mainly involved in skeletal imaging in cases of trauma. This is because of its ability to define the presence and extent of fractures or dislocations and to assess joint abnormalities and associated soft tissues. While cortical bone gives no signal in

MRI, CT provides ready visualization of bony detail and is often used as a follow-up for improved detail to plain film imaging. Bone tumors, in particular, are now usually imaged with CT because of its excellent ability to display bony margins and trabecular patterns. Additionally, it is particularly useful for assessing both bony and soft tissue involvement of tumors. Although CT possesses greater contrast resolution than radiography, much of the role for imaging related soft tissues has been usurped by MRI.

Nuclear medicine retains an advantage not offered by either MRI or CT in skeletal imaging: the ability to look at the entire body at one time in a convenient fashion. It allows ready decision making as to whether any pathology shown is an old injury or a new problem, with activity indicating the bone involved is affected by some new process. Additionally, the bone scan is still the standard of care for examination of metastatic processes.

Bone densitometry, whether performed by a dedicated unit or as an add-on to CT, is also important in evaluation of osteoporosis. Dedicated bone densitometry units readily show bone density, while CT add-ons have an advantage of also showing bony architecture. While providing useful information, the results of bone densitometry may not always be enough to affect the resulting course of treatment.

CONGENITAL AND HEREDITARY DISEASES

Osteogenesis Imperfecta

Osteogenesis imperfecta is a rather rare, but quite serious, congenital disease affecting the newborn skeletal system. Changes in ligaments, skin, sclera, inner ear, and teeth are also noted. With this condition, formation of osseous tissue is deficient and imperfect, leading to an abnormal fragility of bones. Infants afflicted with this disease usually have multiple fractures at birth that heal only to give way to new fractures (Fig. 2-5). This results in limb deformities and may

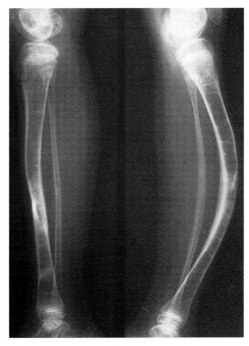

Fig. 2-5 Tibia-fibula radiograph demonstrating bowed lower extremities resulting from osteogenesis imperfecta tarda. This condition was recognized shortly after the child began to walk. (Courtesy the American College of Radiology, Reston, Virginia.)

lead to dwarfism. In milder cases, fractures might not appear for some years after birth and then generally stop once adulthood is reached. In some cases, however, a hearing disorder persists because of abnormal connective tissue around the auditory ossicles.

Achondroplasia

The most common inherited disorder affecting the skeletal system is **achondroplasia,** which results in bone deformity and dwarfism. Because of a disturbance in endochondral bone formation, the cartilage located in the epiphyses of the long bones does not convert to bone in the normal manner. Thus, patients with this type of osteochondrodysplasia present with a normal trunk size and shortened extremities (Fig. 2-6). An adult with achondroplasia is usually no more than 4 feet in height, with lower extremities usually less than half the normal length. Additional clinical manifestations of this disorder include extreme lumbar spine lordosis, bow legs, and a bulky forehead. Occasionally, orthopedic surgery may be necessary in management of complications associated with achondroplasia. In addition, these patients may receive genetic and social counseling.

Osteopetrosis

Osteopetrosis and *marble bone* are terms used to characterize a variety of disorders involving an increase in bone density and defective bone contour, often referred to as *skeletal modeling*. With osteopetrosis, bones are abnormally heavy and compact, but nevertheless brittle. The disorders characterizing osteopetrosis include osteoscleroses, craniotubular (affecting the cranium and tubular long bones) dysplasias, and craniotubular hyperostoses. It is important for the technologist to be aware that both the osteosclerotic and craniotular hyperostotic disorders require an increase in exposure factors to adequately penetrate the bony anatomy because of abnormal bone density (Fig. 2-7). In some cases, adequate radiographic density may never be achieved.

Albers-Schönberg disease is a fairly common form of osteosclerotic osteopetrosis. This benign skeletal anomaly involves increased bone density in conjunction with fairly normal bone contour. If fact, many patients afflicted with Albers-Schönberg disease are asymptomatic, and it is often discovered after radiographing the

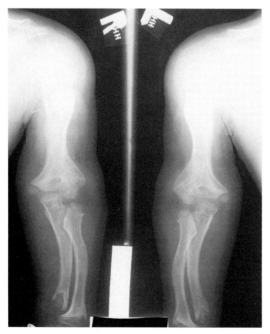

Fig. 2-6 Radiographs of shortened upper extremities caused by a defect in the endochondral bone formation associated with achondroplasia. (Courtesy the American College of Radiology, Reston, Virginia.)

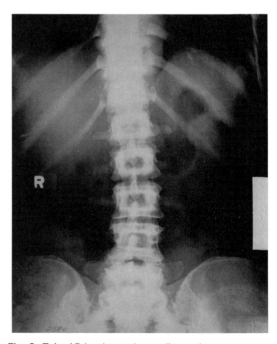

Fig. 2-7 An AP lumbar spine radiograph demonstrating uniform sclerosis of the bone associated with osteopetrosis. (Courtesy the American College of Radiology, Reston, Virginia.)

patient for an unrelated problem. Although this is a hereditary disorder, the bone sclerosis is not radiographically visible at birth. As the individual ages, radiographic manifestations of the osteopetrosis become visible, especially in the region of the cranium and spine; however, general health is unimpaired.

Craniotubular dysplasias are a group of hereditary diseases mainly resulting in abnormal or defective bone contour of the cranium and long bones. Radiographs are useful in demonstrating this alteration in contour, scleroses, and changes within the cortical bone. Craniotubular hyperostoses include a variety of fairly rare hereditary diseases, causing both an increase in bone density and abnormal bone modeling. Both of these craniotubular anomalies present in childhood. Although these disorders do not normally impair the individual's general health,

bony overgrowth may entrap cranial nerves, resulting in some dysfunction such as facial palsy or deafness.

Hand and Foot Malformations

A variety of abnormalities of the fingers and toes may occur during fetal development but can be surgically corrected at birth. Failure of the fingers or toes to separate is called **syndactyly** and gives the physical appearance of webbed digits. **Polydactyly** (Fig. 2-8) refers to the presence of exra digits.

Clubfoot (talipes) is a congenital malformation of the foot that prevents normal weight-bearing. The foot is most commonly turned inward at the ankle. This congenital malformation is more common in males than in females and may occur bilaterally. It is generally corrected by

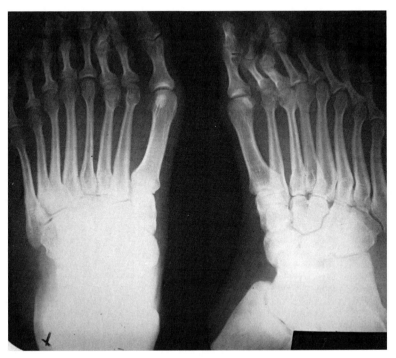

Fig. 2-8 A foot radiograph demonstrating additional digits associated with familial polydactyly. (Courtesy the American College of Radiology, Reston, Virginia.)

casting or splinting the foot in correct anatomic position.

Congenital Dislocation of the Hip

A malformation of the acetabulum often results in **congenital hip dislocations.** Because the acetabulum does not completely form, the head of the femur is displaced superiorly and posteriorly (Fig. 2-9). Many times, the ligaments and tendons responsible for proper placement of the femoral head are also affected. Congenital dislocations of the hip occur more frequently in females than in males. This anomaly is most commonly treated with immobilization through casting or splinting the affected hip.

Vertebral Anomalies

Scoliosis refers to an abnormal lateral curvature of the spine (Fig. 2-10). The lateral curves are usually convex to the right in the thoracic region and to the left in the lumbar region of the spine. Up to 80% of all scolioses are idiopathic, although factors such as connective tissue disease and diet have been implicated. Scoliosis does not generally become visually

apparent until adolescence. It tends to affect females more frequently than males and can generate numerous complications, including cardiopulmonary complications, degenerative spinal arthritis, and fatigue and joint dysfunction syndromes.

Radiography is important in the diagnosis and treatment of scoliosis. Initial evaluation requires initial anteroposterior (AP) or posteroanterior (PA) and lateral standing radiographs with follow-up radiographs on a fairly routine basis. Radiologists use one of several methods to measure the spine's curvature, so consistent quality from one examination to another is important. Good radiation protection techniques are vital because of the large size of the exposure

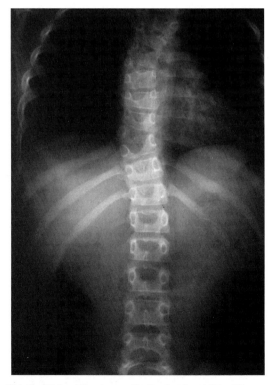

Fig. 2-10 An AP spine radiograph of a child with congenital scoliosis. (Courtesy the American College of Radiology, Reston, Virginia.)

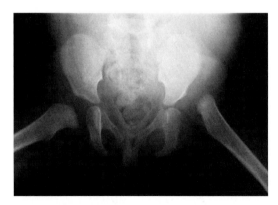

Fig. 2-9 A frog leg lateral projection of the pelvis on an infant demonstrating congenital dislocation of the left hip. (Courtesy the American College of Radiology, Reston, Virginia.)

field, the young age of the patient, and the frequency of the examinations. Special attention is necessary in shielding the breasts of young, female patients during radiographic examination throughout the treatment process. Scoliosis may be corrected surgically or by placing the individual in a brace or body cast. Treatment depends on the site of the deformity and the severity of the curvature.

A **transitional vertebra** is one that takes on the characteristics of both vertebrae on each side of a major division of the spine. Most frequently, such vertebrae occur at the junction between the thoracic and lumbar spine or at the junction between the lumbar spine and the sacrum. The first lumbar vertebra may have rudimentary ribs articulating with the transverse processes (Fig. 2-11), as may the seventh cervical vertebra. A cervical rib most commonly occurs at C7 and may exert pressure on the brachial nerve plexus or the subclavian artery, requiring surgical removal of the rib.

Spina bifida is an incomplete closure of the vertebral canal, which is particularly common in the lumbosacral area (Fig. 2-12). Frequently, such patients have no visible abnormality or neurologic deficit, but failure of bony fusion of the two laminae is visible radiographically (spina bifida occulta). In more severe cases, the spinal cord or nerve root may be involved, which results in varying degrees of paralysis. Treatment of spina bifida is determined based on the extent of the anomaly and requires the services of a variety of physicians.

Cranial Anomalies

The premature or early closure of any of the cranial sutures is called **craniosynostoses.** This congenital anomaly causes an overgrowth of the

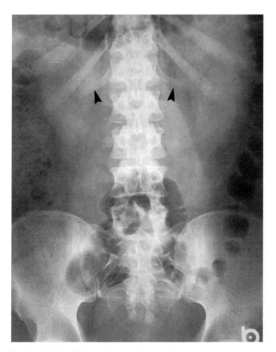

Fig. 2-11 An AP lumbar spine radiograph demonstrating bilateral lumbar ribs. (Courtesy Riverside Methodist Hospitals, Columbus, Ohio.)

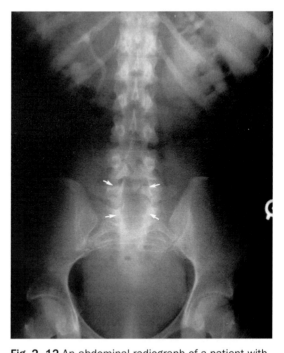

Fig. 2-12 An abdominal radiograph of a patient with spina bifida occulta of the lower lumbar vertebrae. (Courtesy Riverside Methodist Hospitals, Columbus, Ohio.)

unfused sutures to accommodate brain growth, thus altering the shape of the head (Fig. 2-13). Although this defect may be corrected with surgery, brain damage may occur.

Anencephaly is a congenital abnormality in which the brain and cranial vault do not form (Fig. 2-14). In most cases, only the facial bones are formed. This abnormality results in death shortly after birth and may be diagnosed before birth by both sonography and radiography.

INFLAMMATORY DISEASE

Osteomyelitis

Osteomyelitis is an infection of the bone and bone marrow, most often caused by *Staphylococcus* delivered via the bloodstream. It may, however, result from direct infection, such as might occur with an open fracture or from a hospital-acquired surgical infection. In the former case, infants and children are generally affected because of their lowered resistance in combination with the virulence of the organism. Generally, the osteomyelitis develops at the ends of the long bones of the lower limbs in adults and the metaphysis in children.

The acute stage of osteomyelitis is characterized by the formation of an abscess, leading to an inflammatory reaction within the bone that causes a rise in internal bone pressure. Because of the constriction of periosteum, blood vessels compress and thrombose, leading to bone necrosis within 24 to 48 hours. Unfortunately, not until about 10 to 14 days later is new periosteal bone repair evident radiographically to indicate the presence of the disease. Therefore, it is imperative that the condition is recognized clinically and treated with antibiotics and local drainage.

Initially, radiographs may demonstrate soft tissue swelling in the area around the affected bone (Fig. 2-15). Follow-up radiographs may be performed 10 to 14 days after medical treatment to aid in the diagnosis.

With the effective use of antibiotics, osteomyelitis seldom passes the acute stage. When

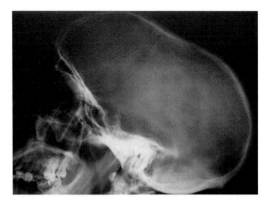

Fig. 2-13 A lateral skull radiograph demonstrating premature closure of the sagittal suture. This results in dolichocephaly and prominent convolutional markings caused by the increased intracranial pressure. (Courtesy the American College of Radiology, Reston, Virginia.)

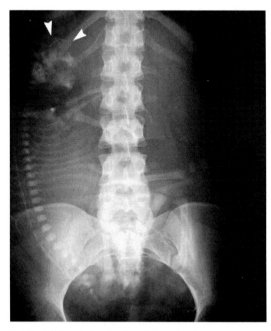

Fig. 2-14 An abdominal radiograph of a pregnant woman carrying a fetus with anencephaly. Notice the lack of the cerebral cranial bones. (Courtesy Riverside Methodist Hospitals, Columbus, Ohio.)

it does, antibiotics in combination with surgical drainage of pus from under the periosteum often result in a complete cure of the bone lesion in a majority of cases. Chronic osteomyelitis, however, is characterized by extensive bone destruction with irregular, sclerotic reaction throughout the bone (Fig. 2-16). A **sequestrum** is the essentially dead, devascularized bone that appears very dense. An **involucrum** is a shell of new supporting bone laid down by the periosteum around the sequestrum. An accurate diagnosis is extremely important to distinguish osteomyelitis from a neoplastic bone disease.

Radiography is not a very sensitive means of diagnosing the condition because a fair amount of destruction must occur before the changes of osteomyelitis are visible radiographically. Nu-

clear medicine bone-scan studies are much more sensitive and demonstrate the bone destruction as a "hot spot" on the final image. In addition, MRI now has a significant role in detection of osteomyelitis.

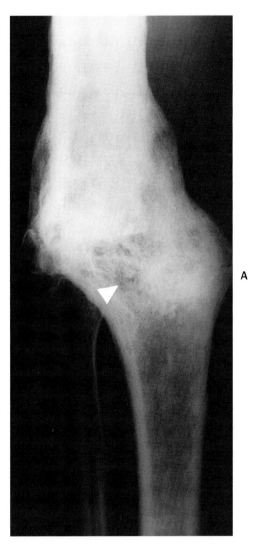

A

Fig. 2-16 A, Chronic osteomyelitis demonstrated in a knee with prior fusion. An involucrum surrounded by fluid densities is seen in the middle of a large intramedullary cavity approximately 3 cm above the fusion site. (Courtesy Riverside Methodist Hospitals, Columbus, Ohio.) *(cont'd)*

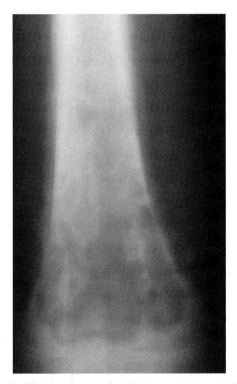

Fig. 2-15 A tomogram of a right knee demonstrating acute osteomyelitis of the femur. The 12-year-old girl complained of swelling and pain. (Courtesy the American College of Radiology, Reston, Virginia.)

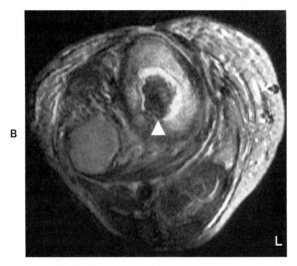

B

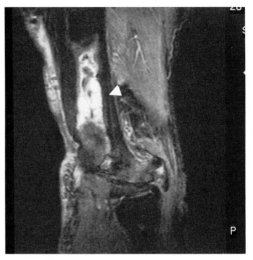

C

L

P

Fig. 2-16 cont'd. **B,** The involucrum as seen in a sagittal MRI on the same patient. **C,** The sequestrum as seen in an axial MRI of the same patient, appearing as very dense bone as a result of devascularization. (Courtesy Riverside Methodist Hospitals, Columbus, Ohio.)

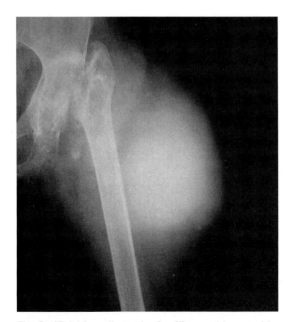

Fig. 2-17 A hip radiograph of a 47-year-old man with extensive destruction of the femoral head and neck caused by tuberculosis of the hip with a cold abscess. (Courtesy the American College of Radiology, Reston, Virginia.)

Tuberculosis

Tuberculosis of the bone is a chronic inflammatory disease, usually more advanced, often, long untreated as compared to pulmonary tuberculosis. Its incidence has sharply declined in the last few decades as the incidence of pulmonary tuberculosis has reduced. It most commonly affects the hip, knee, and spine. Radiographically, the ends of the long bones display a "worm-eaten" appearance, with the disease slowly destroying the epiphyses, spreading to the articular cartilage, and in some cases infecting the joint space (Fig. 2-17). Tuberculosis of the spine is also called *Pott's disease*. Recognized in ancient times, it has been described in Egyptian mummies dating back to 3000 BC. It destroys the spine, causing softening and eventual collapse of the vertebrae, which results in paravertebral abscess formation and exerts abnormal pressure on the spinal cord.

Arthritis

Joint inflammation is known as **arthritis** and may be caused by a variety of etiologic factors.

It can generally be divided into two main types: (1) degenerative, in which pathologic changes begin in the articular cartilage of joints, and (2) inflammatory, in which pathologic changes begin in the synovial membrane of joints. An accurate clinical history is of extreme importance because different types of arthritis are characterized by specific features. For example, it is important to identify the number of joints involved, the location of the joints involved, and the presence of any other disease process. Some types of arthritis involve several joints, while others involve only one joint. In addition, certain types of arthritis have a predilection for specific joints while sparing others. Finally, some types of arthritis are associated with specific disease processes caused by a host of factors, such as bacteria or autoimmune response. Arthritis may be further classified as acute or chronic; the most common forms are chronic and disabling.

ACUTE ARTHRITIS

Acute arthritis is commonly called **pyogenic arthritis** and it is caused by a variety of factors including staphylococci, streptococci, and gonococci. Common clinical symptoms of acute arthritis are pain, redness, and swelling of the affected joint, often accompanied by a fever. Generally, the pyogenic or pus-forming organisms enter the body via a wound, as in the case of an open fracture, or the organisms may spread to the joint from a bone infected with osteomyelitis. Pyogenic arthritis usually responds rapidly to antibiotic therapy. The early radiographic changes demonstrate an increase in joint space, bony destruction, and joint dislocation. Radiographs obtained during the healing stage demonstrate recalcification and sclerosis, often resulting in joint ankylosis.

RHEUMATOID ARTHRITIS

Rheumatoid arthritis may fluctuate in severity and is thought to be an autoimmune disease, triggered by exposure of an immunogenetically susceptible host to an arthritogenic antigen. It is characterized by chronic inflammation and over-

growth of the synovial tissues. As the synovial tissues proliferate, they progressively destroy the cartilage, bone, and supporting structures. In addition, blood chemistry analysis identifies the presence of an autoantibody against gamma globulin, also known as the serologic rheumatoid factor. It usually occurs between the ages of 30 and 40 years and is three times more common in women than in men. Symptoms include pain, swelling, and stiffness of the affected joint with periods of activity or exacerbations and remissions of the disease process.

While any joint may be involved, rheumatoid arthritis typically begins in the peripheral joints, particularly in the small bones of the hands and feet and in the knee. The radiographic changes seen early in this disease are soft tissue swelling and osteoporosis of the affected bones (Fig. 2-18). As the disease progresses, cortical erosion with joint space narrowing occurs because of the

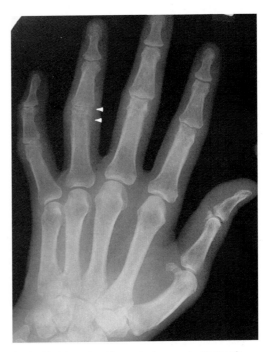

Fig. 2-18 A hand radiograph demonstrating soft tissue joint swelling associated with early rheumatoid arthritis. (Courtesy the American College of Radiology, Reston, Virginia.)

overgrowth of synovial tissue into the articular spaces. This severe damage makes the joint unstable and leads to deformity caused by the displacement of the bones. The late changes of this condition can be quite severe, resulting in bone and cartilage destruction and subluxation or dislocation of the involved joint (Fig. 2-19). Eventually, the joints become ankylosed (fused), which requires surgical intervention. Surgical procedures such as synovium excision, dislocation corrections, joint reconstructions, and prosthetic joint replacements may be performed to improve joint function (Fig. 2-20). Overall, life expectancy is reduced by 3 to 7 years with rheumatoid arthritis, with deaths usually due to complications such as gastrointestinal bleeding related to long-term use of aspirin.

Juvenile rheumatoid arthritis affects about a quarter million American children under 16 years of age and is similar to the adult form of rheumatoid arthritis. There are differences, however, in the pattern of involvement and prognosis. Generally, there is less fibrosis and proliferation than in the adult form. Prognosis is generally good, with fewer than 20% having progressive destructive disease. The majority have long periods of remission without significant joint damage.

Ankylosing Spondylitis

Ankylosing spondylitis (Marie-Strümpell disease) is a progressive form of arthritis, mainly involving the spine, in which joints and articula-

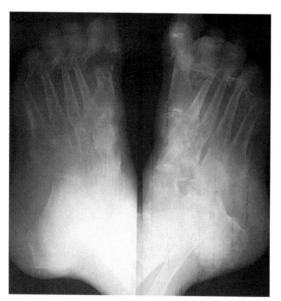

Fig. 2-19 Radiographs of a foot demonstrating subluxations at the metatarsophalangeal joints resulting from late rheumatoid arthritis. (Courtesy the American College of Radiology, Reston, Virginia.)

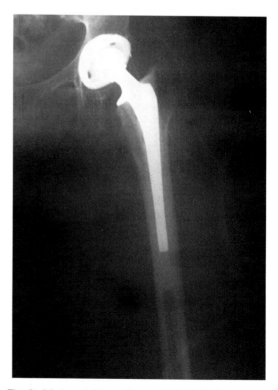

Fig. 2-20 A portable radiograph of a left hip demonstrating proper placement of a prosthetic hip replacement. (Courtesy the Ohio State University Hospitals, Columbus, Ohio.)

tions become ankylosed, especially the sacroiliac joints. It tends to affect males between the ages of 10 and 30 years, with patients presenting with low back pain. Early radiographic changes demonstrate bilateral narrowing and fuzziness of the sacroiliac joints. Eventually, the sacroiliac joints become obliterated, and the condition progresses up the spine. Later radiographic changes show calcification of the bones of the spine with ossification of the vertebral ligaments. The articular cartilage is destroyed, and fibrous adhesions develop. These adhesions lead to bone fusion and calcification of the anulus fibrosis of the intervertebral disks and the anterior and lateral spinal ligaments. The spine becomes a rigid block of bone, giving the condition its characteristic nickname of "bamboo spine" (Figs. 2-21 and 2-22).

Osteoarthritis

The most common type of arthritis is **osteoarthritis,** also known as *degenerative joint disease* (DJD). It affects males and females equally, although patients are usually asymptomatic until they are in their fifties. Osteoarthritis is a disease of cartilage, resulting from a noninflammatory deterioration of the joint cartilage that occurs with the normal wear and tear of aging. It may also be secondary to bone stress associated with trauma. Osteoarthritis generally affects the large, weight-bearing joints of the body such as the hip, where it is particularly disabling (Fig.

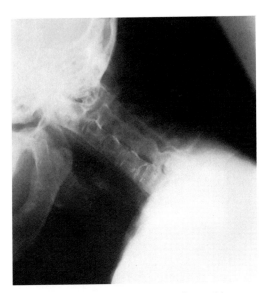

Fig. 2-21 A lateral cervical spine radiographic depicting ankylosing spondylitis with granulation tissue beneath the anterior longitudinal ligament destroying the corners of the contiguous vertebra. (Courtesy the American College of Radiology, Reston, Virginia.)

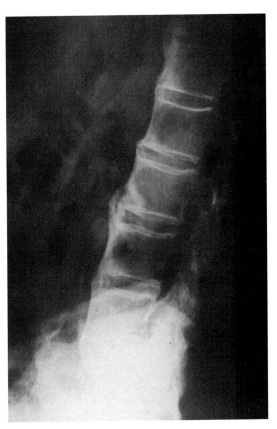

Fig. 2-22 A lateral lumbar spine radiograph on a 64-year-old man with ankylosing spondylitis. Notice the fusion of the vertebrae into a solid block of bone. (Courtesy the Ohio State University Hospitals, Columbus, Ohio.)

2-23), or the interphalangeal joints of the fingers. In joints afflicted with this disease, the articular cartilage degenerates and is gradually worn away, exposing the underlying bone. Radiographically, this loss of articular cartilage appears as a narrowing of the joint space. An overgrowth of articular cartilage occurs on the peripheral surfaces of the joint and often calcifies, which results in **osteophytes** or bone spurs that are visible radiographically (Fig. 2-24). In terms of radiographic diagnosis, the formation of osteophytes is indicative of osteoarthritis, helping to distinguish it from other types of arthritis.

Clinically, an individual with osteoarthritis presents with pain and progressive stiffening of the affected joint. Methods of halting its gradual progression are few; it is second only to cardiovascular disease in causing long-term disability. When possible, treatment consists of surgical prosthetic joint replacement (e.g., hip), which greatly relieves the pain and allows a return of joint mobility.

Inflammation of Associated Joint Structures

The specialized connective tissues that attach muscle to bone are called *tendons*. They are enclosed in a sheath that is susceptible to inflammation, a condition known as **tenosynovitis**. A **ganglion** is a cystic swelling that develops in connection with a tendon sheath, usually on the back of the wrist. Tenosynovitis may spread to the associated tendon, resulting in tendinitis. *Bursae* are sacs lined with a synovial membrane, and they are found in locations where tendons pass over bony prominences. If the bursa becomes inflamed, it is called **bursitis**. Inflammation of these associated structures may be caused by acute or chronic trauma (e.g., housemaid's knee), acute or chronic infection, inflammatory arthritis, gout, and, rarely, pyogenic or tuberculous organisms. These inflammatory conditions are characterized by pain, localized tenderness, and limited

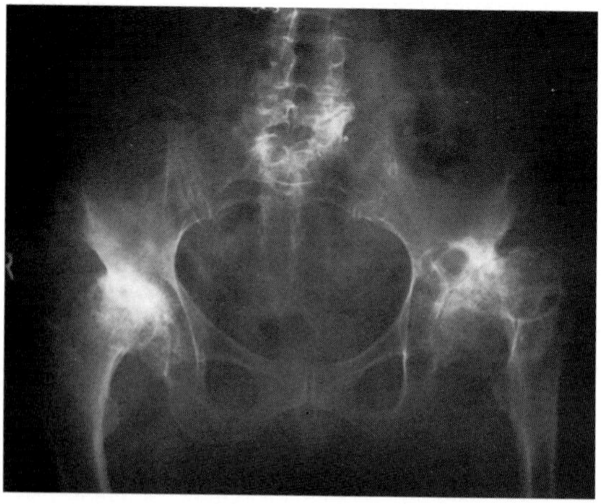

Fig. 2-23 A radiograph of the pelvis demonstrating osteoarthritis of the hip secondary to congenital subluxation. This 68-year-old woman had a history of painful hips and limping. (Courtesy the American College of Radiology, Reston, Virginia.)

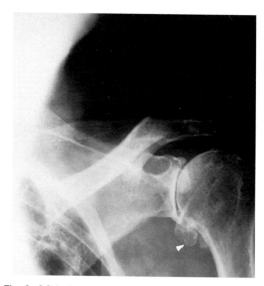

Fig. 2-24 A shoulder radiograph demonstrating the formation of an osteophyte at the inferior lip of the glenoid labrum due to primary osteoarthritis. (Courtesy the American College of Radiology, Reston, Virginia.)

motion of the involved joint. In cases of chronic bursitis, the walls of the bursa become thickened, and calcium deposits may be visible radiographically within the bursa (Fig. 2-25). Chronic tendinitis may also cause the formation of calcium deposits in either the affected tendon or an associated sheath. These calcium deposits that form in the shoulder joint as a result of chronic trauma often cause rotator cuff tears, which can be detected on shoulder arthrogram and magnetic resonance examinations of the shoulder.

Common medical treatment of bursitis and tendinitis include nonsteroidal antiinflammatory agents in combination with analgesics. In severe cases, corticosteroid injections may be used. In cases in which the tendons or bursae ossify, surgical intervention is necessary, especially in conjunction with rotator cuff tears.

Gouty Arthritis

Gouty arthritis is an inherited metabolic disorder in which excess amounts of uric acid are produced and deposited in the joint and adjacent bone. The condition occurs more frequently in males and most commonly affects the metatarsophalangeal joint of the great toe. It is characterized by acute attacks with intervals of remission.

The crystallization of uric acid within the joint causes an acute inflammatory reaction. Large masses of these sodium urate crystalline deposits in joints and other sites are called *tophi*. Bony changes include erosion (Fig. 2-26) with overhanging edges. One long-term complication of gout is the formation of radiolucent kidney stones caused by increased excretion of uric acid by the kidneys. Treatment of gout consists

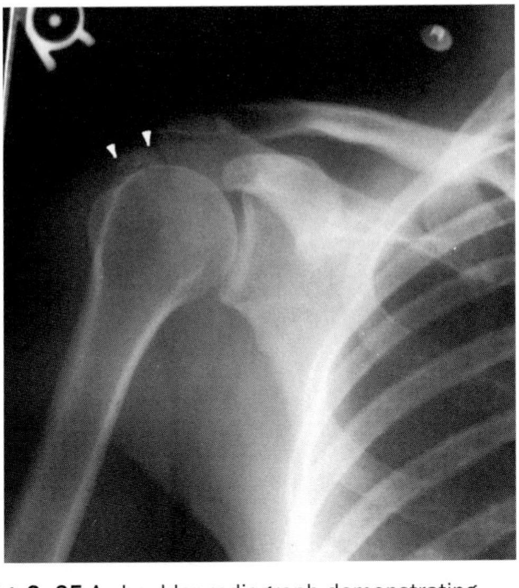

Fig. 2-25 A shoulder radiograph demonstrating radiopaque calcium deposits within the bursa caused by chronic bursitis. (Courtesy Riverside Methodist Hospitals, Columbus, Ohio.)

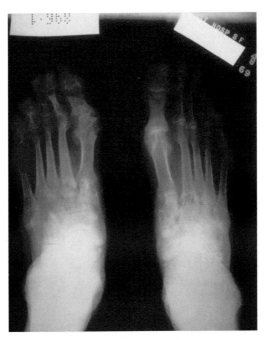

Fig. 2-26 Bilateral feet demonstrates multiple erosions of the bone, some associated with soft tissue tophi, as is consistent with gout. Asymmetry of these lesions helps distinguish them from rheumatoid arthritis. (Courtesy the American College of Radiology, Reston, Virginia.)

of medications either to promote excretion of uric acid by the kidneys or to inhibit the production of uric acid within the body.

METABOLIC DISEASE

Osteoporosis

A prime determinant of radiographic film density is the amount of calcium present in the bone structure. **Osteoporosis** (osteopenia) is an increasingly known metabolic bone disorder common in women past menopause, as well as in the aged as related to problems with protein metabolism. Estimates are that more than half of the women in North America over age 60

have osteoporosis. The disease is characterized by an abnormal decrease in bone density caused by failure of osteoblasts to lay down bony protein matrix. The normal equilibrium associated with osteoid production and withdrawal is quite complicated and depends on a combination of dietary intake and absorption, hormonal interplay, and normal stress or muscular activity. In postmenopausal women, for example, the lack of the hormone estrogen creates a weakened bony matrix, contributing to the development of "porous" bones. As this condition becomes more severe, these bones are subject to compression fractures, as they can literally cave in from the weakness. The bony changes caused by

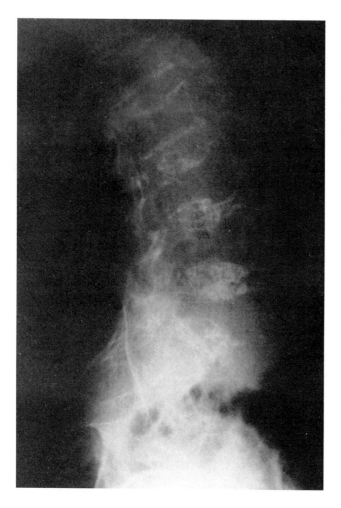

Fig. 2-27 A lateral lumbar spine radiograph of an elderly woman who complained of back pain. The radiograph revealed severe osteoporosis with compression fractures of the vertebrae. (Courtesy Riverside Methodist Hospitals, Columbus, Ohio.)

osteoporosis are best demonstrated in the spine (Fig. 2-27), where decreased bone density stands out clearly against the bony cortex. This condition requires a decrease in exposure technique.

Osteoporosis is by far the most common form of metabolic bone disease and can be differentiated from osteomalacia by examining serum enzyme levels, especially phosphorus. Patients with osteoporosis have normal serum enzyme levels, whereas patients with osteomalacia present with a decrease in serum phosphorus. Treatment generally includes an increase in dietary intake of calcium, vitamin D, and sex hormone supplements.

Osteomalacia

Osteomalacia is a condition caused by a lack of calcium in the tissues and a failure of bone tissue to calcify. This normally results from inadequate

intake or absorption of calcium, phosphorus, or vitamin D. With this condition, the bones remain spongelike, resembling osteoporosis in radiographic appearance. Laboratory analysis and other testing are necessary to differentiate the diagnosis. If osteomalacia occurs before growth plate closure, it is known as **rickets** (Fig. 2-28). Proper nutritional education is vital to populations susceptible to osteomalacia. Adequate calcium, phosphorus, and vitamin D intake can prevent or frequently cure this disorder.

Paget's Disease (Osteitis Deformans)

Paget's disease is a metabolic disorder of unknown etiology that is fairly common in the elderly population, affecting men twice as frequently as women. It usually begins in the fifth decade of life and may affect one or more bones, most commonly the pelvis, spine, skull (Fig. 2-29), and the long bones (Fig.

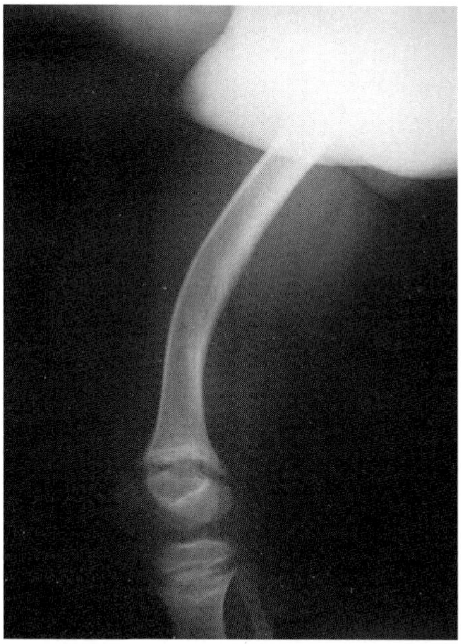

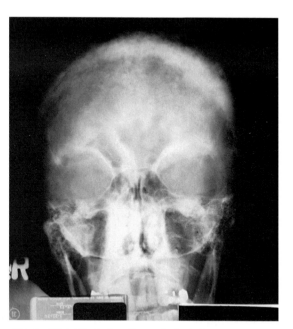

Fig. 2-28 A radiograph of a femur of a child diagnosed with vitamin D–resistant rickets. Notice the bowing of the extremity. (Courtesy the American College of Radiology, Reston, Virginia.)

Fig. 2-29 A PA skull radiograph depicting an advanced proliferative phase of Paget's disease. Notice the changes within the inner and outer tables of the skull. (Courtesy the American College of Radiology, Reston, Virginia.)

2-30). Paget's disease is characterized by two stages in which the bone undergoes continuous destruction, called the *osteolytic stage*, and simultaneous replacement by abnormally soft and poorly mineralized material, called the *osteoblastic stage*. The osteoid material that replaces the normal bone tissue is very bulky and porous, with exceptional vascularity. Although this osteoid matrix is thicker than the normal bone, its softness often leads to weight-bearing, stress-induced deformities and fractures. As the skull enlarges, additional complications may occur because of impingement of the cranial nerves. These complications include hearing and vision disturbances. In addition, individuals with Paget's disease have an increased risk of developing osteogenic sarcoma, a malignant neoplastic disease of the skeletal system. Radionuclide bone scans readily detect Paget's disease, even in its very early stages. Radiographically, the affected bones typically demonstrate cortical thickening with a coarse, thickened trabecular

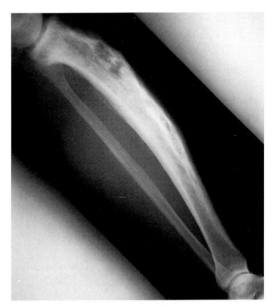

Fig. 2-30 A radiograph of the tibia of the patient in demonstrating the effect of advanced proliferative Paget's disease on the tibia. (Courtesy the American College of Radiology, Reston, Virginia.)

pattern. Mixed areas of radiolucent osteolysis and radiopaque osteosclerosis may be seen. Blood chemistry results indicate very high alkaline phosphatase levels with normal serum calcium and phosphorus. There is no known cure for this disease. Most cases are mild and asymptomatic; no treatment is necessary. In symptomatic cases, medications are administered to decrease bone resorption.

Hyperparathyroidism

Hyperparathyroidism is a fairly common disease of the endocrine system, but it is discussed in this chapter because of its effect on the skeletal system. This disease is often very mild and may go undetected for a long time. Like all metabolic bone diseases, the entire skeleton is affected in hyperparathyroidism, with some sites more affected than others.

Remember that the skeletal system is involved in the balance of serum calcium and phosphorus levels and that the body strives to keep this ratio constant. Hyperparathyroidism applies to any disorder that disrupts the calcium-phosphate ratio and results in an elevated level of parathyroid hormone (PTH). Excess PTH secretion overstimulates the osteoclasts that are responsible for bone removal, thus leading to bone destruction. This osteoclastic activity results in a decreased bone density, so a decrease in radiographic exposure is necessary to produce a high-quality radiographic image.

There are basically three types of hyperparathyroidism: primary hyperparathyroidism, secondary hyperparathyroidism, and a third type caused by ectopic production of a parathyroid-like hormone. Treatment varies with each specific cause of hyperparathyroidism and is very complex.

Primary hyperparathyroidism arises from an adenoma, carcinoma, or hyperplasia of the parathyroid gland and may be treated surgically. The excess production of PTH causes bone destruction, an increased absorption of calcium by the intestines and kidneys, and an increase in urine calcium, which predisposes the individual to renal stones. The net effect of these reactions to the high level of PTH is an increase in serum calcium with a decrease in serum phosphate. Individuals affected with primary hyperparathyroidism may first present with symptoms of renal colic, but radiographic investigation demonstrates subperiosteal bone resorption, especially in the diaphyses of the phalanges and clavicles. Bone resorption is also radiographically evident in the teeth.

Secondary hyperparathyroidism (Fig. 2-31) represents a response to hypocalcemia, hyperphosphatemia, or hypomagnesemia. It is caused by a very complex metabolic disorder that is beyond the scope of this text and is most commonly seen in individuals with chronic renal disease. Decreased renal function leads to a loss of the kidneys' ability to produce vitamin D and compromises their ability to excrete phosphate.

Acromegaly

Although **acromegaly** is an endocrine disorder caused by a disturbance of the pituitary gland, it is briefly mentioned in this chapter because of its effect on the skeletal system. This disorder is caused by excessive secretion of growth hormones in the adult, which is often due to a pituitary adenoma. Acromegaly is a slowly progressive disease that may be diagnosed years after the individual is symptomatic. An increase in growth hormone in the adult produces a thickening and coarsening on the bones because the epiphyses have closed and the bone cannot grow in length. Radiographic studies demonstrate an enlarged sella turcica and changes in the skull, often obliterating the diploë found between the inner and outer tables of the cortical bone. Individuals with acromegaly present with a prominent forehead and jaw, widened teeth, abnormally large, spadelike hands (Fig. 2-32), and a coarsening of

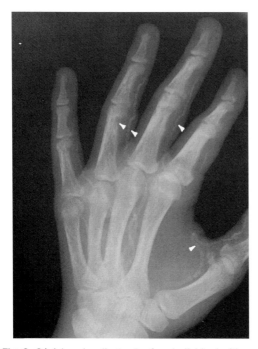

Fig. 2–31 A hand radiograph of an individual with secondary hyperparathyroidism. Notice the subperiosteal resorption of bone and calcification of the arteries of the hand. (Courtesy the American College of Radiology, Reston, Virginia.)

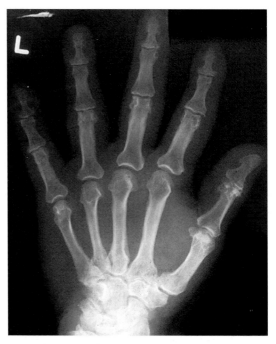

Fig. 2–32 A hand radiograph of an individual diagnosed with acromegaly. Notice the spadelike appearance of the hand. (Courtesy the American College of Radiology, Reston, Virginia.)

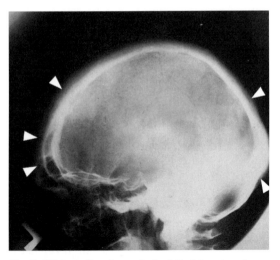

Fig. 2-33 A skull radiograph depicting the changes caused by acromegaly. (Courtesy the American College of Radiology, Reston, Virginia.)

Table 2-1   Anatomic Components of the Scotty Dog

Dog Part	Anatomic Component
Eye	Pedicle
Nose	Transverse process
Ear	Superior articular process
Foreleg	Inferior articular process
Neck	Pars interarticularis
Body	Lamina

facial features (Fig. 2-33). This disorder is frequently treated with a combination of surgery and radiation therapy to eradicate the adenoma.

VERTEBRAL COLUMN

The causes of vertebral column injuries include direct trauma, hyperextension-flexion injuries (whiplash), osteoporosis, or metastatic destruction. **Whiplash** is a broad term encompassing soft tissue neck injuries from a variety of causes. Pain in the posterior neck is a primary manifestation, either dull or sharp, and may radiate. Imaging of whiplash injuries is limited to soft tissue studies, with exclusion of fractures and dislocations the first priority. Loss of lordosis is the most common finding on postwhiplash radiographs.

Radiographic indications of spinal column injuries include the interruption of smooth, continuous lines formed by the vertebrae stacking on each other. Also, the vertebral bodies may lose some height, or the interspace may narrow. Muscle spasm as a result of trauma may cause a reversal or straightening of the normal spinal curvatures.

Perhaps the most common condition of the vertebral column is generalized back pain, typically in the lumbar area. Such back pain may not always result from bony involvement. Disk disease can cause muscle spasm with pain referral throughout the back. Finally, back pain may be secondary to referred pain from the hip.

Spondylolysis exists when there is a cleft, or breaking down, of the body of a vertebra between the superior and inferior articular processes (pars interarticularis). Typically, this occurs in the arch of the fifth lumbar vertebra as a result of developmental or congenital anomaly rather than as related to acute trauma. It appears radiographically as a "collar" or "broken neck" on the "Scotty dog" (Table 2-1) appearance and is demonstrated on an oblique projection of the lumbar spine (Fig. 2-34). When forward slippage of the vertebral column off a vertebra occurs because of spondylolysis, it is known as **spondylolisthesis.** The patient with this condition may present symptoms identical to those of a herniated disk. Approximately 90% of such slippage commonly occurs at the L5-S1 junction and is best detected on a lateral projection (Fig. 2-35). Conservative medical management (e.g., rest, chiropractic manipulative therapy) is the preferred choice for treatment prior to surgical fusion.

NEOPLASTIC DISEASE

Many varieties of bone tumors exist and are seen in patients of all ages. The most common benign tumors are osteoma, osteochondroma, and giant cell tumor. The primary malignant bone tumors are osteosarcoma, Ewing's tumor, and multiple myeloma (discussed in the hemopoietic system).

The diagnosis of a bony abnormality is often made radiographically on the basis of the patient's age, pattern of bone destruction, the location of the tumor, and its position within the bone. In terms of age, benign tumors most often occur within the first three decades of life; a bone tumor in the elderly is likely to be malignant. The pattern of bony destruction in benign lesions is to expand the bone and demonstrate sharp, sclerotic margins. Malignant neoplasms often infiltrate, permeate, and destroy anatomic margins. The location of a tumor is also important. For example, half of all osteosarcomas

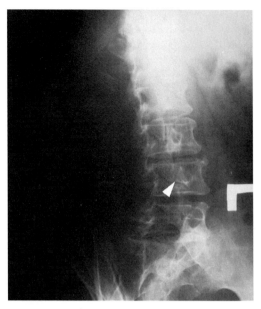

Fig. 2-34 An oblique radiograph of the lumbar spine demonstrating spondylolysis of the fourth and fifth lumbar spine on the left side. Notice the "break in the Scotty dog's neck." (Courtesy the American College of Radiology, Reston, Virginia.)

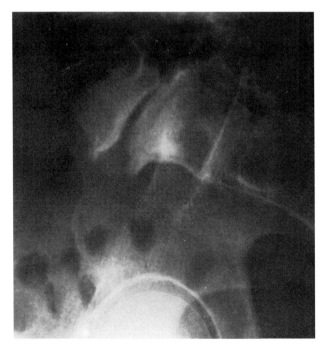

Fig. 2-35 An L5-S1 spot radiograph of a female complaining of low back pain, demonstrating spondylolisthesis of this joint. (Courtesy Riverside Methodist Hospitals, Columbus, Ohio.)

appear in the distal femoral or proximal tibial metaphysis. Similarly, chondrosarcomas tend to involve the trunk, shoulder girdle, and proximal long bones.

Radiographic studies contribute greatly to the diagnosis and management of bone tumor patients. Plain films are used to disclose the lesions and show the growth characteristics that assist in determining their benign or malignant nature. In conjunction with conventional tomography and CT, plain radiographs identify malignant growth patterns and the proper site for biopsy. Sometimes, seemingly unrelated examinations, such as a barium enema or chest radiograph, are ordered by the physician to rule out distant metastases.

Osteochondroma (Exostosis)

The most common benign bone tumor is the **osteochondroma** (Fig. 2-36), typically affecting males three times more often than females. An osteochondroma arises from the growth zone between the epiphysis vand diaphysis of long bones, also called the *metaphysis*. Most commonly, it involves the lower femur or upper tibia and is capped by growing cartilage at-

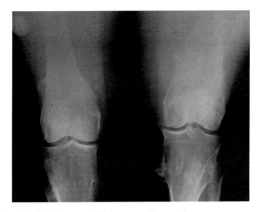

Fig. 2-36 Bilateral AP knee radiographs demonstrating osteochondroma with exostoses within the knee joint. (Courtesy the American College of Radiology, Reston, Virginia.)

tached to the skeleton by a bony stalk. The cortex of an osteochondroma blends with the normal bone, and the growth tends to protrude up and away from the nearest joint, most commonly the knee. **Exostoses** or excessive bone growth may appear as singular or multiple lesions and are normally diagnosed in childhood or adolescence. Multiple exostoses is a hereditary disorder and usually appears at an earlier age than the single-lesion osteochondroma. In addition, multiple exostoses may transform to malignant neoplasms such as chondrosarcoma. Many times, osteochondromas are asymptomatic unless the affected long bone is traumatized, which results in a pathologic fracture of the diseased bone.

Osteoma

An **osteoma** is a less frequent benign growth most commonly located in the skull. These lesions are composed of very dense, well-circumscribed, normal bone tissue that usually projects into the orbits or paranasal sinuses. They are generally slow-growing tumors of little significance unless they cause obstruction, impinge on the brain or eye, or interfere with the oral cavity. A term associated with osteoma of the skull is **hyperostosis frontalis interna** (Fig. 2-37).

Endochondroma

An **endochondroma** is a slow-growing benign tumor composed of cartilage. It grows in the marrow space and most commonly affects the small bones of the hands and feet in individuals between the ages of 10 and 30 years. These benign tumors do not invade the surrounding tissue as they grow; however, they do expand the cortical bone, causing thinning. Radiographically, endochondromas appear as radiolucent lesions containing small, stippled calcifications (Fig. 2-38). The erosion of the cortex may cause pain and swelling and increase the incidence of pathologic fractures.

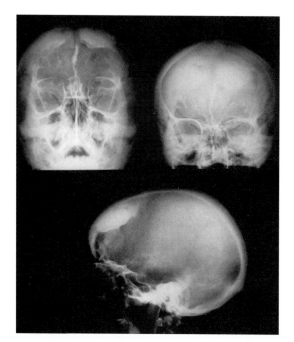

Fig. 2-37 Various skull projections demonstrating hyperostosis frontalis interna. (Courtesy the American College of Radiology, Reston, Virginia.)

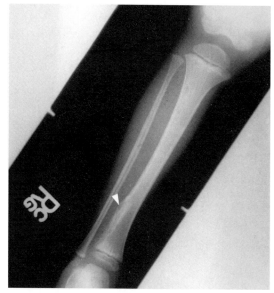

Fig. 2-38 An AP tibia-fibula radiograph demonstrating an endochondroma of the distal tibia as evidenced by small, scattered, well-defined, oval lucent defects. (Courtesy the American College of Radiology, Reston, Virginia.)

Multiple growths, termed *endochondromatosis,* may also occur in childhood and, like multiple osteochondromas, may undergo malignant transformation.

Simple Bone Cyst

A **simple bone cyst** is a wall of fibrous tissue filled with fluid. These frequently occur in the long bones of children, most commonly in the humerus (Fig. 2-39) and proximal femur. Eighty percent of all simple bone cysts occur between 3 and 14 years of age, and twice as often in boys as in girls. The cyst is usually first noticed when the patient presents with pain caused by the increased tumor growth or as a result of a pathologic fracture.

Radiographically, simple bone cysts appear radiolucent with well-defined margins from the normal bone surrounding the lesion (Fig. 2-40). Occasionally, the cyst may be surrounded by a thin rim of sclerotic bone. Small cysts tend to heal and obliterate themselves; larger cysts require surgical intervention. The benign bone cyst is treated by surgical excision and packing with bone chips to obtain complete healing.

Osteoid Osteoma and Osteoblastoma

Other common benign tumors of the skeletal system are the **osteoid osteoma** and the **osteoblastoma.** Similar in histologic features, they differ in size, origin, and symptoms. Osteoid osteomas are less than 2 cm in dimension, while osteoblastomas are larger. Osteoblastomas more frequently involve the spine, and pain may not be present. Further, they are not associated with a marked bony reaction.

A

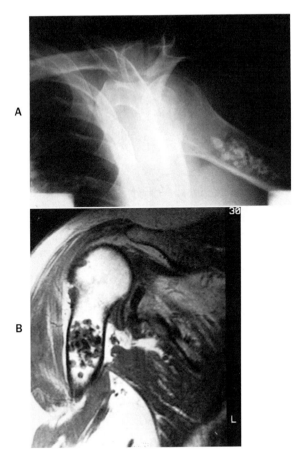

B

Fig. 2-39 A, A conventional shoulder radiograph in a 66-year-old man demonstrates calcification in the proximal diaphysis of the right humerus. **B,** Follow-up MRI demonstrates an intramedullary lesion without breakthrough of the cortex, consistent with an enchondoma. (Courtesy Riverside Methodist Hospitals, Columbus, Ohio.)

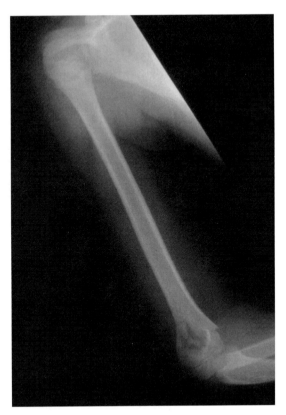

Fig. 2-40 An AP radiograph demonstrating a well-circumscribed radiolucency consistent with a simple bone cyst. (Courtesy Riverside Methodist Hospitals, Columbus, Ohio.)

Osteoid osteomas occur twice as often in males than in females and almost always develop before the age of 30 years. Osteoid osteomas are most commonly found in the femur, tibia, or spine of the young adult. They arise within the cortical bone and erode the underlying bone tissue, resulting in a lytic lesion called a *nidus.* The area of erosion is surrounded by a zone of dense, sclerotic bone, making the radiographic appearance of osteoid osteomas very distinctive (Fig. 2-41). In some cases, however, the rim of hypertrophied bone may obscure the lytic center, requiring the use of tomography to better visualize the nidus. Radionuclide bone scans are also of value in identifying and localizing osteoid osteomas. The erosion of the surrounding tissue causes extreme pain, often at night, which is readily relieved by aspirin. Treatment of an osteoid osteoma requires surgical removal of the nidus.

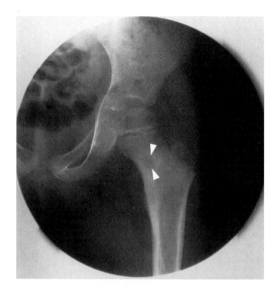

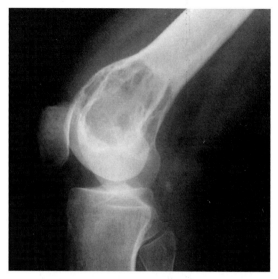

Fig. 2-41 An AP hip radiograph of a 7-year-old girl who complained of a 2-month history of aching pain. The radiograph demonstrates an osteoid osteoma as evidenced by the well-defined defect in the cortical area of the femoral neck. (Courtesy the American College of Radiology, Reston, Virginia.)

Fig. 2-42 A lateral knee radiograph of a 30-year-old man who complained of a painful knee for approximately 2 months. The radiograph demonstrates a benign osteoclastoma of the knee. (Courtesy the American College of Radiology, Reston, Virginia.)

Osteoclastoma (Giant Cell Tumor)

Osteoclastoma refers to a group of tumors characterized by the presence of numerous, multinucleated osteoclastic giant cells. Unlike the previously mentioned neoplastic diseases, giant cell tumors may be either benign or malignant. Approximately 50% of osteoclastomas are benign, 35% recur after surgical excision, and 15% are aggressively malignant from the beginning. This neoplasm affects the sexes equally and is found in individuals between the ages of 20 to 30 years. Anatomically, this disease tends to affect the ends or epiphyses of long bones, especially the lower femur, upper tibia, and lower radius. It begins in the medullary canal and expands outward, producing a club-like deformity of the end of the long bone. In addition, soft tissue extensions may be present, but giant cell tumor does not involve the joint space.

Clinical signs and symptoms of an osteoclastoma are nonspecific and include pain, tenderness, an occasional palpable mass, and an occasional pathologic fracture. Because this is an osteoclastic disease process, bone and cartilage formation generally do not occur in these lesions; therefore, the technologist must decrease exposure factors to avoid overpenetration of the affected bone. Radiographically, a giant cell tumor presents as a mass of osteolytic or cystic areas surrounded by a thin shell of bone, giving it the classic "soap bubble" appearance (Fig. 2-42). Treatment of an osteoclastoma consists of surgical excision and bone grafting.

Osteosarcoma (Osteogenic Sarcoma)

Except for myeloma, the most common primary malignancy of the skeleton is the **osteosarcoma,**

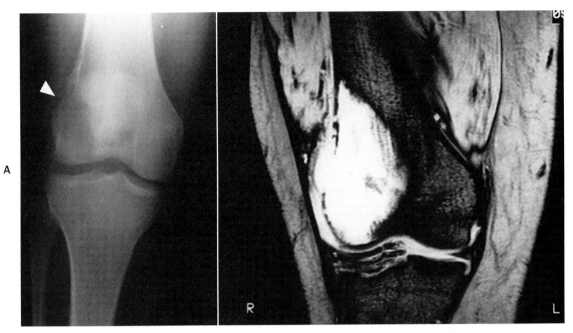

Fig. 2-43 A, An AP radiograph of the right knee demonstrates a tumor in the distal lateral femoral condyle. Interruption of the cortex and reactive sclerotic bone changes are suspect for metastatic disease or primary malignancy. **B,** Follow-up MRI of the knee reveals an osteosarcoma that has replaced the distal femoral condyle. (Courtesy Riverside Methodist Hospitals, Columbus, Ohio.)

which arises from osteoblasts. This neoplasm is most frequently found in the metaphyses of long bones, with approximately 50% affecting the knee (Fig. 2-43). Osteosarcoma can occur at any age, but 75% occur in patients younger than 20 years old. It is occasionally seen in older individuals with Paget's disease or following high-level radiation exposure to the bone. Clinically, the patient may present with pain and swelling.

Osteosarcoma is a highly malignant disease with a poor prognosis because lung metastasis almost always occurs via the bloodstream. This metastatic lung disease may appear as multiple, rounded, calcified shadows within the lung fields on a conventional chest radiograph. If the chest radiograph is clear, CT of the chest often

demonstrates micrometastases, as they are commonly present in the lungs before the primary osteosarcoma is discovered. Secondary growths or spread to other bones is very rare with osteosarcoma. Treatment of osteosarcoma includes amputation of the limb followed by chemotherapy. The 5-year survival rate has improved with advances in treatment from 20% to about 60% in recent years.

As the tumor grows from the metaphysis, it lifts the periosteum from the cortical bone and lays down spicules of new bone radiating out from the origin, which gives the radiographic appearance of a sunray or sunburst. This appearance is due to the radiopaque and radiolucent changes within the newly created space between the cortex of the metaphysis and the displaced

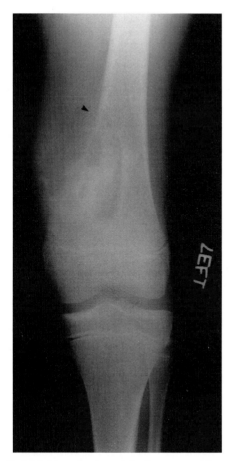

Fig. 2-44 A PA projection of the knee on a 14-year-old boy with painful swelling above the left knee. The radiograph demonstrated cortical destruction along the posteromedial margin of the distal femur consistent with an osteosarcoma of the left femur. (Courtesy the American College of Radiology, Reston, Virginia.)

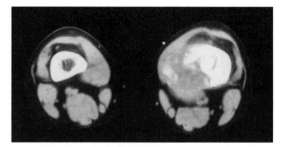

Fig. 2-45 An MRI of the left femur of the patient in Fig. 2-44, MRI is helpful in determining the medullary extension of the osteosarcoma. (Courtesy the American College of Radiology, Reston, Virginia.)

periosteum. However, radiographic findings (Figs. 2-44 and 2-45) vary greatly in appearance because some osteosarcoma tumors produce very little osteoid tissue and contain no calcifications, and others are densely opaque. In both cases, the radiograph would not display the characteristic sunray appearance. Accurate diagnosis must be made through biopsy of the questionable lesion.

Ewing's Sarcoma

Another primary malignant bone tumor is a **Ewing's sarcoma.** This neoplasm occurs at a younger age than any other primary malignant bone neoplasm, usually between the ages of 5 to 15 years and rarely after age 30. It is also more common in males than in females and shows a predilection for whites, with blacks rarely affected.

Unlike osteosarcoma, Ewing's sarcoma arises from the medullary canal and involves the bone more diffusely, giving rise to uniform thickening of the bone. These lesions tend to be very extensive, often involving the entire shaft of a long bone. Also unlike osteogenic sarcoma, Ewing's sarcoma does not begin at the end of a long bone. It does, however, tend to affect the extremities and pelvis. Although Ewing's sarcoma is a fairly rare disease, it is extremely malignant. Increasingly effective chemotherapy has improved the prognosis to a 75% 5-year survival rate. Clinical symptoms are nonspecific and include pain and tenderness of the affected area. The lesions undergo a combination of bone formation in the early stages and destruction in the later stages, with new bone being

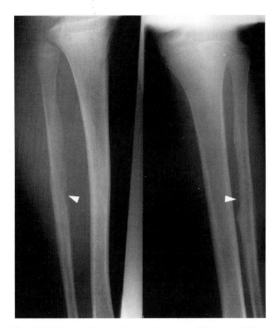

Fig. 2-46 Lower leg radiographs on a 12-year-old boy complaining of the left leg pain demonstrating a Ewing's sarcoma of the tibia as indicated by the lytic defect in the proximal diaphysis of the fibula.
(Courtesy the American College of Radiology, Reston, Virginia.)

formed on the surface (Fig. 2-46). This process often gives a classic onionskin or laminated appearance radiographically.

Chondrosarcoma

A **chondrosarcoma** is a malignant tumor of cartilaginous origin and is composed of atypical cartilage. It is only about half as common as osteosarcoma and comprises approximately 10% of all malignant tumors of the skeletal system. Common locations for chondrosarcoma are the pelvis, shoulder, and ribs. Men are three times more likely than women to develop chondrosarcoma, and it is more common in older adults. As mentioned earlier in this chapter, benign exostoses and multiple endochondromas may be transformed into chondrosarcomas.

However, this type of change accounts for only about 10% of the cases, with approximately 90% of chondrosarcomas arising afresh without prior cartilaginous lesions. Chondrosarcomas may be bulky, and they tend to destroy the bone as they extend through the cortex into the surrounding soft tissue. These lesions have the ability to implant or seed into the surrounding soft tissue, so careful excision is a necessity. While neither radiation therapy nor chemotherapy is particularly effective in the treatment of chondrosarcomas, adequate excision leads to a good prognosis, with a 5-year survival rate of 50% to 90%.

Metastases from Other Sites

Virtually any type of cancer can metastasize to bone; metastatic disease from carcinomas is the most common malignant tumor of the skeleton, with secondary bone tumors of any origin far outnumbering primary bone tumors. Patients presenting with skeletal metastases are usually past the fourth decade in age. Principal signs are pain and pathologic fracture.

The bones of the skeletal system that contain red bone marrow are the major bones affected by the metastatic disease because of their good vascularization (Fig. 2-47). These include flat bones (such as the ribs, sternum, pelvis, and skull), the vertebrae, and the upper ends of the femora and humeri. The spine is the most common site for metastasis to occur, accounting for about 40% of all metastatic lesions. Radionuclide bone scans are more accurate than conventional radiography in detection of metastasis. Three percent to 5% bone destruction renders a "hot spot," while plain films require at least 30% loss of bone for metastasis to be detected visually. Radiographically, signs of bone metastasis include alteration of bone density and architecture. These can be osteolytic, osteoblastic, or mixed. Osteolytic metastases account for 75% of all metastatic lesions.

Certain characteristics help distinguish between a primary malignant neoplasm and a sec-

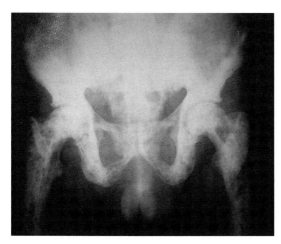

Fig. 2–47 An AP pelvis radiograph on an elderly man diagnosed with carcinoma of the prostate. There is diffuse metastatic disease to the pelvis from the prostatic primary. (Courtesy the American College of Radiology, Reston, Virginia.)

ondary one. Periosteal response is much more common with primary malignant tumors. Soft tissue masses are common in primary tumors and rare in metastases. Lesions longer than 10 cm often represent a primary malignant tumor; most metastatic tumors range between 2 and 4 cm in length. Tumors that expand bone are primary in nature, with rare exception. Most primary tumors are solitary, while metastatic lesions are usually multiple. Definitive diagnosis is obtained through biopsy.

The most common primary sites for metastatic bone cancer are the breast, lung, prostate, kidney, thyroid, and bowel, with the tumor spreading via proximity (direct extension), the bloodstream, or the lymphatic system. Treatment of metastatic disease is dependent on the primary disease, but radiation therapy in combination with either chemotherapy or hormone therapy is commonly used to manage such patients. Bone scans are used to follow the progress of therapy; a reduction in uptake on serial scans is a positive sign.

QUESTIONS

1. Specialized cells responsible of the formation of bone are termed:
   a. chondroblasts   c. osteoclasts
   b. osteoblasts   d. both b and c

2. A freely movable joint is classified as:
   a. amphiarthrodial   c. synarthrodial
   b. diarthrodial   d. triarthrodial

3. Bone marrow is located anatomically within the:
   a. cortex   c. periosteum
   b. medullary canal   d. trabeculae

4. The end portion of a long bone is referred to as the:
   a. epiphysis   c. diploë
   b. diaphysis   d. metaphysis

5. The human body normally contains:
   a. 156 bones   c. 197 bones
   b. 175 bones   d. 206 bones

6. The most common inherited disorder that results in dwarfism is:
   a. achondroplasia
   b. Albers-Schönberg disease
   c. osteogenesis imperfecta
   d. spina bifida

7. The term *marble bone* is often associated with the skeletal disorder:
   a. achondroplasia   c. osteopetrosis
   b. osteomalacia   d. osteoporosis

8. The formation of extra digits is termed:
   a. adactyly   c. syndactyly
   b. polydactyly   d. talipes

9. An abnormal lateral curvature of the spine is referred to as:
   a. ankylosing spondylitis
   b. scoliosis
   c. spondylolisthesis
   d. spondylolysis

10. Osteomyelitis is a disease of the skeletal system that is:
    a. arthritic   c. inflammatory
    b. congenital   d. neoplastic

11. The most common type of arthritis affecting both sexes equally is:
    a. ankylosing spondylitis
    b. gout
    c. osteoarthritis
    d. rheumatoid arthritis

12. The type of arthritis believed to be an autoimmune disease is:
    a. bursitis   c. osteoarthritis
    b. gout   d. rheumatoid arthritis

13. Rickets, which affects children, is a type of:
    a. hyperparathyroidism
    b. osteomalacia
    c. osteopetrosis
    d. osteoporosis

14. The most common benign bone tumor is the:
    a. endochondroma   c. osteoma
    b. osteoid osteoma   d. osteochondroma

15. All of the following are malignant neoplasms of the skeletal system *except:*
    a. chondrosarcoma
    b. Ewing's sarcoma
    c. osteosarcoma
    d. osteoma

16. A 60-year-old patient who was discharged from the hospital following knee replacement continued to complain of generalized pain in the area of the knee for several days. If you're this patient's physician, what imaging test might you order and why?

17. A 35-year-old woman presents to her family physician with complaints of swelling that comes and goes in her hands. What might be your initial suspicion?

18. Describe the mechanism behind the development of osteoporosis.

19. A male construction worker presents to his physician with lower back pain. What might a couple of causes be that are unrelated to the bony vertebral column?

20. In diagnosing bone tumors, what are some of the characteristics taken into consideration?.

Chapter 3

The Respiratory System

Anatomy and Physiology Review
Imaging Considerations
    Exposure factor conditions
    Position and projection
    The standard chest radiograph
    Other chest studies
    Soft tissues of the chest
    Bony structures of the chest
    The mediastinum
Chest Tubes, Vascular Access Lines, and
    Catheters
Congenital and Hereditary Diseases
    Cystic fibrosis
    Hyaline membrane disease

Inflammatory Diseases
    Pneumonias
    Bronchiectasis
    Tuberculosis
    Chronic obstructive pulmonary disease
    Pneumoconioses
    Fungal diseases
    Lung abscess
    Pleurisy
    Pleural effusion
    Sinusitis
Neoplastic Diseases
    Bronchial adenomas
    Bronchogenic carcinoma
    Metastases from other sites

Upon completion of Chapter 3, the reader should be able to:

- Describe the anatomic components of the respiratory system.

- Distinguish between the results obtained and uses for the various projections of the chest.

- Describe the various types of tubes, vascular access lines and catheters used in relation to the respiratory system.

- Characterize a given condition as congenital, inflammatory, or neoplastic.

- Identify the pathogenesis of the chest pathologies cited and the typical treatments for them.

- Describe, in general, the radiographic appearance of each of the given pathologies.

KEY TERMS

Mediastinal emphysema
Subcutaneous emphysema
Cystic fibrosis
Respiratory distress
 syndrome
Pneumonia
Pneumococcal lobar
 pneumonia
Staphylococcal pneumonia
Streptococcal pneumonia

Legionnaires' disease
Mycoplasma pneumonia
Aspiration pneumonia
Viral pneumonia
Bronchiectasis
Tuberculosis
Miliary tuberculosis
Chronic Obstructive
 Pulmonary Disease
 (COPD)

Chronic bronchitis
Emphysema
Pulmonary edema
Pneumoconioses
Pleural effusion
Sinusitis
Bronchial adenoma
Bronchogenic carcinoma

ANATOMY AND PHYSIOLOGY REVIEW

The respiratory system distributes air for the gas exchange with the circulatory system. This system is usually subdivided into the upper respiratory tract—the nose, mouth, pharynx, and larynx—and the lower respiratory tract—the trachea, bronchi, alveoli, and lungs (Fig. 3-1). The thoracic cavity comprises the right and left pleural cavities and the mediastinum. The parietal pleura lines the thoracic cavity, while the visceral pleura adheres directly to the lung tissue.

Anatomically, the mediastinum is divided into anterior, middle, and posterior portions. The anterior mediastinum contains the thyroid and thymus glands. The middle mediastinum contains the heart and great vessels, esophagus, and trachea. The posterior mediastinum contains the descending aorta and spine.

The anatomic bony structures of the thorax assist in both inspiration and expiration. These bony structures include the ribs, sternum, and thoracic vertebrae.

The paranasal sinuses are lined with respiratory epithelium and communicate with the nasal cavities, hence their inclusion in this chapter. The maxillary and ethmoid sinuses are the only paranasal sinuses present at birth. The frontal sinuses generally develop shortly after birth and are fully developed by the age of 10 years. The sphenoid sinus begins to develop around the age of 2 or 3 years and is fully developed by late adolescence.

IMAGING CONSIDERATIONS

The examination most frequently performed in any radiology department is the chest radiograph. Although this examination may seem "routine," chest radiography provides important information about the soft tissues, bone, pleura, and mediastinum, in addition to the lung tissue.

Exposure Factor Conditions

Correct exposure factor selection is critical because it may hide or appear to create pathologic findings. This is particularly true for serial

A

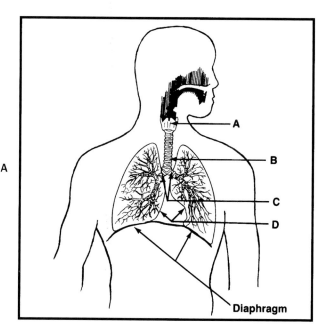

Fig. 3-1 A, The respiratory system. **B,** The trachea and its bifurcation at the carina. (From Bontrager KL: *Textbook of radiographic positioning and related anatomy,* ed 3, St Louis, 1993, Mosby.)

B

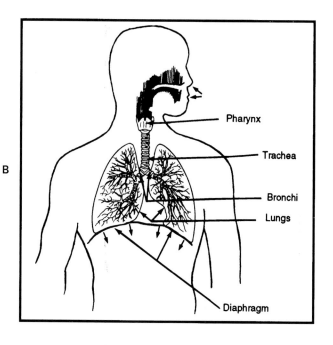

Continued

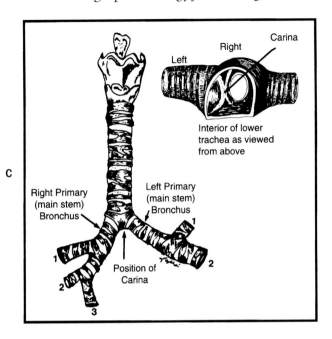

C

Fig. 3-1 cont'd C, The secondary bronchi and alveoli. (From Bontrager KL: *Textbook of radiographic positioning and related anatomy,* ed 3, St Louis, 1993, Mosby.)

portable radiographs since the interpreting physician relies heavily on consistent exposure conditions to analyze the change in pathology after treatment. Institutions use various manual recording techniques for portables so that different technologists can use similar exposure conditions. Mobile automatic exposure control (AEC) devices are also available for portable situations and offer the advantage of exposure consistency associated with conventional AEC. Their use is a bit trickier in portable conditions, however, given the reduced number of sensors. Finally, the emergence of computed radiography (as described later) offers the potential to eliminate exposure repeats caused by the inadequacy or inconsistency of technical factors.

Some sources describe pathologies, including those in the chest, as additive (harder than normal to penetrate) or subtractive (easier than normal to penetrate). In the respiratory system, any condition that adds fluid or tissue to the normally aerated chest (e.g., pneumonia) requires an increase in exposure to afford proper pene-

tration. Similarly, any condition that increases the aeration of the chest (e.g., emphysema) reduces the amount of exposure required for proper densities to be achieved. Most experts agree that manipulation of the milliampere seconds (mAs) is the best approach for exposure adjustments since kilovoltage peak (kVp) changes affect image contrast, making it more difficult for the clinician to compare films.

The use of AEC facilitates consistent radiographic exposures but requires careful analysis of the clinical history and conscious thought about the type of disease present and its location to ensure truly optimal diagnostic-quality radiographs. Activation of the ionization chamber, for example, over an area of significant aeration or *consolidation* (tissue or fluid accumulation) can result in excessive or insufficient exposure, respectively, necessitating a repeat exposure. Again, experience with AEC, combined with careful thought in selecting the proper ionization chambers, can eliminate these mistakes.

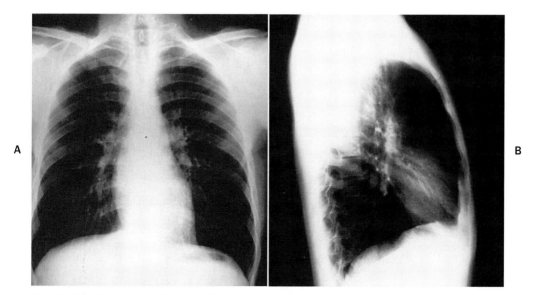

Fig. 3–2 **A,** Normal erect PA chest. **B,** Normal erect lateral chest. (Courtesy the Ohio State University Medical Center, Columbus, Ohio.)

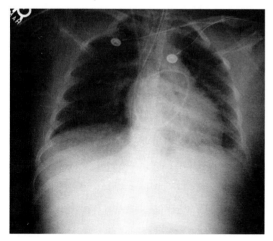

Fig. 3–3 Recumbent AP chest demonstrating obscuring of the lower lung fields. (Courtesy Riverside Methodist Hospitals, Columbus, Ohio.)

Position and Projection

Patient position and projection are also critical exposure conditions that may distort the final image. *Position* refers to the arrangement of the patient's body (e.g., erect, supine, recumbent), while *projection* refers to the path of the x-ray beam (e.g., anteroposterior [AP], meaning entering through the body's anterior surface and exiting the posterior surface). The standard projections for chest radiography are the posteroanterior (PA) and left lateral (Fig. 3-2). Each of these serves to place the heart closest to the film, since it lies in the anterior part of the chest and mostly to the left side. When combined with a standard 72-inch source-to-image distance (SID), magnification of the heart is minimized.

The Standard Chest Radiograph

On a normal erect PA chest image, the costophrenic and cardiophrenic angles are demonstrated with the right hemidiaphragm appearing 1 to 2 cm higher than the left because of the liver. When a patient is radiographed in a recumbent position, the lower lung fields may be obscured because of abdominal pressure raising the level of the diaphragm (Fig. 3-3).

Other projections of the thorax are used less frequently than the PA and left lateral chest radiographs. The AP projection is the method of choice for portable radiography when the patient is too ill to tolerate a visit to the department and assume an erect position. As much as possible, it is important that portable or mobile chest radiographs be taken in an erect position to demonstrate any air-fluid levels present. Maintenance of the beam perpendicular to the plane of the image receptor is most important to avoid any foreshortening of the heart. Further, use of the 72–inch SID is most important for portable radiography to minimize magnification created by the heart, which is located further from the image receptor in the AP projection.

The AP or PA projections of the patient lying in a lateral decubitus position are also useful under specific conditions, such as diagnosing free air in the pleural space or pleural fluid. For example, for a right lateral decubitus chest radiograph, the patient lies on his or her right side. In this position, any fluid present tends to layer out along the edge of the lung field on the dependent side, which enhances its visibility, whereas the free air rises toward the left side.

For evaluation of the standard PA chest radiograph, the size and radiolucency of both lungs should be compared. Criteria for adequate inspiration and penetration of chest radiographs vary from institution to institution; however, a rule of thumb is that adequate inspiration should provide visualization of 10 posterior ribs within the lung field. Additionally, all thoracic vertebrae and intervertebral disk spaces should be faintly visible through the mediastinum on an adequately penetrated chest radiograph. The average movement of the lungs and diaphragm between inspiration and expiration is approximately 3 cm (Fig. 3-4).

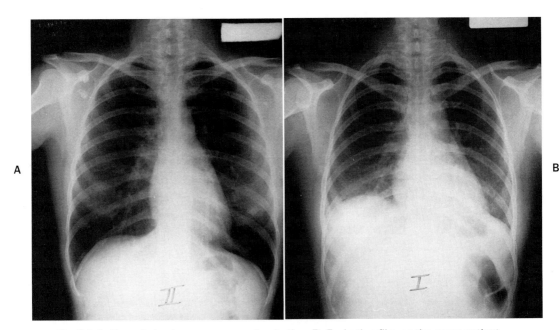

Fig. 3-4 **A,** Normal chest appearance on inspiration. **B,** Expiration film on the same patient demonstrates elevation of the diaphragm and a heart that is more transverse and appears larger. (Courtesy Riverside Methodist Hospitals, Columbus, Ohio.)

Other Chest Studies

Oblique projections are useful in separating superimposed structures such as the sternum, esophagus, and thoracic spine. A lordotic chest

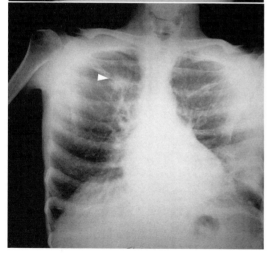

radiograph is useful in demonstrating the apical regions of the lung, which are normally obscured by bony structures on the standard PA projection (Fig. 3-5). Certain diseases (e.g., tuberculosis) have a predilection for the apices. Fluoroscopy of the chest is rarely performed today, but it may be used to appraise the movements of the diaphragm or to assist the physician in biopsy procedures. It may also be performed in differentiating a lung nodule from a pseudonodule and in evaluating cardiac, especially valvular, calcification. Tomography of the chest is useful in the diagnosis of cavities and calcifications in the chest, but has been largely supplanted by computed tomography.

Computed tomography (CT) is becoming the method of choice for evaluation of pulmonary adenopathy (Fig. 3-6). Standard radiographs are only about 50% sensitive to chest disease, typically displaying advanced pathologic conditions. In many cases, they are becoming a screening technique for CT analysis of questionable chest pathology. However, the excellent

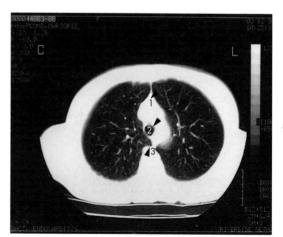

Fig. 3-5 A, PA chest radiograph reveals a suspicious density behind the right clavicle. **B,** Lordotic chest radiograph more clearly reveals coin lesion previously obscured by the right clavicle, later revealed to be cancer. (Courtesy the American College of Radiology, Reston, Virginia.)

Fig. 3-6 A, Normal CT of the chest in the upper lungs with "lung windows", demonstrating *1,* the anterior junction line (sometimes seen on chest radiographs), *2,* the trachea, and *3,* the esophageal recess.(Courtesy Riverside Methodist Hospitals, Columbus, Ohio.) *Continued*

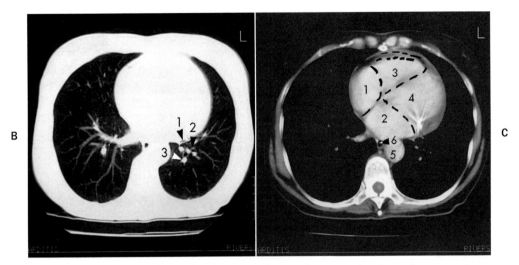

Fig. 3-6 cont'd B, CT view of the chest in the midlungs, demonstrating *1,* a pulmonary vein (distinguished from an artery because of its oval shape), *2,* bronchi, and *3,* an artery (with characteristic rounded shape). **C,** A third CT view of the same chest at the same level as **B,** with a window level adjusted to demonstrate the heart and surrounding structures. Seen are the heart's chambers, *1,* right atrium, *2,* left atrium, *3,* right ventricle, *4,* and left ventricle, as well as other structures, including *5,* the aorta, and *6,* the esophagus (fitting in the esophageal recess). The azygos vein is the small rounded density immediately inferior to the esophagus. Also seen are a small pericardial effusion immediately above the right ventricle. The star-shaped calcification in the left atrium is a mitral anulus calcification. (Courtesy Riverside Methodist Hospitals, Columbus, Ohio.)

specificity of CT can be a problem because most people have granulomatous disease, which is often benign. A rule of thumb for evaluating the character of a visualized nodule relates to its size: those less than 1 cm in size are usually benign, and those larger than 1 cm may be malignant. Also, the presence of calcium within a nodule is a reasonable indication of benignancy, particularly in the middle of the lesion or diffusely within the nodule, but eccentric calcification may indicate malignancy.

The emergence of thin-cut CT, in which slice thicknesses range from 1 to 1.5 mm, holds great promise for evaluation of interstitial lung disease. This typical role of conventional radiography may be supplanted in time by the developing CT techniques, as the role of traditional tomography

has greatly declined in pulmonary evaluations. Spiral or helical CT now also offers the advantage of imaging the entire chest with one breath hold, which allows better evaluation of the chest, especially the diaphragm area. In the past, areas near the diaphragm may or may not have been fully imaged because of variances in the patient's breathing pattern. In addition, the advent of dynamic scanning, made possible with a bolus injection of iodinated contrast agents via an automatic injector, has greatly enhanced CT's role in chest imaging. Magnetic resonance imaging (MRI) is not currently useful in evaluation of pulmonary lesions because of the associated motion. It does have use in mediastinal evaluation to separate adenopathy from vasculature, although this is usually done first by CT.

Perfusion and ventilation scans, as performed in nuclear medicine, are also useful in evaluating chest disease, particularly in the case of obstructive disease and pulmonary emboli. Injection of a radionuclide into the venous system for a perfusion causes it to become trapped in the pulmonary circulation, allowing for gamma camera visualization of its distribution. In a ventilation scan, the patient inhales a radioactive gas (such as xenon) and holds his or her breath while an image is taken of the gas distribution throughout the lungs (Fig. 3-7).

Computed radiography has emerged over the past few years as an imaging modality important in chest radiography (Fig. 3-8), particularly in portable situations such as the

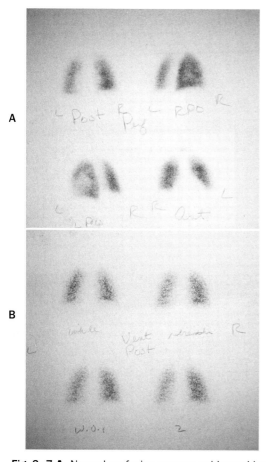

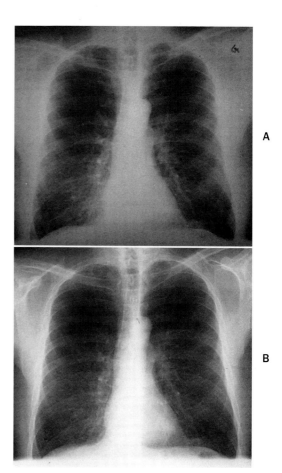

Fig. 3-7 **A,** Normal perfusion scan as evidenced by the sharply defined pleural margins and lung apices. **B,** A ventilation scan with radioactive xenon. The gas "washout" is not entirely normal in the right lung, as seen on the lower right image, where the lungs are not of uniform density. This suggests a partial obstruction of the right mainstream bronchus.
(Courtesy Riverside Methodist Hospitals, Columbus, Ohio.)

Fig. 3-8 **A,** PA chest radiograph taken on a patient, demonstrating proper exposure conditions for comparison to a chest radiograph taken with computed radiography. **B,** Computed radiograph on same patient produced with photostimulable phosphor plate technology, demonstrating nearly 33% dose reduction with increased scale of contrast.
(Courtesy Fuji Medical Systems, Stamford, Connecticut.)

intensive care unit. Most current applications feature photostimulable phosphor plate technology as a replacement for the typical film-screen combination, with trade-offs of significant improvements in film latitude and reduced patient dosages but somewhat less resolving capability than a conventional film-screen image. Precise positioning of the thorax is critical, but the improvement in exposure latitude possible with computed radiography does allow elimination of most repeat radiographs for poor exposure technique—a common complaint of radiologists reading these critical films. In combination with teleradiology and electronic image review capabilities, significant advantages emerge, including the ability to maintain several days of on-line storage at the patient care site, elimination of lost films, and increased availability of the images. Computed radiography is rapidly emerging as a technique important in chest radiography and may gradually become the method of choice for digitizing much of the remaining analog imaging in modern radiography.

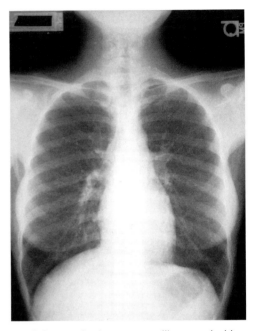

Fig. 3-9 Breast shadows are readily recognizable on the normal PA chest radiograph. (Courtesy Riverside Methodist Hospitals, Columbus, Ohio.)

Soft Tissues of the Chest

Various soft tissue densities are present on chest radiographs. They may vary with patient age, sex, and pathologic conditions. The pectoral muscles are normally demonstrated overlying and extending beyond the lung fields. Radiographs of both men and women demonstrate breast shadows in the midchest region (Fig. 3-9). These shadows are normally homogeneous in appearance, and female breasts may obscure the costophrenic angles. Elevation of the breasts may be necessary to better demonstrate the bases of the lungs. Surgical removal of one or both breasts is also evident on a chest radiograph; breast prostheses, which appear as well-defined, circular radiopaque densities, are also evident. Nipple shadows may be visible at the level of the fourth or fifth anterior rib spaces and may occasionally mimic nodules or masses in the chest. These soft tissue structures may be differentiated with nipple markers or oblique projections of the chest.

Bony Structures of the Chest

The ribs, sternum, and thoracic spine enclose the thoracic cavity. These structures assist the technologist in the assessment of the technical adequacy of chest radiographs. Congenital anomalies of the ribs may be demonstrated (Fig. 3-10), as well as calcified costal cartilages. This calcification generally occurs in patients in their late twenties and beyond. Rib fractures may be seen (Fig. 3-11), sometimes with an accompanying pneumothorax. A depressed sternum (pectus excavatum) may also be demonstrated, possibly displacing the heart (Fig. 3-12). The thoracic spine may be assessed for scoliosis, which can affect the chest cavity, and kyphosis or compression fractures of the vertebrae.

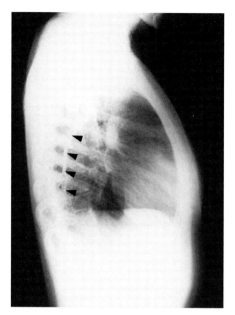

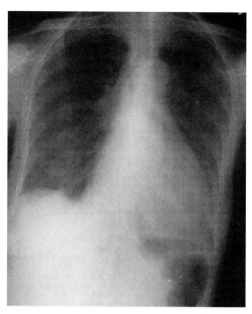

Fig. 3-10 Congenital intrathoracic rib seen as curving, tubular density in the posterior thorax. Usually, these ribs are attached at one or both ends of a posterior rib and lie extrapleurally inside the thoracic cage. (Courtesy the American College of Radiology, Reston, Virginia.)

Fig. 3-11 Rib fractures of the eighth, ninth, and tenth posterior ribs with right apical pneumothorax. (Courtesy the Ohio State University Medical Center, Columbus, Ohio.)

A

B

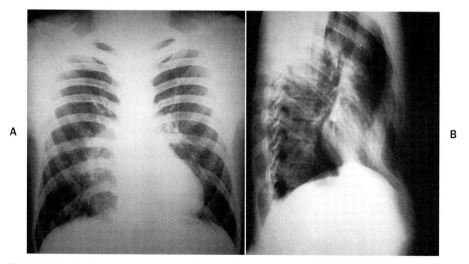

Fig. 3-12 A, Pectus excavatum on a 23-year-old man, indicated by vague density in medial portion of right lower lung field and obscuring of right heart margin. **B,** Lateral projection demonstrating pectus excavatum, including compression of heart toward spine. (Courtesy the American College of Radiology, Reston, Virginia.)

The Mediastinum

The mediastinum contains all thoracic organs except the lungs. The heart occupies a large portion of the mediastinum, and its shape varies with age, degree of respiration, and patient position. Other organs contained within the mediastinum include the thyroid and thymus glands and nervous and lymphatic tissues.

Radiographically, the mediastinum is divided into three sections. Anterior mediastinal masses generally arise from the thyroid gland, thymus gland, or lymphatic tissue. Middle mediastinal masses are commonly lymphatic tissue, and posterior mediastinal masses usually arise from nervous or bony tissue.

In infants, the mediastinum appears wide because the thymus is normally large in a healthy infant. On frontal projections, it may extend beyond the heart borders and caudally to the diaphragm, while on a lateral projection it may fill the anterior portion of the mediastinum, which is normally radiolucent later in life. This radiographic appearance is readily visible on both PA and lateral views and is referred to as the *sail sign* because of its characteristic appearance (Fig. 3-13). Diagnosis is difficult because the width of the upper mediastinum varies greatly with the phase of respiration. A crying child may present an opportune moment for the technologist to make an exposure, but the resultant Valsalva maneuver adds to the distortion of the thymus. True mediastinal masses are rare in infants and generally represent congenital malformations or neoplasms. In the elderly mediastinum, the aorta dilates, and the aortic knob becomes much more visible.

Mediastinal emphysema (pneumomediastinum) occurs when there has been a disruption in the esophagus or airway and air is trapped in the mediastinum (Fig. 3-14). It may result from chest trauma, endoscopy, or violent vomiting. When unaccompanied by a pneumothorax, spontaneous mediastinal emphysema is usually self-limited, subsiding in a few days without complication. Air in the

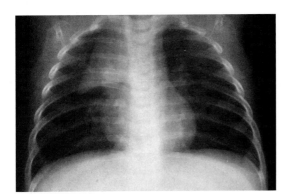

Fig. 3-13 Normal enlargement of the thymus in a 3-month-old infant demonstrates the "sail sign," evidenced by the uniform density increase in the right upper lung area. (Courtesy the American College of Radiology, Reston, Virginia.)

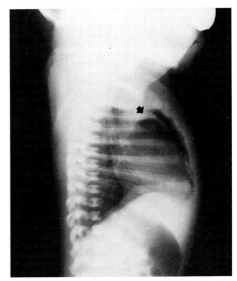

Fig. 3-14 Pneumomediastinum in a lateral chest projection of a full-term newborn, evidenced by air in the normally dense retrosternal space, with sharp outlining of the heart's anterior border. (Courtesy the American College of Radiology, Reston, Virginia.)

mediastinum from rupture of the esophagus (usually from vomiting) or a major bronchus (usually from trauma) is more serious and requires prompt diagnosis and surgical intervention. An esophogram may be performed with a water-soluble contrast agent to verify that a leak has not occurred.

When the pneumomediastinum is extensive, air may pass from the mediastinum into the subcutaneous tissues of the chest or neck, resulting in **subcutaneous emphysema** (Fig. 3-15). Diagnosis of this may be made by feeling air bubbles in the skin of the chest or the neck.

Glandular enlargements of the thyroid gland are demonstrated by a displacement or narrowing of the trachea. The thyroid gland is usually located superior to the lung apices, but an ectopic thyroid gland may also displace the trachea.

Clinical manifestations of an ectopic thyroid gland are often absent, and the mass may be discovered accidentally when chest radiography is performed for some other purpose. Nuclear medicine studies are the modality of choice for detecting thyroid dysfunction and location.

CHEST TUBES, VASCULAR ACCESS LINES, AND CATHETERS

A variety of tubes, lines, and catheters can be placed in relation to particular parts of the respiratory system. It is important for the technologist to be familiar with each of these and exercise great caution in attempting patient movement with any of these in place. It is best to have assistance from another technologist or nursing personnel to ensure the lines and tubes are free of any obstructions before patient movement occurs. Further, the technologist who is unsure whether the patient is allowed to sit erect should always ask the patient's nurse. The x-ray tube, image receptor, and exposure technique should be established before the patient is moved. Patients in critical care units often can be erect for only a short period because of the instability of their blood pressure. Finally, it is necessary to cover cassettes with a plastic bag to limit infection transfer and keep the cold cassette surface from touching the patient's back.

An *endotracheal* (ET) *tube* is a large plastic tube inserted through the patient's nose or mouth into the trachea. It helps to manage the patient's airway, allows frequent suctioning, and allows mechanical ventilation. Its proper position is below the vocal cords and above the carina, the bifurcation of the trachea (Fig. 3-16). Movement of a patient with an endotracheal tube should be done with great caution because inadvertent displacement or extubation may leave the patient without a patent airway.

A *chest tube* is a large plastic tube inserted through the chest wall between the ribs. It allows drainage of air (e.g., pneumothorax) or fluid (e.g., pleural effusion or hemothorax)

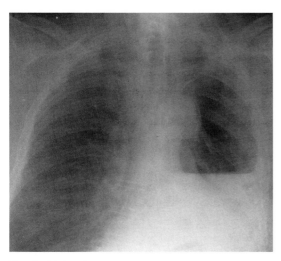

Fig. 3–15 Significant subcutaneous emphysema seen extending along the left chest wall and the left side of the neck, following a left pneumonectomy. (Courtesy the Ohio State University Medical Center, Columbus, Ohio.)

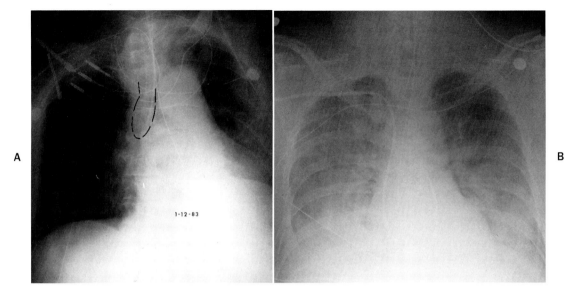

Fig. 3-16 **A.** Incorrect endotracheal (ET) tube placement creates shift of heart and mediastinum to the left with loss of air volume in the left lung. The ET tube tip lies in the proximal right main stem bronchus inferior to the carina. **B,** Correct placement of the endotracheal tube demonstrating balanced lung ventilation. (Courtesy the Ohio State University Medical Center, Columbus, Ohio.)

from the thoracic cavity (Fig. 3-17). Those placed lower on the chest wall are usually for fluid drainage; those placed higher are usually for air removal. After open heart surgery, a chest tube may be placed in the mediastinum for proper fluid drainage. Its location is midline, just below the sternum. The collection device attached to the chest tube must be kept below the level of the chest to allow for proper drainage.

Central venous pressure (CVP) *lines* are usually inserted via the subclavian vein, but they can also be placed through the jugular vein, antecubital vein, or femoral vein. Proper insertion places the tip of the CVP catheter in the distal superior vena cava (SVC) (Fig. 3-18). This catheter provides an alternative injection site to compensate for loss of peripheral infusion sites or to allow for infusion of massive volumes of fluids. In addition, it allows for measurement of

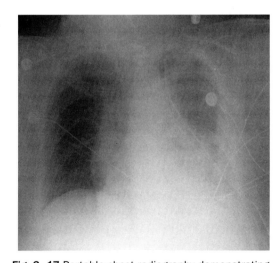

Fig. 3-17 Portable chest radiography demonstrating proper chest tube placement in the left lung near the apex. (Courtesy the Ohio State University Medical Center, Columbus, Ohio.)

central venous pressure, which indicates the patient's fluid status and provides function information about the heart's right side. However, pulmonary artery catheters have largely supplanted the use CVP lines for these purposes because they provide even greater accuracy in measurements.

A *pulmonary artery catheter* (Swan-Ganz catheter) is usually inserted via the subclavian vein, but other injection sites include the antecubital vein, jugular vein, and femoral vein. It is a multilumen catheter that serves to evaluate cardiac function. The pulmonary artery catheter measures pulmonary wedge pressure, reflecting left atrial pressure. It does not enter the heart's left side but is positioned in the pulmonary artery (Fig. 3-19). Inflation of the balloon at the tip of the catheter allows the tube to float into a smaller pulmonary artery capillary. Diagnosis and management of heart failure resulting from myocardial infarction and cardiogenic shock represent the most common use of the catheter.

A *Hickman catheter* is usually inserted via the subclavian vein. The tip of the catheter lies in the superior vena cava (Fig. 3-20). Its purpose is to allow multiple tapping for injection of various

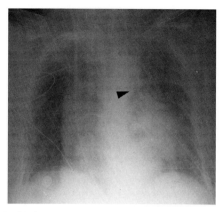

Fig. 3–19 Swan-Ganz catheter placement from the right IJ with the tip in the proximal right pulmonary artery near the takeoff of the truncus anterior. (Courtesy the Ohio State University Medical Center, Columbus, Ohio.)

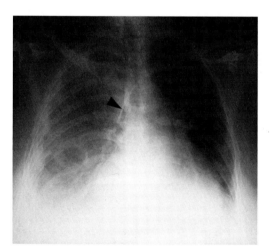

Fig. 3–18 Proper CVP line placement is demonstrated with the tip in the superior vena cava. Bilateral pleural effusions and cardiomegaly are also noted in this 71-year-old man. (Courtesy Riverside Methodist Hospitals, Columbus, Ohio.)

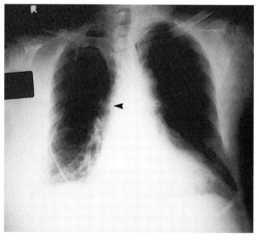

Fig. 3–20 Correct placement of a Hickman catheter within the superior vena cava as demonstrated on this portable chest radiograph of a 73–year-old woman. (Courtesy Riverside Methodist Hospitals, Columbus, Ohio.)

agents, typically chemotherapeutics. Patients on whom these catheters are used typically have poor peripheral venous access because of the toxic effects of chemotherapeutic drugs. Location in the subclavian vein provides ready access to the venous circulation and its blood flow return to the heart and a relatively clean site.

An *intra-aortic balloon pump* (IABP) catheter is a specialized device typically inserted in surgery or at the bedside in critical care units. A 40-cc balloon at the distal end of the catheter allows inflation and deflation by a pump to provide mechanical support of the left ventricle and thus the systemic circulation. Proper placement of the catheter is below the subclavian artery and above the renal arteries (Fig. 3-21). Particular caution should be used in moving these patients because movement may cause the balloon to float downward, possibly blocking the lower circulation.

Ventricular pacing electrodes may be placed for temporary or permanent purposes. Temporary pacing electrodes are inserted via the ante-cubital vein into the right ventricle. They provide electrical pacing of the heart in patients experiencing a very slow heart rate (i.e., *brady-cardia*) as a substitute for misfiring of the heart's normal electrical system. Also, patients who have had open heart surgery may have these electrodes placed directly on the heart's surface and brought externally beneath the sternum at midline as a temporary precaution against heart arrhythmia problems. Permanent electrodes are used for permanent heart pacing needs. The pacemaker generator is inserted under the skin below the right clavicle, with the electrodes placed into the right ventricle (Fig. 3-22).

CONGENITAL AND HEREDITARY DISEASES

Cystic Fibrosis

Cystic fibrosis is a generalized disorder resulting from a genetic defect transmitted as an autosomal recessive gene that affects the function of ex-

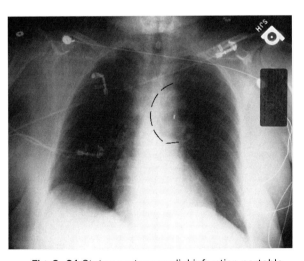

Fig. 3-21 Status postmyocardial infarction portable chest demonstrates proper placement of an intraaortic balloon pump in the descending thoracic aorta of this 76-year-old woman. (Courtesy Riverside Methodist Hospitals, Columbus, Ohio.)

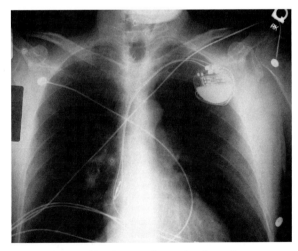

Fig. 3-22 Portable chest radiograph taken after pacemaker insertion demonstrates one pacemaker lead wire in the superior vena cava and the other near the apex of the right ventricle in this 52-year-old man. (Courtesy Riverside Methodist Hospitals, Columbus, Ohio.)

ocrine glands. It involves many organs in addition to the respiratory system, such as the salivary glands, small bowel, pancreas, biliary tract, female cervix, and male genital system. Although the basic cause of the disorder remains unknown, its complications are well defined. In the respiratory system, gradually increasing secretions from hypertrophy of bronchial glands lead to obstruction of the bronchial system. The resultant plugging promotes staphylococcal infection, followed by more tissue damage, as well as atelectasis (collapse of lung tissue) and emphysema. Once the cycle is in motion, it is difficult to stop.

The disease remains the most common lethal genetic disease for white children, despite increasing life spans of 20 years or more because of improved treatments. Its diagnosis rests largely on certain clinical and laboratory findings, most notably elevated sodium and chloride levels in sweat. Radiographs taken over a period of years demonstrate gradually worsening structural abnormalities. Early changes of

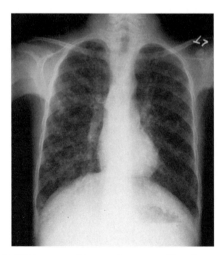

Fig. 3–23 Increased lung volume resulting from generalized obstructive disease and air trapping, which is characteristic of cystic fibrosis, as seen in this 9-year-old boy. Also seen are areas of irregular aeration with cystic and nodular densities. (Courtesy the American College of Radiology, Reston, Virginia.)

bronchial thickening and hyperinflation (Fig. 3-23) progress to extensive bronchiectasis, cyst formation, scarring, and overinflation of the lung and chest wall. Chest radiographs are useful in revealing the origin and extent of the many respiratory complications (e.g., pneumonia) that plague cystic fibrosis patients. Treatment methods include antimicrobial drugs to combat infection, bronchodilators administered through inhalers, and respiratory physical therapy. Expert psychological guidance is also important in helping affected patients adjust to limitations to their quality of life.

Hyaline Membrane Disease

Also known as **respiratory distress syndrome,** hyaline membrane disease affects infants and is a disorder of prematurity. Incomplete maturation of the surfactant-producing system causes unstable alveoli, the structures in which gas exchanges occur in the lungs. Infants are particularly in need of a low surface tension in the alveoli, and surfactant (an agent that lowers surface tension) provides this. Its deficiency results in alveolar collapse with widespread atelectasis. Chest radiographs demonstrate the *air-bronchogram sign,* characterized by bronchi surrounded by non aerated alveoli (Fig. 3-24). Treatment consists of maintenance of a proper thermal environment and satisfactory levels of tissue oxygenation, which is monitored frequently via arterial blood gas measurements.

INFLAMMATORY DISEASES

Pneumonias

Pneumonia is the most frequent type of lung infection, resulting in an inflammation of the lung and compromised pulmonary function. The main causes of pneumonia are bacteria, viruses, and mycoplasms. Radiograph-ically, pneumonias appear as soft, patchy, ill-defined alveolar infiltrates or pulmonary densities. Alveolar infiltration results

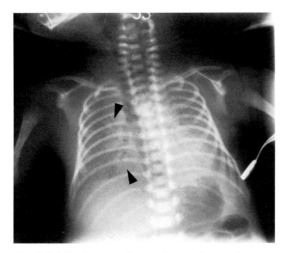

Fig. 3-24 Hyaline membrane disease in a preterm infant as shown by the uniform opacity of the lungs. Air-filled bronchi also are seen in contrast to the poorly aerated lungs. (Courtesy the American College of Radiology, Reston, Virginia.)

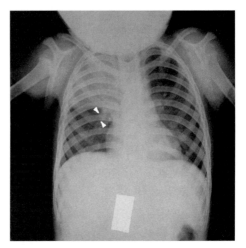

Fig. 3-25 Pneumococcal pneumonia with "air-bronchogram sign" in right lung created by consolidation within the lung that serves to outline the air-filled bronchi. The air-filled esophagus lies to the left of the spine. (Courtesy the American College of Radiology, Reston, Virginia.)

when the alveolar air spaces are filled with fluid or cells.

Pneumococcal lobar pneumonia is the most common bacterial pneumonia. This type of infection can affect anyone at any age and is generally preceded by an upper respiratory infection. Pneumococcal bacteria is present in healthy throats. When the body defenses are weakened, the bacteria multiply, work their way into the lungs, and inflame the alveoli. This disease is usually accompanied by chills, a cough, and a fever. Pneumococcal pneumonia generally affects the alveoli of an entire lobe of a lung, without affecting the bronchi themselves (Figs. 3-25 and 3-26). Chest radiographs demonstrate a collection of fluid in one or more lobes, with a lateral view serving to identify the degree of segmental involvement. Pleural fluid can often be seen in lateral decubitus views. Antibiotics (typically penicillin) and bed rest are the treatment for pneumococcal pneumonia, which is usually resolved in approximately 1 week.

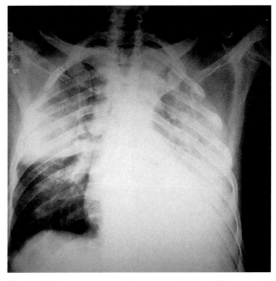

Fig. 3-26 Pneumococcal pneumonia in a 35-year-old man with severe head injuries. This relatively severe case demonstrates replacement of air by exudate and pus. (Courtesy the American College of Radiology, Reston, Virginia.)

Far less frequent types of bacterial pneumonia are **staphylococcal and streptococcal pneumonia**. Staphylococcal pneumonia occurs sporadically except during epidemics of influenza, when secondary infection with staphylococci is common. It is severe and may be fatal, especially in infants. A *pneumatocele,* a thin-walled, air-containing cyst, is the characteristic radiographic lesion and is more typically seen in children. These may enlarge and form abscesses in the later stages of the disease. Another characteristic sign is patchy, spreading areas localized in and around the bronchi (Fig. 3-27). Drug therapy with particular chemotherapeutic agents is the treatment of choice.

Streptococcal pneumonias are even rarer, accounting for less than 1% of all hospital admissions for acute bacterial pneumonia. The radiographic appearance is localized around the bronchi, usually of the lower lobes. Appropriate antibiotic therapy is the treatment of choice for this condition.

Legionnaires' disease is the name given to a severe bacterial pneumonia that became known after causing the deaths of four people attending an American Legion convention in Philadelphia in 1976. It is thought to be responsible for less than 10% of all pneumonia cases in the United States. The causative bacteria (*Legionella pneumophila*) was unknown at the time of the 1976 outbreak, and its explosive effects attracted significant attention. *Legionella pneumophila* thrives in warm, moist places and was believed to be transmitted through heating-cooling systems. Clinically, patients complain of malaise, muscular aches, chest pain with a nonproductive cough, and occasional vomiting and diarrhea. Its radiographic appearance is similar to bacterial pneumonia, with patchy infiltrates throughout the lungs (Fig. 3-28). Treatment consists

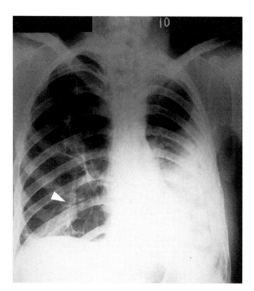

Fig. 3-27 Staphylococcal pneumonia in a 20-year-old man indicated by multiple large pneumatoceles in right lung and consolidation of the left lower lobe of the lung. An empyema in the lower left lung was later drained surgically. (Courtesy the American College of Radiology, Reston, Virginia.)

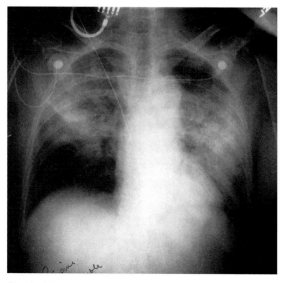

Fig. 3-28 Legionnaires' disease in a 55-year-old woman showing rounded opacities in the upper half of the right lung and lower two thirds of the left lung. (Courtesy the American College of Radiology, Reston, Virginia.)

primarily of antibiotic (erythromycin) administration and oxygen therapy.

Mycoplasma pneumonia is caused by mycoplasmas, the smallest group of living organisms. They have characteristics of both bacteria and viruses. Because they do not have a typical bacterial cell wall, there was confusion among the scientific community in the past in reference to their classification. Today they are classified as bacteria. Mycoplasma pneumonia is most common in older children and young adults. Radiographically, this disease demonstrates as a fine reticular pattern in a segmental distribution, followed by patchy areas of air space consolidation. In severe cases, the radiographic appearance may mimic tuberculosis. The morbidity rate associated with mycoplasma pneumonia is very low, even when the disease is not treated.

Aspiration (chemical) **pneumonia** is caused by acid vomitus aspirated into the lower respiratory tract, resulting in a chemical pneumonitis. It may follow anesthesia, alcoholic intoxication, or stroke that causes by loss of the cough reflex. Chest radiographs reveal edema produced by the irritation of the air passages (Fig. 3-29), appearing as densities radiating from one or both hila into the dependent segments. The treatment of aspiration pneumonia is strictly supportive, including correction of hypoxia, control of secretions, and replacement of fluids. Further infection is treated by antimicrobial drugs based on laboratory results.

Viral (interstitial) **pneumonia** can be caused by various viruses, most commonly influenza. It is more common than bacterial pneumonia but less severe. This disease is spread by an infected person shedding the virus to a nonimmune individual. Most cases of viral pneumonia are mild, and the radiographic findings are often minimal. The diagnosis of this disease is based on clinical findings and serologic tests. Symptoms include a dry cough and fever. Complications include secondary bacterial infections, termed *superinfections,* which result from a low-

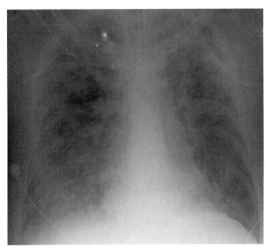

Fig 3-29 Aspiration pneumonia following aspiration of gastric contents. (Courtesy the Ohio State University Medical Center, Columbus, Ohio.)

ered resistance brought on by the inflammatory response to the virus. Otherwise, treatment of viral pneumonia usually focuses on relief of symptoms because viral infections do not respond to antibiotic agents.

Bronchiectasis

Bronchiectasis is a permanent, abnormal dilatation of one or more large bronchi as a result of destruction of the elastic and muscular components of the bronchial wall (Fig. 3-30). The basic pathogenesis is either congenital or an acquired weakness, typically following inflammation of the bronchial walls because of a viral or bacterial infection. The weakened wall allows the bronchus to become dilated, forming a saclike structure that is a haven for infection. As infection grows, the bronchial wall is destroyed, resulting in an abscess.

Tuberculosis

Tuberculosis is an infection caused by inhalation of *Mycobacterium tuberculosis.* Although it

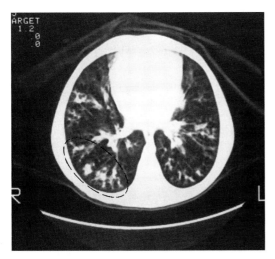

Fig. 3-30 Bronchiectatic changes are seen peripherally on this CT of the lungs from the 9-year-old patient with cystic fibrosis in Fig. 3–23. Compare the size of these bronchi with those seen in the normal chest CT (Fig. 3–5). (Courtesy the American College of Radiology, Reston, Virginia.)

generally affects the lungs, it may also affect other areas of the body. Of great concern worldwide is an alarming increase in tuberculosis, including its rise in the United States, where it was once considered nearly eradicated. An estimated 1.7 billion people worldwide (including 10 million Americans) carry the tuberculosis bacteria. Eight million develop active disease annually, and 3 million of them die.

Early pulmonary tuberculosis is asymptomatic, with signs appearing when the lesion is large enough to be seen on a chest radiograph. Lesions are most commonly seen in the apical region of the chest (Fig. 3-31); therefore, the apical lordotic projection of the chest is useful in the evaluation of tuberculosis. Tuberculosis may follow three possible courses: (1) healing with scarring of the lung tissue, (2) fibrocaseous tuberculosis, or (3) acute tuberculous pneumonia.

If the patient is in good health and the dose of the bacteria is fairly small, healing with scar-

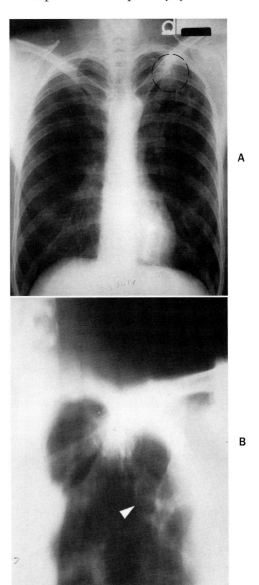

Fig. 3-31 A, Tuberculosis of left upper lobe in a 49-year-old male admitted with esophagitis and dull pain in the left subclavicular region. Subsequent tomography demonstrated a tuberculous, cavitary lesion. **B,** Routine linear tomography of the left upper lobe reveals the tuberculous cavitary lesion. (Courtesy the American College of Radiology, Reston, Virginia.)

ring of the lung tissue is the most common result of infection. The presence of tuberculous scars may be demonstrated radiographically in the apex of one or both lungs. These scars result from the body's immune system surrounding the bacilli with fibrous tissue, which invades and destroys the infectious agent.

Fibrocaseous tuberculosis is usually the disease's course if the patient demonstrates active signs of tuberculosis. Necrosis is a prominent feature of the disease because its infiltration affects lung parenchyma. This infiltration may expand and produce the formation of a cavity *(cavitation)* (Fig. 3-32). Chest tomograms demonstrate the extent of these cavities. If these cavities spread to communicate with the bronchus, the bacteria is spread throughout the lung.

In a few cases, the infection overwhelms the immune system and progresses through the lungs at a rapid rate to cause acute tuberculous pneumonia. The body does not develop fibrous tissue to surround the bacteria, so the infection spreads quickly. Without medical treatment, acute tuberculous pneumonia may result in death within a few months.

If the bloodstream picks up the tuberculosis, large numbers of bacteria are carried throughout the body, resulting in **miliary tuberculosis.** This type of tuberculosis is really a complication of one of the three courses described previously. *Miliary* refers to its characteristic resemblance to millet seeds, which are small, white grains (Fig. 3-33).

A positive response to intradermal injection of purified protein derivative (the Mantoux test) is the primary means of diagnosing tuberculosis. Because reading the results of this test is more art than science, further testing may be necessary to confirm the diagnosis. Patients with pulmonary tuberculosis are contagious and should be placed in respiratory isolation. The bacteria are spread through sputum and airborne droplets expelled upon coughing. Modern treatment of tuberculosis consists primarily of various chemotherapeutic agents. Historical

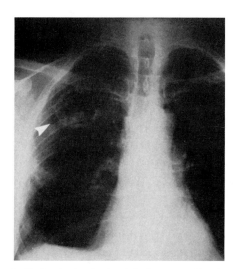

Fig. 3-32 Cavitation in the right lung resulting from expansion of tubercular lesion. (Courtesy Riverside Methodist Hospitals, Columbus, Ohio.)

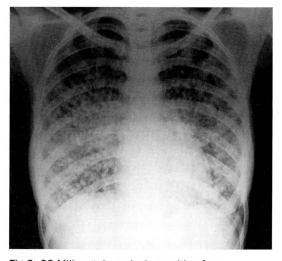

Fig 3-33 Miliary tuberculosis resulting from hematogenous spread of tuberculosis, demonstrating small, distinct nodules throughout the lung fields. (Courtesy the American College of Radiology, Reston, Virginia.)

treatments of bed rest, collapse therapy (i.e., artificial reduction in lung volume by one of several methods, including an artificial pneumothorax), and placement in a sanitarium are no longer practiced.

Chronic Obstructive Pulmonary Disease

Chronic obstructive pulmonary disease (COPD) refers to a group of disorders that cause chronic airway obstruction. The most common forms are chronic bronchitis and emphysema, which frequently coexist and may be associated with varying degrees of asthma and bronchiectasis—two other causes of airway obstruction.

Since it may be difficult to determine whether the pulmonary obstruction is due to bronchitis, emphysema, or a combination of the two diseases, the designation of chronic obstructive pulmonary disease is commonly used. This disease is irreversible and results in limited airflow and decreased elastic recoil in the case of emphysema. Statistics show the mortality rate of COPD doubling approximately every 5 years.

Chronic bronchitis most often arises from long-term, heavy cigarette smoking or prolonged exposure to high levels of industrial air pollution, which irritates the mucous lining of the bronchial tree and increases susceptibility to both bacterial and viral infections. Chronic exposure to these respiratory irritants leads to hyperplasia of the mucus glands, hypertrophy of the smooth muscle, and thickening of the bronchial wall.

Persistent cough and *expectoration* (expulsion of mucus or phlegm from the throat) are the primary symptoms of chronic bronchitis. The effects of the disease develop slowly and progressively over months and years, gradually resulting in bronchial obstruction from excess secretion of mucus. Eventually, the lungs remain in a chronically inflated state because more air is inhaled than is exhaled. Additional signs and symptoms of chronic bronchitis include wheezing, shortness of breath, and arterial hypoxemia

leading to right heart hypertrophy and failure (*cor pulmonale*). No dependable radiographic criteria exist for a definitive diagnosis of chronic bronchitis.

Chest radiographs may demonstrate hyperinflation of the lungs. Elimination of the causative agent (e.g., cigarettes) is an important first step in treatment. Antibiotics can reduce the presence of infection; bronchodilators are used to reduce bronchospasm.

Emphysema is a condition in which the lung's alveoli become distended, usually from loss of elasticity or interference with expiration. It is characterized by an increase in the air spaces distal to the terminal bronchioles, with destruction of the alveolar walls.

The primary symptom of emphysema is dyspnea, which at first occurs only during exertion but eventually even at rest. In the early stages of emphysema, the patient may present with a normal chest radiograph. However, as the disease progresses, hyperinflation results (Fig. 3-34). It

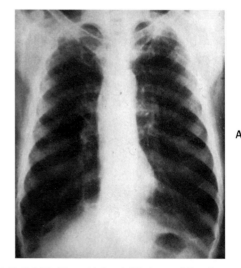

A

Fig. 3–34 PA *(A)* and lateral *(B)* views of the chest demonstrate pulmonary emphysema, a form of COPD, with its characteristic hyperinflation of the lungs, increased radiolucence, and barrel-shaped chest. (Courtesy Riverside Methodist Hospitals, Columbus, Ohio.) *Continued*

B

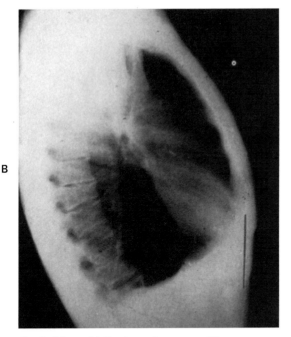

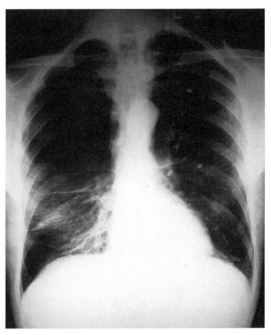

Fig. 3-34 cont'd. For legend see page 67.

Fig. 3-35 Pulmonary emphysema with a giant emphysematous bleb occupying the upper half of the right lung. (Courtesy the American College of Radiology, Reston, Virginia.)

appears radiographically as a depressed or flattened diaphragm, abnormally radiolucent lungs, and an increased retrosternal air space (barrel-shaped chest). Large *bullae,* or blisters filled with air, may be visible on conventional chest radiographs (Fig. 3-35), but smaller lesions are best demonstrated by CT examinations of the chest.

Treatment of emphysema is much like that for chronic bronchitis. Goals are to improve symptoms, treat any reversible elements (e.g., infection), and prevent further progression of the disease as possible.

Because these two forms of COPD represent chronic deterioration of the pulmonary system, the continued problems eventually lead to heart failure. The heart begins to wear out over time in its effort to overcompensate blood flow for the decreased airflow caused by COPD. Eventually, **pulmonary edema** results and, if the patient lives long enough, cor pulmonale. These conditions are both discussed in Chapter 8.

Pneumoconioses

Pneumoconioses are occupational diseases in which inhalation of foreign inorganic dust results in pulmonary fibrosis. The size of the dust particle inhaled is of particular. Most occupationally generated dusts and those occurring naturally are too large to cause pneumoconioses. Dusts greater than 10 microns are filtered out in the nasal passages or the mucous lining of the tracheobronchial tree; those smaller than 1 micron generally remain sus-

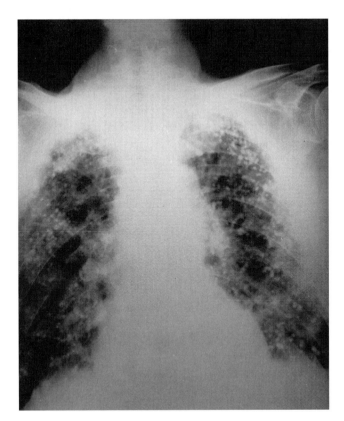

Fig. 3-36 "Eggshell calcifications" of silicosis in hilar and mediastinal lymph nodes of 70-year-old male stonecutter. Multiple small calcifications are also distributed throughout the lungs. (Courtesy the American College of Radiology, Reston, Virginia.)

pended in air and are exhaled. Those most likely to be trapped are 1 to 5 microns. In addition to the size criterion, exposure to a substance capable of causing disease and for a sufficient duration are factors required to cause a pneumoconiosis.

Radiography assists in the detection and follow-up of this disease group. Lesions produced by the different pneumoconioses vary, but may include nodules, cavitation, and pleural thickening. The three primary types of pneumoconioses are silicosis, anthracosis, and asbestosis. Treatment centers on preventing infection, relieving any respiratory symptoms, and maintaining adequate oxygenation.

Silicosis results from inhaling silica (quartz) dust and is common among miners, grinders, and sandblasters. It is the most widespread and most serious type of pneumoconiosis. Phagocytes located within the bronchioles carry the silica dust into the septa of the alveoli. In response to the foreign dust particles, the alveoli form large amounts of fibrous, connective tissue, thus destroying the normal lung tissue. This disease is clearly visible on conventional chest radiographs as multiple small, rounded, opaque nodules throughout the lungs, resulting from the creation of the fibrous tissue. Sometimes these calcifications are peripheral "eggshell calcifications" (Fig. 3-36). With the

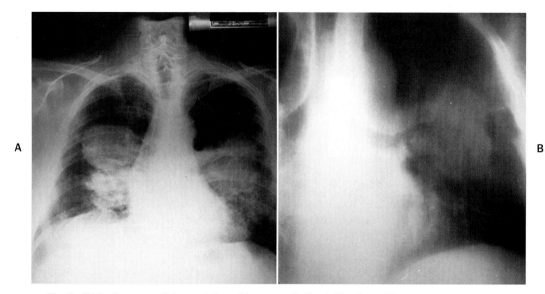

A

B

Fig. 3-37 A, Large, perihilar nodules without eggshell calcifications. Thoracotomy revealed heavy anthracotic pigmentation, with two largest nodules containing black fluid, consistent with anthracosis. **B,** Tomography of left hilar nodule in patient subsequently found to have anthracosis reveals air-bronchogram sign. (Courtesy the American College of Radiology, Reston, Virginia.)

exception of a lung transplant, there is no treatment for silicosis. Therefore, prevention through protective masks and adequate ventilation is the key to controlling this occupational disease.

Anthracosis (Black lung disease) results from inhalation of coal dust (Fig. 3-37). As the coal dust is deposited in the lungs, "coal macules" develop around the bronchioles and cause their dilation. This dilation does not affect the alveoli or the airflow.

Asbestosis results from the inhalation of asbestos dust, which can cause chronic injury to the lungs. Asbestos dust is found in building materials and insulation. Radiographically, diaphragmatic pleural calcifications suggest asbestosis. Pleural changes in asbestosis are considered far more striking than parenchymal changes. Pleural thickening may also be present. Exposure to asbestos dust has been shown to increase the chance of developing mesothelioma, a rare malignant neoplasm of the pleura.

Fungal Diseases

Histoplasmosis is a systemic fungal infection caused by a fungus that thrives in soil, especially that fueled by bird or bat excreta. Fungi are plants without chlorophyll and are widely found in nature. Histoplasmosis is particularly endemic to the Ohio and Mississippi River valleys. Most cases are so mild that they go undiagnosed. Disseminated histoplasmosis that leads to cavitary formations is more serious. Dyspnea, cough, and fatigue may persist for months or even years, but recovery most often occurs. Chest radiographs eventually may reveal small calcifications as a late manifestation of the disease, although these do not usually appear for 4 or 5 years. Fewer than 1% of those who acquire histoplasmosis require treatment because most forms of the disease are self-limiting and may evade diagnosis.

Coccidioidomycosis is also a systemic, fungal infection. It is caused by a fungus that thrives in semiarid soil, particularly the southwestern United States and northern Mexico. Infective spores in the soil become airborne from winds, digging, or other disruption. For this reason, agriculture and construction workers are particularly at risk. Like histoplasmosis, most infections are mild, usually self-limited, and may go unrecognized. The most common radiographic finding, if present, is a small area of pulmonary consolidation (Fig. 3-38). Lesions may form nodules of varying size that can simulate a malignant nodule, thus requiring biopsy or surgical excision. The typical treatment is bed rest, since most occurrences are mild.

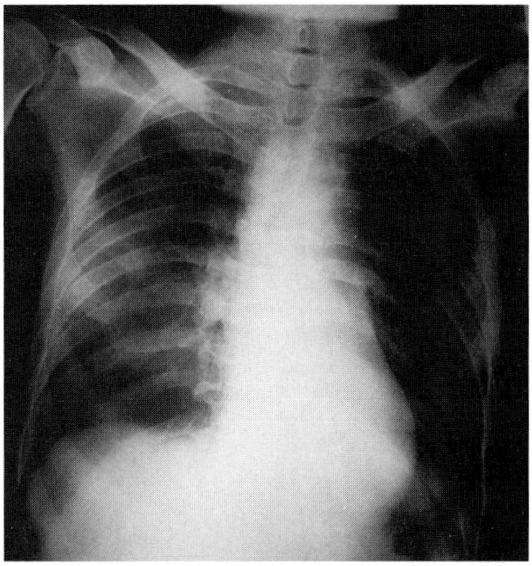

Fig. 3-38 Coccidioidomycosis with diffuse fine miliary infiltration, especially in right lung. (Courtesy the American College of Radiology, Reston, Virginia.)

Lung Abscess

A *lung abscess* is a localized area of dead (necrotic) lung tissue surrounded by inflammatory debris. These abscesses may result from periodontal disease, pneumonia, neoplasms, or other organisms that invade the lungs. Lung abscess is more common in the right lung because of the vertical orientation of the right main bronchus. Clinical manifestations of a lung abscess include fever, cough, expectoration of pus, and foul sputum. Radiographically, an abscess generally appears as a consolidation that becomes globular in shape as pus accumulates (Fig. 3-39), or it may appear as a round, thick-walled capsule containing air and fluid. Computed tomography may be used to detect cavity formations. *Empyemas* consist of an accumulation of pus in the pleural cavity, usually caused by some primary lung infection. They may be caused by the invasion of a lung abscess, resulting in a bronchopleural fistula.

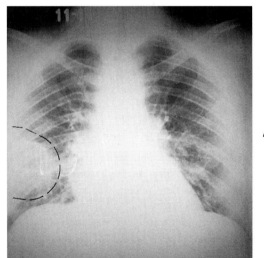

Fig. 3-39 A, Tuberculous abscess in a 33-year-old man seen in the lateral segment of the right middle lobe before treatment. (Courtesy the American College of Radiology, Reston, Virginia.) *Continued*

A

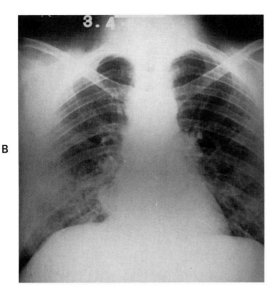

B

Fig. 3–39 cont'd **B,** Aggressive chemotherapeutic management reduced the tuberculous abscess significantly in size after 7 weeks of treatment. (Courtesy the American College of Radiology, Reston, Virginia.)

Treatment of an abscess and empyema centers on treatment of the primary condition causing it, including antibiotic therapy and possible drainage of fluids.

Pleurisy

Inflammation of the pleura is loosely termed *pleurisy,* a word often used to indicate inconsequential thoracic pain. True pleurisy is often indicative of serious conditions such as pneumonia, pulmonary embolism, tuberculosis, or malignant disease. Pain, varying in intensity, is usually distributed to one side or the other and along the intercostal nerve roots. Since the parietal layer of the pleura contains sensory receptors (while the visceral layer does not), pain indicates that the parietal layer is involved in the inflammatory process.

Chest radiographs do not generally demonstrate pleurisy, but they are helpful in confirming the presence of pleural fluid associated with the disease. Diagnosis and treatment of any underlying condition are important in relieving the symptoms of pleurisy.

Pleural Effusion

Pleural effusion results when excess fluid collects in the pleural cavity. It is a frequent manifestation of serious thoracic disease, usually pulmonary or cardiac in origin. It should be regarded not as a disease entity but rather as a sign of an important underlying condition. Pleural effusion may be caused by inflammation, renal disease, surgery, or chest trauma. A pleural effusion containing blood is called a *hemothorax.* The radiographic signs of pleural effusion include a blunting of the costophrenic angles (Fig. 3-40), which is often best demonstrated on an erect lateral chest radiograph. Lateral decubitus chest radiographs are also valuable (Fig. 3-41). Thoracocentesis, sometimes with fluoroscopic or sonographic guidance, is used to remove excess fluids for symptom alleviation and laboratory analysis.

Sinusitis

The communication with the nasal cavities subjects the paranasal sinuses to infection and inflammation called **sinusitis.** The ethmoid sinuses tend to be the most commonly affected because of their proximity to the nose. Common causes are exposure to extremes in humidity and temperature and a deviated septum. The symptoms of sinusitis include nasal discharge and headache.

Radiography is important in the diagnosis of sinusitis. Upright sinus radiographs demonstrate increased density and possible air-fluid levels in the affected sinuses (Fig. 3-42). This increased density results from both mucosal swelling and fluid accumulation. Computed tomography is also useful in demonstrating sinusitis (Fig. 3-43). Chronic sinusitis may cause nasal polyps.

Treatment of sinusitis typically involves antibiotic therapy and analgesics for pain relief. A

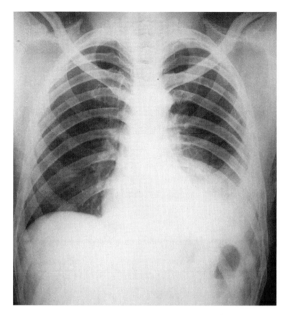

Fig. 3-40 Left pleural effusion on erect PA chest of 40-year-old male recovering from acute pancreatitis. (Courtesy the American College of Radiology, Reston, Virginia.)

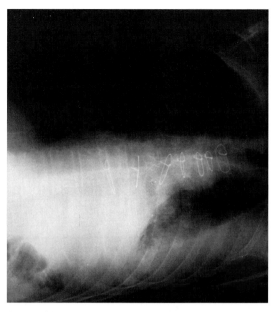

Fig. 3-41 Left lateral decubitus chest shows free pleural fluid layering out against the chest wall. AEC for correct density in area of interest has resulted in overexposure of the superior right lung. (Courtesy Riverside Methodist Hospitals, Columbus, Ohio.)

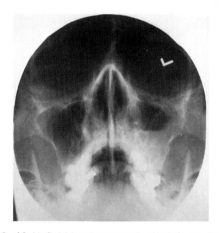

Fig. 3-42 Air-fluid level present in the left maxillary sinus reflects sinusitis in this 26-year-old woman, secondary to an oral-antral fistula. (Courtesy the American College of Radiology, Reston, Virginia.)

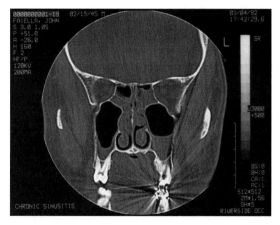

Fig. 3-43 Coronal CT view of the sinuses reveals sinusitis as shown by air-fluid levels in the maxillary sinuses and significant amounts of fluid in the maxillary sinuses. Obstruction seen in the nasal cavity is the cause of this sinusitis. (Courtesy Riverside Methodist Hospitals, Columbus, Ohio.)

deviated septum that contributes to sinusitis can be corrected surgically, if necessary.

NEOPLASTIC DISEASES

Bronchial Adenomas

Bronchial adenomas are usually considered benign but are included in the World Health Organization's classification of "lung cancer" because they tend to invade local tissues, sometimes metastasize, and are treated much like other malignant neoplasms. The radiographic appearance of this neoplasm shows opacity (Fig. 3-44), bronchial narrowing, and possible collapse of the affected segment of the lung. Bronchial obstruction is the most common presentation.

Bronchogenic Carcinoma

Bronchogenic carcinoma is the most common fatal primary malignancy in the United States. There are four main types: squamous cell, small (oat) cell, large cell, and adenocarcinoma. These tumors arise in the major bronchi near the hilar area and metastasize via lymph nodes, the

bloodstream, or both. The most common radiographic presentation of this neoplasm is airway obstruction of unilateral hilar mass (Fig. 3-45). As the tumor grows, it may occlude the bronchus, producing atelectasis and pneumonitis. These secondary effects provide more opacity radiographically than the actual tumor. Computed tomography is also used in the diagnosis of small lesions that are not visualized with conventional chest radiography.

The second most common radiographic presentation of a neoplasm consists of a solitary radiopaque lung nodule, sometimes called a *coin* lesion. Computed tomography is used in the evaluation of lung nodules and calcium deposits within these lesions. Malignant lesions are rarely calcified, whereas benign lesions generally have a calcified center. Fluoroscopy also aids in the diagnosis of neoplasms of the lung. The patient may undergo percutaneous lung biopsy bronchoscopy or brush biopsy. In the latter procedure, a device with tiny brushes is introduced through a bronchoscope or bronchial catheter to procure cells and tissues under fluoroscopic guidance. Although rarely used, pulmonary arteriography may assess ob-

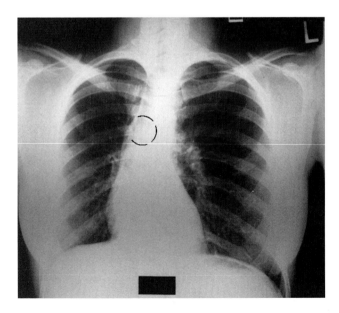

Fig. 3-44 Rounded marble-size density within the lumen of the right mainstem bronchus, along with clinical history indicative of bronchial adenoma. (Courtesy the American College of Radiology, Reston, Virginia.)

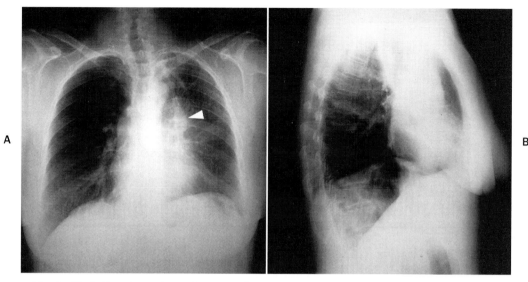

A   B

Fig. 3-45 A, Bronchogenic carcinoma on PA projection indicated by large nodular density in the left hilum. **B,** Lateral projection demonstrates decreased translucency of left upper lobe, indicative of collapse due to bronchogenic carcinoma. (Courtesy the American College of Radiology, Reston, Virginia.)

struction of a pulmonary artery caused by an invasive tumor.

The prognosis is very poor for bronchogenic carcinoma, with a 5-year survival rate of only 12% to 14%. Cigarette smoking is by far the most important etiologic factor. Exposure to potentially carcinogenic substances from air pollution and occupational exposure is also an etiologic factor. This disease process may be treated with surgery, chemotherapy, radiation therapy, or any combination of the three modalities.

Metastases from Other Sites

Pulmonary metastases are much more common than primary lung neoplasms. Many malignancies develop pulmonary metastases, which are detectable on a chest radiograph (Fig. 3-46). The most common primary sites for these tumors are the breast, gastrointestinal tract, female reproductive system, and the kidneys.

Malignancy is spread to the lungs from a primary site via five different routes: (1) through

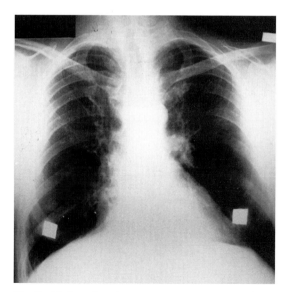

Fig. 3-46 Questionable densities seen on routine chest radiograph resulted in application of nipple markers. Film with markers demonstrated lesions above, which were found to be metastases secondary to colon carcinoma. (Courtesy the American College of Radiology, Reston, Virginia.)

the bloodstream in hematogenous metastases, (2) through the lymph system in lymphogenous metastases, (3) by direct extension in local invasion, (4) through the tracheobronchial system in bronchogenic metastases, and, rarely, by (5) direct implantation from biopsies or other surgical procedures. Radiographically, these metastatic lesions appear as single or multiple rounded opacities throughout the lungs (Fig. 3-47). Again, CT is more sensitive than conventional chest radiography in the detection of small metastatic lesions.

As in the case of bronchogenic carcinoma, treatment of pulmonary metastases is accomplished through surgery, chemotherapy, radiation therapy, or a combination of them, depending on the type of tumor and its likely primary site. For example, hormonal therapy of prostatic and breast carcinoma can cause pulmonary lesions to resolve. The field of oncology is growing, with new treatment options in research and ongoing development.

QUESTIONS

1. Bony structures such as the clavicles can be removed from the apices of the lungs by use of what radiographic position?
   a. AP
   b. lateral decubitus
   c. lordotic
   d. 45-degree oblique

2. The "sail sign" in an infant is commonly associated with enlargement of the:
   a. heart
   b. pulmonary arteries
   c. thymus
   d. thyroid

3. Which of the following types of tubes is readily visible on a chest radiograph and serves to maintain an adequate airway in a pulmonary-compromised patient?
   a. chest tube
   b. CVP line
   c. endotracheal tube
   d. Swan-Ganz catheter
   e. none of the above

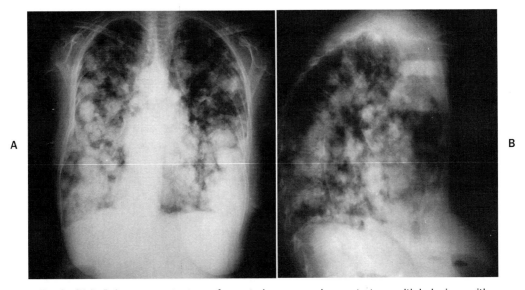

Fig. 3-47 A, Pulmonary metastases from uterine cancer demonstrates multiple lesions with characteristic "cotton ball" appearance. **B,** Lateral projection of pulmonary metastases resulting from uterine cancer. (Courtesy Riverside Methodist Hospitals, Columbus, Ohio.)

4. An infant born after only 6 months of gestation may likely suffer from:
   a. cystic fibrosis
   b. hyalinephysema membrane disease
   c. mediastinal emphysema
   d. pectus excavatum

5. Which of the following is the most common type of bacterial pneumonia?
   a. aspiration
   b. Legionnaires'
   c. pneumococcal
   d. streptococcal

6. A thin-walled, air-containing cyst within the thorax is most likely a(n):
   a. air-bronchogram
   b. alveoli
   c. mycoplasma
   d. pneumatocele

7. Loss of elasticity of the bronchial walls as a result of bacterial infection can result in:
   a. bronchiectasis
   b. bronchogenic carcinoma
   c. pneumococcal pneumonia
   d. tuberculosis

8. Pulmonary fibrosis resulting from occupationally inhaled dusts is characteristic of:
   a. atelectasis
   b. chronic bronchitis
   c. pleural effusion
   d. pneumoconiosis

9. An accumulation of pus in the pleural cavity is known as a(n):
   a. coin lesion
   b. empyema
   c. pleural effusion
   d. pleurisy

10. The most common etiologic factor in brochogenic carcinoma is:
    a. automobile emissions
    b. cigarette smoking
    c. dust
    d. Iatrogenic treatment

11. Explain how technical exposure factors must be changed to compensate for additive and subtractive pathologies of the chest. Give one example of each type of pathology.

12. Specify the reasons chest radiographs should be obtained in an erect position at a 72-inch SID.

13. What specialized radiographic projection of the chest is utilized to demonstrate tuberculosis? Why is this projection of benefit?

14. Chronic obstructive pulmonary disease includes both emphysema and chronic bronchitis. Compare and contrast these two pathologic conditions, and explain how both can be considered COPD.

15. Metastasis to the lungs from other primary tumors occurs via five routes. What are they?

Chapter 4

The Abdomen and Gastrointestinal System

Anatomy and Physiology Review
  The abdomen
  The gastrointestinal system
Imaging Considerations
  The abdomen
  The gastrointestinal system
    The esophagus
    The stomach
    The small bowel
    The large bowel
    Other studies
  Abdominal tubes and catheters
Congenital and Hereditary Anomalies
  Atresia
    Bowel atresia
  Hypertrophic pyloric stenosis
  Malrotation
  Imperforate anus
Inflammatory Diseases
  Esophageal strictures
  Peptic ulcer
  Gastroenteritis
  Malabsorption syndrome

  Regional enteritis
  Appendicitis
  Ulcerative colitis
Esophageal Varices
Degenerative Diseases
  Herniation
  Hiatal hernia
Bowel Obstructions
  Mechanical bowel obstruction
  Paralytic ileus
Neurogenic Diseases
  Achalasia
  Hirschprung's disease
Diverticular Diseases
  Esophageal diverticula
  Colonic diverticula
Neoplastic Diseases
  Tumors of the esophagus
  Tumors of the stomach
  Small-bowel neoplasms
  Colonic polyps
  Colon cancer

Upon completion of Chapter 4, the reader should be able to:

- Describe the anatomic components of the abdomen and gastrointestinal system and how they are visualized radiographically.

- Compare and contrast the various imaging modalities used in evaluation of the abdomen and its contents.

- Identify the tubes and catheters related to the gastrointestinal system by type, and briefly explain their use.

- Characterize a given condition as congenital, inflammatory, neurogenic, or neoplastic.

- Identify the pathogenesis of the gastrointestinal pathologies cited and typical treatments for them.

- Describe, in general, the radiographic appearance of each of the given pathologies.

KEY TERMS

Endoscopy	Gastroenteritis	Gallstone ileus
Dysphagia	Regional enteritis	Volvulus
Colostomy	Appendicitis	Intussusception
Ileostomy	Ulcerative colitis	Achalasia
Atresia	Esophageal varices	Hirschsprung's disease
Hypertrophic pyloric stenosis	Hernia	Diverticulum
Malrotation	Hiatal hernia	Diverticulitis
Imperforate anus	Mechanical bowel	Leiomyoma
Reflux esophagitis	obstruction	Adenocarcinoma
Peptic ulcer	Paralytic ileus	

ANATOMY AND PHYSIOLOGY REVIEW

The Abdomen

The abdomen comprises the abdominal and pelvic cavities and is often divided into nine anatomic regions: right hypochondriac, epigastric, left hypochondriac, and right lumbar, umbilical, left lumbar, right iliac, hypogastric, and left iliac (Fig. 4-1). It may also be described in terms of quadrants: right-upper (RUQ), right-lower (RLQ), left-upper (LUQ), and left-lower (LLQ) (Fig. 4-2). The abdominal cavity contains organs of the digestive system (stomach and intestines), the hepatobiliary system (liver, gallbladder, and pancreas), the urinary system (kidneys and ureters), and the circulatory system (spleen). The pelvic cavity contains the bladder,

portions of the intestines, and the reproductive organs.

The abdominal cavity is lined by the peritoneum, a serous membrane. (Fig. 4-3, *A*). The serous lining attached to the abdominal organs is the visceral peritoneum. The peritoneum attached directly to the abdominal wall is the parietal peritoneum. The mesentery is a double fold of parietal peritoneum projecting from the posterior abdominal wall in the lumbar region (Fig. 4-3, *B*). Most of the small bowel is attached to the outer edge of the mesentery.

The greater omentum is a double fold of peritoneum that attaches to the duodenum, stomach, and transverse colon. It hangs loosely over the intestines. The lesser omentum is a fold of peritoneum that attaches the liver to the

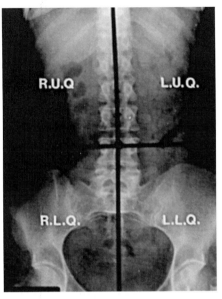

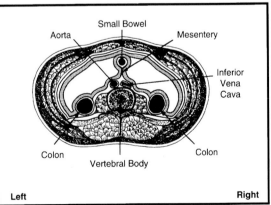

Fig. 4-1 The nine regions of the abdomen. (From Bontrager KL: *Textbook of radiographic positioning and related anatomy*, ed 3, St Louis, 1993, Mosby.)

Fig. 4-2 The four quadrants of the abdomen. (From Bontrager KL: *Textbook of radiographic positioning and related anatomy*, ed 3, St Louis, 1993, Mosby.)

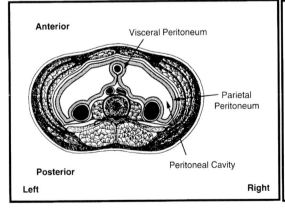

Fig. 4-3 A, A cross-sectional drawing of the abdomen demonstrates the peritoneum; **B,** a cross-sectional drawing of the lower abdomen demonstrates the mesentery. (From Bontrager KL: *Textbook of radiographic positioning and related anatomy*, ed 3, St Louis, 1993, Mosby.)

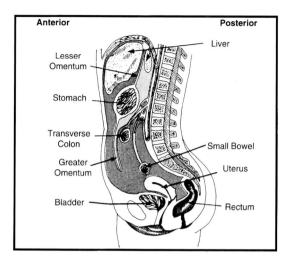

Fig. 4–4 A cross-sectional drawing of the abdominal cavity demonstrates the omentum. (From Bontrager KL: *Textbook of radiographic positioning and related anatomy,* ed 3, St Louis, 1993, Mosby.)

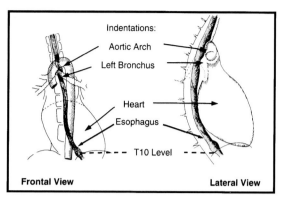

Fig. 4–5 The esophagus in the mediastinum. (From Bontrager KL: *Textbook of radiographic positioning and related anatomy,* ed 3, St Louis, 1993, Mosby.)

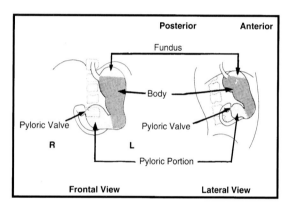

Fig. 4–6 The stomach depicted in its average orientation when empty. (From Bontrager KL: *Textbook of radiographic positioning and related anatomy,* ed 3, St Louis, 1993, Mosby.)

lesser curvature of the stomach and the duodenum (Fig. 4-4).

The Gastrointestinal System

A major portion of the gastrointestinal (GI) system is the alimentary tract, which serves to digest and absorb food. Extending from the mouth to the anus, the alimentary tract comprises the mouth, pharynx, esophagus, stomach, small and large bowel, and rectum.

The esophagus is the first part of the GI system. It is approximately 10 to 12 inches long and extends from the posterior pharynx to the stomach (Fig. 4-5). The upper esophagus is midline, but it courses to the left to pass behind the aortic arch, which indents the esophagus. Other indentations occur at the level of the left mainstem bronchus and at the gastroesophageal junction. As it passes downward, the esophagus follows the curvature of the thoracic spine and thoracic descending aorta.

The stomach occupies the body's left-upper quadrant, with the cardiac orifice at the level of the tenth or eleventh thoracic vertebra and the pyloric canal just to the right of the first or second lumbar vertebra (Fig. 4-6). Peristalsis churns the gastric content and propels it toward the pylorus. Gastric emptying of liquids is accounted for by the peristalsis initiated in the fundus of the stomach; gastric emptying of solids requires a to-and-fro action of the antrum and pylorus. In the presence of masses, inflammation, or diabetes, the peristaltic activity may be diminished. When filled with barium, the curvatures of the stomach visualize as generally smooth contours. The rugae appear as longitudinal ridges within the stomach.

The small bowel includes the duodenum, jejunum, and the ileum. It arises from the stomach at the duodenal bulb and courses to the ileocecal valve (Fig. 4-7), over a length of nearly 21 feet. The duodenal C-loop moves posteriorly from the gastric antrum to its ending at the ligament of Treitz. The jejunum begins here and coils in the left-upper quadrant before terminating into the ileum in the right-upper quadrant. The ileum then courses through the right- and left-lower quadrants to terminate at the ileocecal junction. When filled with barium, the segments of the small bowel are distinguishable by their appearance. Duodenal mucosa is indicated by its transverse rigid appearance. Jejunal mucosa appears delicate and feathery. Ileal folds look like those of the duodenum, though not as large.

The large bowel extends from the terminal ileum to the anus for a length of about 6 feet (Fig. 4-8). Its distinct regions are the cecum, the orifices for the terminal ileum and the appendix, the ascending colon and hepatic flexure, the transverse colon and the splenic flexure, the descending colon, sigmoid, rectum, and anus. The cecum is usually retroperitoneal, and anterior

and lies against the abdominal wall. The ascending colon is also retroperitoneal and becomes more posterior as it ascends to lie adjacent to the undersurface of the liver. The hepatic flexure, transverse colon, and splenic flexure are all intraperitoneal. They lie more anteriorly and are attached to the posterior abdominal wall by the mesocolon, a double layer of peritoneum. The descending colon is retroperitoneal, moving posteriorly as it descends. The peritoneal sigmoid colon lies in the pelvis and is quite mobile. Structures located anterior to it include the bladder and the female uterus. Posterior structures include the iliac arteries and sacral nerves. The rectum is extraperitoneal, beginning at the third sacral segment and following the sacrococcygeal curve to the anus. The valves of Houston are prominent transverse folds in the distal rectum where it dilates. The anus forms the distal 1 to 2 inches of the large bowel and contains no peritoneal covering.

IMAGING CONSIDERATIONS

The Abdomen

Abdominal radiography is often performed for survey purposes, without contrast agents. The

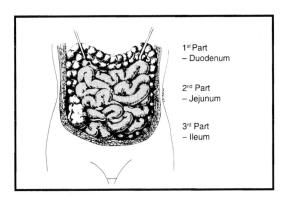

Fig. 4-7 The small bowel and its divisions. (From Bontrager KL: *Textbook of radiographic positioning and related anatomy*, ed 3, St Louis, 1993, Mosby.)

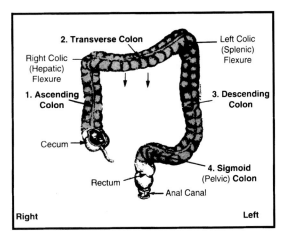

Fig. 4-8 The colon and its four parts. (From Bontrager KL: *Textbook of radiographic positioning and related anatomy*, ed 3, St Louis, 1993, Mosby.)

usual starting point is a "KUB," which refers to a supine film taken to include the kidneys, ureters, and bladder. The frequency of abnormal findings on a plain abdominal radiograph is fairly low and nonspecific but are of most value in patients complaining of severe abdominal tenderness and to rule out bowel obstructions and perforations. In addition, plain abdomen radiographs are invaluable in assessing the placement of various tubes and catheters, as discussed later in this chapter.

The AP projections of the abdomen are generally taken in the supine position. Such a radiograph allows an examination of the air distribution within the bowels and of the size of the viscera, serves to evaluate vascular and other types of calcifications and body or soft tissue trauma, and, finally, serves as a preliminary radiograph for other procedures.

On the initial inspection of the abdomen radiograph, the technologist should verify that the technique chosen is correct or diagnostic, that motion is nonexistent, and that the anatomy under consideration has been properly visualized. As with other body areas, an evaluation of the abdomen should be done systematically. This should include an inspection of the renal outlines, ureters, psoas muscles, spleen, liver, gallbladder, and peritoneal fat stripes.

In a normal abdomen (Fig. 4-9), varying amounts of gas and fecal material are always present in an unprepared patient. The liver, kidney, spleen, and psoas muscle shadows are variably outlined because of the lucent layer of fat surrounding them. Properitoneal fat stripes are visible as radiolucencies extending laterally from the costal margins down to the iliac crests. The aorta and pancreas are not normally seen unless they are calcified, as might be expected in an elderly patient in the case of the aorta or in a patient with chronic calcific pancreatitis. The inferior margin of the liver should lie at or above the level of the right twelfth rib. The left kidney is usually slightly higher than the right kidney because of the presence of the liver superior to it. In terms of renal size, the kidneys are generally

the length of three vertebrae in children over 1 year of age. As the child becomes an adult, the kidneys are about the length of two and a half vertebrae.

Few, if any, air-fluid levels are present in the normal patient who is radiographed in the erect position. Limited fluid levels in the small and large bowel, however, may be considered normal. Fluid levels are abnormal when they are seen in dilated bowel loops or when they are numerous.

The intestinal gas pattern can be confusing to the diagnostician. In infants and children, gas may be scattered throughout the bowel, but in adults gas is normally seen only in the stomach and colon. Small-bowel gas in an adult, therefore, may indicate a pathologic process. In some patients, gas may be recognizable only on erect films because of the presence of intraluminal fluid.

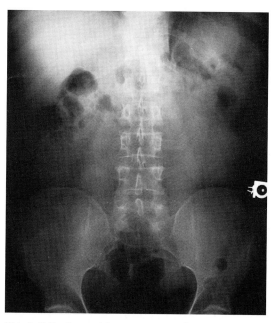

Fig. 4-9 Radiographic appearance of a normal abdomen, demonstrating kidney shadows, liver shadow, psoas muscles, and transverse processes of the lumbar spine. (Courtesy Riverside Methodist Hospitals, Columbus, Ohio.)

The Gastrointestinal System

Some contents of the abdomen can be seen without contrast media, as explained. However, most of the GI tract cannot be examined directly. The internal surfaces of both ends can be visualized through **endoscopy,** the use of lighted instruments with optics to visualize disease of the esophagus, stomach and duodenum, rectum and distal colon, and occasionally the terminal ileum. Endoscopy is becoming more common in health care as the instrument technology continues to improve and allows more detailed studies and improved patient comfort. Abnormal areas can be visualized, biopsied, and examined histologically. Those areas that cannot be directly examined are studied radiographically.

Radiographic investigation of the GI system is commonly a combination of fluoroscopy and radiography. Fluoroscopy provides dynamic information, whereas radiographs provide a permanent static record of the examination. Radiographic examination of the GI system requires positive and negative contrast agents for visualization of the body parts. Barium sulfate is generally used as the positive contrast agent but is contraindicated in cases of GI tract perforation. If a perforated bowel is suspected, a water-soluble contrast agent should be used. Although infrequently used alone, a negative contrast agent (e.g., air or carbon dioxide) may be used to distend the stomach and bowel for better visualization of the mucosal lining. A combination of both positive and negative contrast agents is commonly used so that the thicker barium sulfate adheres to the mucosa while the CO_2 expands the stomach or bowel, thus allowing optimal visualization of small variances in the walls of the gastrointestinal organs.

THE ESOPHAGUS

Most upper GI studies begin with the patient in an erect position to evaluate air-fluid levels in the alimentary tract. An esophageal study may be performed to demonstrate anomalies and abnormalities of the esophagus. Transport of the food or liquid bolus through swallowing is the sole function of the esophagus. If it is studied as part of a GI tract examination, thin barium sulfate may be used. Thick barium sulfate is used if the esophagus is the single object of study. Most patients presenting for a traditional esophagram have a chief complaint of **dysphagia,** or difficult swallowing. The causes for dysphagia are numerous and are discussed later in this chapter.

Radiographs are typically taken of a barium-filled esophagus in an erect or prone position. They include a PA, right lateral, and right anterior oblique (RAO) (Fig. 4-10) to visualize the esophagus between the spine and the heart.

During fluoroscopy, the radiologist can visualize mechanical problems presented while the patient is swallowing the barium sulfate mixture. Esophageal studies are also used to study the contour of the heart, as described in Chapter 9.

THE STOMACH

One of radiology's most common procedures is an "upper GI," in which barium sulfate flows from the esophagus and into the stomach and small bowel. Once the barium reaches the stomach, the radiologist evaluates the stomach contour, position, rugae, and the peristaltic changes occurring as the stomach fills and empties.

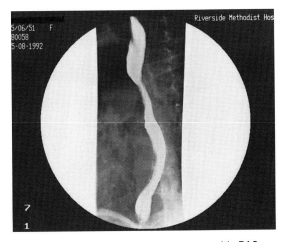

Fig. 4-10 Normal esophagus as seen on this RAO digital spot film on a 21-year-old woman. (Courtesy Riverside Methodist Hospitals, Columbus, Ohio.)

In the event the radiologist wishes to diminish peristalsis, glucagon is given to relax the stomach musculature. In many instances, a gas-producing substance (CO_2 crystals) is used with the barium sulfate to produce a double-contrast examination. The purpose is to expand the stomach and promote coating of the stomach mucosa. The duodenal bulb is studied as it fills with barium sulfate and empties into the small bowel. Compression may be used for better visualization of specific anatomic areas of the upper GI tract.

A series of radiographs is taken after fluoroscopy, with the projections differing from one institution to another. Typical patient positions include a recumbent PA projection to demonstrate the entire stomach and duodenal bulb, RAO to highlight the pyloric canal and duodenal bulb (Fig. 4-11), right lateral to show the duodenal bulb and loop, and the LPO to demonstrate the gastric fundus. Proper positioning relates significantly to the patient's body habitus. Generally, the more hypersthenic a patient is, the higher and more transverse the stomach tends to lie. For other body habiti (i.e., sthenic, hyposthenic, and asthenic), the stomach is more J-shaped, lying lower and closer to the spine.

THE SMALL BOWEL

In some instances, the barium sulfate mixture may be followed as it progresses through the small intestines. Radiographs are exposed at set intervals to determine GI motility and to demonstrate abnormalities within the small bowel. Once the contrast agent reaches the ileocecal valve, the small-bowel study is complete, typically within 2 to 3 hours (Fig. 4-12).

The small intestines may also be studied radiographically by means of *enteroclysis*, a small-bowel enema. This is accomplished by advancing an intestinal tube through the patient's mouth to the end of the duodenum at the ligament of Treitz. Contrast agents, both positive and negative (barium sulfate and methylcellulose, respectively), are directly injected into the small bowel.

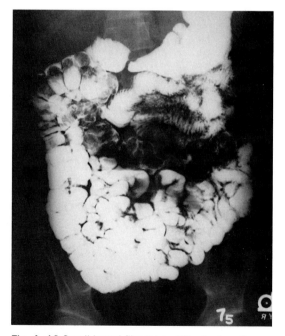

Fig. 4-12 Small bowel film taken 75 minutes after the examination began on this 18-year-old man, demonstrating passage through the ileocecal valve into the colon, with no mucosal abnormalities or dilated loops of small bowel. (Courtesy Riverside Methodist Hospitals, Columbus, Ohio.)

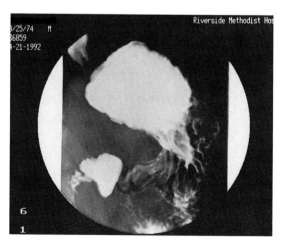

Fig. 4-11 Normal stomach as seen on this digital spot film on an 18-year-old man. (Courtesy Riverside Methodist Hospitals, Columbus, Ohio.)

THE LARGE BOWEL

The lower GI tract is examined by administering a barium enema through the rectum. This examination demonstrates abnormalities of the large bowel and intraluminal neoplasms. The barium enema can be performed in a single-contrast fashion with only barium or as a double-contrast study utilizing barium sulfate in combination with a negative contrast agent (e.g., air). The negative contrast agent distends the lumen, allowing improved visualization of the mucosal lining (Fig. 4-13), especially small polyps and intraluminal tumors. In either case, the radiologist typically exposes a series of spot films with the patient in various positions to highlight certain areas of the colon (e.g., flexures). The technologist may also expose a series of radiographs per the radiologist's instructions (Fig. 4-14). Following evacuation of the barium sulfate mixture, the technologist takes a "postevacuation" radiograph to visualize colon contraction and demonstrate mucosa.

If a patient has had a surgical enterostomy procedure, the contrast media may be administered through the opening in the abdominal wall to the specific area of the GI system. A **colostomy** is a procedure in which a stoma is surgically created to the abdominal wall to allow drainage of bowel contents into a closed pouch hung outside the body. Those in the sigmoid and descending colon are most frequently placed because of rectal or sigmoid cancer. Those placed in the transverse or ascending colon are often for indications that allow the colostomy to be placed for temporary purposes for diversion of flow of colonic contents (e.g., sigmoid diverticulitis, rectovaginal fistula, colon obstruction).

Ileostomies are similar openings but placed from the ileum, with the most common indication being ulcerative colitis. As with colostomies, patient problems with ileostomies include proper skin protection and odor control. Proper fit of the appliance for drainage is essential to

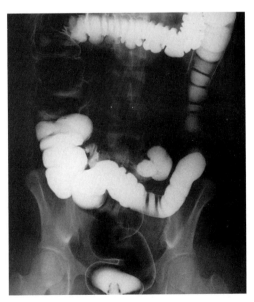

Fig. 4-13 Normal air-contrast enema on this 19-year-old woman with a history of low hemoglobin, as demonstrated on this PA projection. (Courtesy Riverside Methodist Hospitals, Columbus, Ohio.)

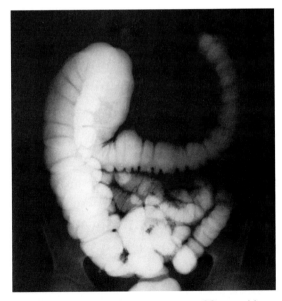

Fig. 4-14 Normal barium enema on a 23-year-old woman with a history of irritable bowel and severe constipation as demonstrated on this PA projection. (Courtesy Riverside Methodist Hospitals, Columbus, Ohio.)

prevent problems caused by excoriating digestive enzymes. Other enterostomies (i.e., jejunostomies and duodenostomies) are more rarely used and only under very specific circumstances because of the loss of electrolytes that occurs before their absorption through the small bowel. These patients often require total parenteral nutrition (TPN) to maintain life.

If a patient has had a surgical enterostomy procedure, the contrast agent may be administered through the opening in the abdominal wall to the specific area of the GI system (Fig. 4-15).

OTHER STUDIES

Computed tomography (CT) is an important modality in abdominal survey examination, as well as in the examination of the GI system. Because CT can visualize small differences in tissue density, it clearly demonstrates abdominal organs that are normally not apparent on conventional abdominal radiographs without the use of contrast agents. With the advent of spiral CT

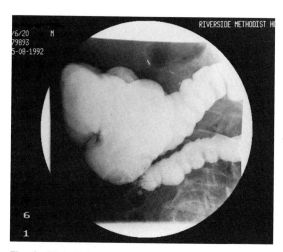

Fig. 4–15 A digital spot film of an enema through a colostomy in the descending colon on this 72-year-old man. The ostomy is clearly indicated by its circular opening into the bowel. Also visible is a small diverticulum just adjacent to the colostomy site and an inverted cecum. (Courtesy Riverside Methodist Hospitals, Columbus, Ohio.)

technology, small abnormalities lying within the upper abdomen that may have been missed with conventional CT methods are consistently demonstrated because one scan is obtained with one breath hold. With conventional CT, the patient breathed between exposures, and often the depth of inspiration was inconsistent, resulting in poorer visualization of structure in the upper abdomen close to the diaphragm.

Upon CT examination, the liver, spleen, pancreas, and kidneys appear as homogeneous soft tissue densities, making any alteration in the density from pathologic conditions readily visible, even without contrast media. Abscesses and solid and cystic masses all have a respective range of densities between water and normal soft tissue densities. The CT is also quite useful in the evaluation of retroperitoneal pathologies such as lymph node enlargement resulting from neoplastic disease or infection. Finally, it has become the accepted modality for following the progress of GI malignancies and also plays a role in the diagnosis of inflammatory conditions (e.g., abscess).

Routine CT examination of the abdomen requires good opacification of the bowel and vascular structures. Poorly opacified bowel loops may be mistaken for abdominal masses. Patients must be given an oral contrast agent such as barium sulfate or a water-soluble iodinated contrast agent approximately 45 minutes to 1 hour prior to the abdominal CT scan. This time allows the contrast agent to reach the distal ileum prior to examination. If pelvic pathology is suspected, a barium enema prior to the scan may also be indicated.

The role of magnetic resonance imaging (MRI) in the abdomen and GI tract is still evolving, as current scan times and bowel motion are still limiting factors, although emerging developments may allow it to play a larger role. Along with ultrasound, CT and MRI are useful in demonstrating the presence of any retroperitoneal masses that may impinge on the GI tract. In nuclear medicine, GI bleed scans are useful in demonstrating GI bleeding and help direct angiographers to the site of bleeding if therapeutic intervention is to be performed.

Digital fluoroscopy has emerged as a substantive improvement over traditional fluoroscopy for a number of reasons. Sophisticated on-line image processing allows enhancement of selective image quality parameters relevant to diagnosis that is not possible with conventional spot-film devices. Radiologists can view the images throughout the procedure rather than waiting for film processing at the end of the study. This immediate availability has altered the practice of fluoroscopy in terms of its speed and efficiency. Hard-copy film production is available at the touch of a button with no interruptions for changing cassettes. Anatomic motion can be captured as it occurs, instead of depending on the radiologist's synchronization of the timing of filming with, for example, esophageal swallowing. Serial filming capability further enhances this capacity and allows several images per second to be exposed. Diagnosis is often made in midprocedure, allowing hard copies to be produced later for historical purposes. Fewer hard copies are necessary and film costs are consequently reduced. The radiation dose is therefore also reduced.

As earlier noted, endoscopy is the use of tubular fiber optic devices to look inside the GI tract and other hollow organs or cavities of the body. As its sophistication and specificity have increased, it is assuming a greater role in diagnosis and therapy of the GI tract. Upper endoscopy is capable of seeing down into the esophagus, stomach, duodenum (including the ampulla of Vater), and even the proximal jejunum. Colonoscopy can allow visualization retrograde through the rectum as far as the terminal ileum. The small bowel is still largely out of reach through endoscopy. Photographic views of the interior of the body provide readily diagnosable information (Figs. 4-16 and 4-17). Therapeutic applications of endoscopy are numerous. They include polyp removal, injection and thermal method to stop hemorrhaging, sclerosing and banding of esophageal varices, le-

sion biopsy, sealing of tracheoesophageal fistulas, stone removal, esophageal prosthesis insertion, and laser tumor removal (both generally for palliative purposes). In addition, enteric wall stents have been used to open colon lesions in nonoperative malignancies.

Abdominal Tubes and Catheters

As with the chest, a variety of tubes and catheters can be placed within particular portions of the abdomen. The technologist must be familiar with each type of tube and exercise great caution in attempting to move patients with abdominal tubes in place. The technologist should also ask the patient's nurse or consult the chart before altering the patient's position. In addition, some abdominal tubes and catheters allow entry into body systems that are normally sterile and require special care to avoid infection.

Gastric tubes may be placed (generally through the nose) for a variety of diagnostic and therapeutic purposes. They may be indicated for aspiration of gastric contents, to help control nausea and vomiting, for decompression and removal of gastric contents because of bowel dysfunction or surgery, and for nutritional support tube feedings (gastric gavage) or medication administration. A *Levin tube* is the most common nasogastric tube. It is a fairly small, single-lumen tube with a plain tip, and it may be visualized radiographically. Proper placement is commonly assessed through aspiration of gastric juices and listening for proper placement within the stomach via a stethoscope. If a nasogastric tube is placed for feeding, the patient's head must remain elevated to prevent the tube from becoming displaced, leading to aspiration of the gastric contents. If an emergent condition exists that requires large amounts of gastric contents to be aspirated quickly (gastric lavage), an *Ewald* or *Edlich tube* may be used. These tubes are placed through the mouth, are wider than a Levin tube, and contain several openings that allow quicker aspiration. A *Levacuator tube* may also

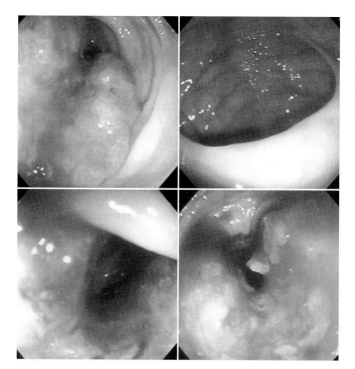

Fig. 4–16 Endoscopic image of a sigmoid colon mass in a 72-year-old woman visible as a mass bulging into the lumen of the colon. (Courtesy Riverside Methodist Hospitals, Columbus, Ohio.)

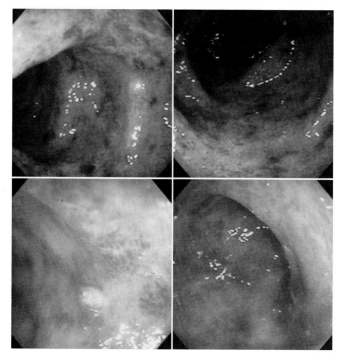

Fig. 4–17 Endoscopic image of diffuse colitis with a bacterial etiology in this 40-year-old man indicated by the splotchiness of the bowel mucosa. (Courtesy Riverside Methodist Hospitals, Columbus, Ohio.)

be used for evacuation of gastric contents. This is a wide, double-lumen tube placed through the patient's mouth. The larger lumen is used for gastric lavage, while the smaller lumen allows instillation of an irrigant.

An *enteral tube* is a small-caliber tube used to deliver a liquid diet directly to the duodenum or jejunum. It most commonly has a weighted end to hold the tube in the proper placement. The *Dobhoff tube* is a common radiopaque enteral tube (Fig. 4-18).

Nasoenteric decompression tubes are used to remove gas and fluids in the prevention and treatment of abdominal distention. These tubes have a balloon or rubber bag at one end filled with air, mercury, or water to stimulate peristalsis and facilitate passage through the pylorus into the intestinal tract. The *Miller-Abbott tube* is a common type of double-lumen decompression tube. It is passed through the nose, phar-

ynx, and esophagus with the balloon uninflated. Once the end of the tube reaches the stomach, the balloon is inflated and the tube is pulled back until it stops at the cardiac sphincter. The patient is then placed on his or her right side in a semierect position, and the air is withdrawn from the balloon and replaced with mercury. Progress of the tube is assessed by taking abdominal radiographs at regular intervals. *Harris* and *Cantor tubes* are other types of decompression tubes. Unlike the Miller-Abbott tube, however, the Cantor (Fig. 4-19) and Harris tubes contain a single lumen.

Levin tubes or *Foley catheters* may also be surgically placed in any portion of the GI system. A gastrostomy tube indicates the tube is placed in the stomach, whereas a duodenostomy tube or jejunostomy tube is specific to that portion of the intestines. A percutaneous endoscopic gastrostomy (PEG) tube is frequently placed

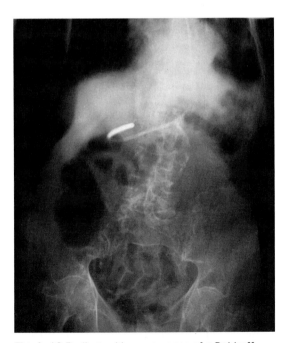

Fig. 4-18 Radiographic appearance of a Dobhoff tube being checked for placement in this 93-year-old woman. It is placed in the antrum of the stomach. Also seen are extensiver vascular calcifications. (Courtesy Riverside Methodist Hopitals, Columbus, Ohio.)

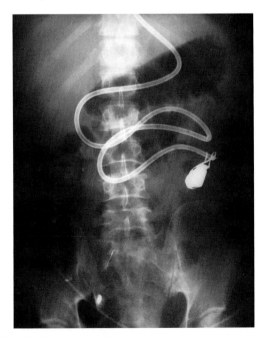

Fig. 4-19 Radiographic appearance of a Cantor tube. Placed 4 hours earlier in this 50-year-old man with a mechanical bowel obstruction, it is now advanced into the second portion of the duodenum. (Courtesy Riverside Methodist Hospitals, Columbus, Ohio.)

endoscopically. These tubes provide a direct route for administering liquid feedings.

CONGENITAL AND HEREDITARY ANOMALIES

Atresia

Atresia is a congenital absence or closure of a normal body orifice or tubular organ. *Esophageal atresia* is a congenital anomaly in which the esophagus fails to develop past some point, resulting in a discontinuation of the esophagus (Fig. 4-20). The symptoms of esophageal atresia are visible soon after birth and include excessive salivation, choking, gagging, dyspnea, and cyanosis. Diagnosis of this congenital anomaly may be established by inability to pass a nasogastric tube into the stomach. If a radiopaque nasogastric tube is utilized, the terminal end of the pouch may be demonstrated radiographically with a chest radiograph without the use of a contrast agent. Immediate surgery is required to alleviate the problem, and preoperative care must be taken to prevent aspiration pneumonia. The infant may not receive oral feedings, and continuous suction is necessary to prevent aspiration. Under most circumstances, this increased risk of aspiration contraindicates the use of a contrast agent to visualize the extent of the atresia.

Usually coincident with atresia is a tracheoesophageal fistula. This consists of an atresia at the level of the fourth thoracic vertebra with a fistula—an abnormal tubelike passage from one structure to another—to the trachea (Fig. 4-21).

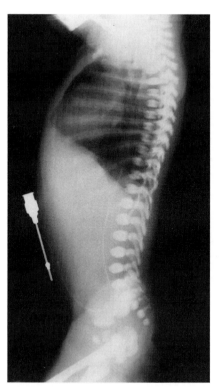

Fig. 4-20 Lack of any GI air below the diaphragm indicates an isolated esophageal atresia. (Courtesy the American College of Radiology, Reston, Virginia.)

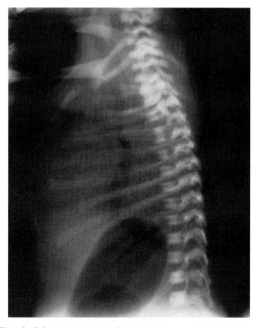

Fig. 4-21 Lateral view of the chest on a 1-day-old premature infant demonstrates distention of the distal esophagus with air and in continuity with the trachea. Marked gastric distention is also present. Appearance is consistent with esophageal atresia and a tracheoesophageal fistula. (Courtesy the American College of Radiology, Reston, Virginia.)

In addition, a gastrostomy tube may be placed in the infant's stomach to prevent reflux of gastric secretions into the trachea through the fistula. Such a condition is incompatible with life for more than 2 to 3 days, but the prognosis is good if the infant is handled appropriately prior to surgery to prevent aspiration.

BOWEL ATRESIA

Ileal atresia, a congenital discontinuation of the ileum, is the most frequent type of bowel atresia, followed by duodenal atresia. This anomaly presents a few days after birth. The most common signs and symptoms of ileal atresia are abdominal distention and the inability of the infant to pass stool. Eventually the infant regurgitates feedings. Treatment consists of surgery to resect the atretic portion of the bowel and reconnect the bowel proximal and distal to the discontinuation. In some cases, the proximal ileum may be grossly dilated, requiring the surgeon to perform a double-barrel ileostomy. Once the lumen of the proximal ileum returns to a more normal size, the ileostomy is reversed and the bowel anastomosis can be performed.

Duodenal atresia is a congenital anomaly in which the lumen of the duodenum does not exist, resulting in complete obstruction of the GI tract at the duodenum. Although rare (1 in approximately 20,000 births), it is evident soon after birth when vomiting begins and the epigastrium becomes distended. A radiographic indication of duodenal atresia is the "double bubble sign." Gaseous distention of the stomach creates one bubble, and gas in the proximal duodenum creates a second bubble (Fig. 4-22). Like esophageal atresia, oral feedings should be withheld in infants with duodenal atresia. Nasogastric decompression of the stomach is indicated to prevent vomiting and possible aspiration of

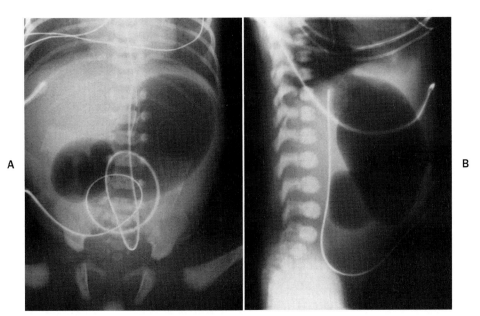

Fig. 4-22 A, Marked distention of the stomach and duodenal bulb with bowel gas distal to the duodenum. Visualization of the classic "double bubble sign" indicates duodenal atresia.
B, The "double bubble sign" in a lateral projection of the same 1-day-old infant. (A Courtesy Riverside Methodist Hospitals, Columbus, Ohio; B Courtesy the American College of Radiology, Reston, Virginia.)

the gastric contents. Treatment consists of surgery to open the duodenum for connection to the pylorus. During surgery, it is common to examine the other areas of the small and large bowel for other sites of atresia and malrotation, which often accompany duodenal atresia.

Colonic atresia is a congenital failure of development of the distal rectum and anus, which can occur to a variable extent (Fig. 4-23). A frequent complication is fistula formation to the genitourinary system, which often can be repaired surgically.

Prognosis is excellent after surgical intervention for all three types of bowel atresia.

Hypertrophic Pyloric Stenosis

Hypertrophic pyloric stenosis is a congenital anomaly of the stomach where the pyloric canal leading out of the stomach is greatly narrowed because of hypertrophy of the pyloric sphincter (Fig. 4-24). It is the most common indication for surgery in infants. Its exact etiology is unknown, but it seems genetically related. It occurs 3 to 4 times more often in male children and most often in the first-born male. Typically, the first sign of the condition is projectile vomiting at 3 to 5 weeks of age. These infants often become dehydrated and fail to gain weight. An

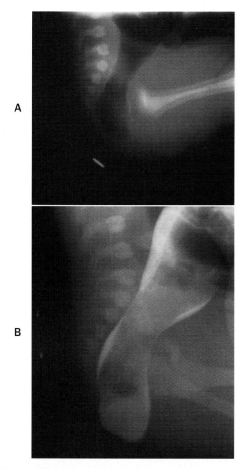

A

B

Fig. 4-23 **A,** Visualization of the rectal air column extending to within centimeters of the perineum (indicated by lead marker) in a 15-hour-old newborn with abdominal distention; **B,** A transperineal percutaneous water-soluble contrast study of the rectum reveals a blind distal colon pouch, evidence of colonic atresia. No genitourinary fistulas were noted, as is common with this condition. (**A** and **B** Courtesy the American College of Radiology, Reston, Virginia.)

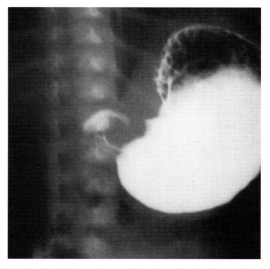

Fig. 4-24 A thin column of barium flowing from the stomach into the pylorus in this 1-month-old boy with projectile vomiting indicates hypertrophic pyloric stenosis. (Courtesy the American College of Radiology, Reston, Virginia.)

upper GI study demonstrates delayed gastric emptying, accompanied by a classic string sign, as the barium trickles through the narrowed, elongated pyloric canal. A surgical procedure is used to incise the hypertrophied muscle fibers and thus increases the opening of the pyloric channel. These infants generally are able to begin normal feedings within a few days after the surgical procedure.

Malrotation

Aberrations of the normal process of intestinal rotation in utero can result in the anomalous position of the small and large bowel, with abnormal fixations predisposing the patient to internal herniation and volvulus.

Malrotation exists when the intestines are not in their normal position (Fig. 4-25), which occurs in an equal male-to-female ratio. There are varying degrees of malrotation of the intestinal tract, ranging from failure of fixation of the cecum in the right-lower quadrant to complete transposition of the bowel, a condition in which the small bowel is on the right and the colon is on the left. Malrotation of the bowel is clearly visible on a barium enema because in all cases the cecum is not located in the right-lower quadrant of the abdomen. Such errors of fixation are often symptomless, but they may lead to bowel volvulus, or incarceration of bowel in an internal hernia. In some instances, the patient may present with clinical signs of bowel obstruction, as discussed later in this chapter. Surgery is the choice for correction of a volvulus or bowel incarceration, with resection of the involved bowel required to relieve infarction of the intestine.

Complete reversal of all abdominal organs, although rare, is known as *situs inversus*.

Imperforate Anus

Imperforate anus is a congenital disorder in which there is no anal opening to the exterior. This condition is corrected surgically shortly after birth.

INFLAMMATORY DISEASES

Esophageal Strictures

Esophageal strictures can occur in varying degrees, with the symptoms displayed differing according to the amount of obstruction produced. Strictures can be secondary to the ingestion of caustic materials such as strong acids or alkalines (Fig. 4-26) or from any factor that inflames the mucosa and creates scarring. Common types of caustics include household cleansers and detergents containing sulfuric acid and sodium hydroxide. These caustic agents burn the esophagus and cause edema, swelling, and possibly perforation. Endoscopy is usually performed to assess the damage to the esophagus, and the esophageal lesions are treated with corticosteroid therapy.

Strictures can be differentiated radiographically from normal peristalsis by their unchanging

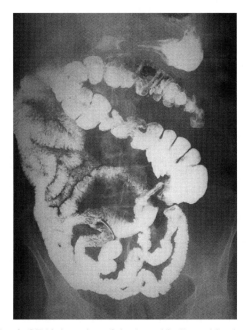

Fig. 4–25 Malrotation of the bowel indicated by the position of the small bowel in the right abdomen and the colon in the left. Note how the terminal ileum enters the cecum from the right. (Courtesy the American College of Radiology, Reston, Virginia.)

appearance; peristalsis is transitory. The mucosa of a benign stricture appears normal with a smooth contour; the contour of a malignant stricture typically appears ragged. Esophageal strictures require repeated dilation with special, mercury-filled tubes of varying diameters to maintain proper patency. Common tubes for this purpose include Hurst and Maloney dilators and pneumatic balloon dilators that are passed over a wire.

Reflux esophagitis, the backward flow of gastric acids into the esophagus, is the primary cause of esophageal inflammation. Reflux is not necessarily abnormal, and heartburn, or symptomatic reflux, has been experienced by most people. It is only when the normal event leads to chronic symptoms and complications, such as a stricture, that it becomes of concern. Esophageal manometry to determine the pressure in the upper and lower esophageal sphincters, pH monitoring of the esophagus, an acid perfusion (Berstein) test, and esophagoscopy are performed, in addition to barium swallow radiographs, to help confirm the diagnosis of gastroesophageal reflux. Treatment includes antacids to wash gastric acids out of the esophagus for pain relief and medical therapy with a variety of medicines to inhibit their production or prokinetic agents to enhance motility.

Surgery as a treatment is the last option for those whose symptoms have failed to respond to medical therapy.

Peptic Ulcer

A **peptic ulcer** is an erosion of the mucous membrane of the lower end of the esophagus, stomach, or duodenum. The most likely site of development of a peptic ulcer is in the duodenal bulb and on the lesser curvature of the stomach. This abnormality affects approximately 10% of the adult population of the United States. Duodenal ulcers are found in adults of all ages and are almost always benign. Gastric ulcers affect individuals primarily over 40 years of age and require careful evaluation and follow-up because a small percentage of gastric ulcers are malignant.

Current studies suggest that peptic ulcers result from a combination of hereditary and environmental factors. Environmental agents include smoking, alcohol, coffee, certain medications such as aspirin and nonsteroidal antiinflammatory drugs, and the bacteria *Helicobacter pylori*. This is a gram-negative, spiral-shaped bacillus identified in 1983. Researchers are fairly certain that *H. pylori* is responsible for chronic antral gastritis; however, the relationship between this bacteria and peptic ulcers is still uncertain. It is believed that peptic acid and the presence of *H. pylori* have a synergistic effect on the development of duodenal ulcers.

The pathogenesis of peptic ulcers varies with location. Duodenal ulcers are believed to result from a hypersecretion of peptic acid, which normally functions to digest meat and other proteins that reach the stomach. A small, superficial erosion of the mucosa, whose cause is not yet fully understood, becomes larger as the gastric acid

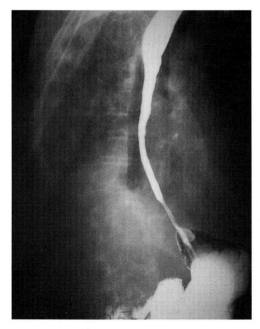

Fig. 4-26 Long-standing esophageal stricture in a 78-year-old man due to accidental ingestion of a caustic agent at age 3. (Courtesy the American College of Radiology, Reston, Virginia.)

and pepsin begin digesting deeper tissues. Unlike duodenal ulcers, gastric ulcers are believed to result from a decreased mucosal resistance that allows the stomach mucosa to self-digest. Normally, the gastric mucosa is protected by a gel-like barrier comprised of bicarbonate and a water-insoluble mucous gel. Certain drugs such as aspirin have also been shown to contribute to the development of gastric ulcers by inhibiting prostaglandin sythesis which impairs healing.

The main symptom of a peptic ulcer is pain, usually above the epigastrium and radiating to all parts of the abdomen. Food ingestion or antacids provide temporary relief, but the pain usually returns when the stomach is empty. In some patients, food may actually increase pain as it stimulates peristalsis, which irritates the ulcer.

Intermittent healing in the midst of continuing digestion leads to considerable scarring at the base of the ulcer. Based on the pattern of scarring, certain radiographic features suggest the benign or malignant nature of an ulcer. Approximately 95% of gastric ulcers are benign and generally display as radiating, spikelike wheels of mucosal folds that run to the edge of the crater (Fig. 4-27). Seen en face, the edge of this ulcer appears round and regular (Fig. 4-28). Also, benign ulcers usually occur on the lesser curvature and rarely on the greater curvature of the stomach. Malignant ulcers, by contrast, show mucosal folds that are obliterated at some distance from the edge of the ulcer crater edge. In profile, such an ulcer does not usually project beyond the original lumen, as does a benign ulcer. Seen en face, the edge of the malignant ulcer is irregular. As mentioned earlier, ulcers can occur anywhere, but those in the proximal stomach and on the greater curvature are particularly suspect for malignancy.

Ulcers should respond to treatment within a few weeks if they are benign. Medication may be given to minimize acid production and intestinal spasm. Dietary adjustments are made to minimize irritating food substances (e.g., coffee, alcohol, and aspirin). Failure of such medical therapies may necessitate surgery for complications of ulcers, such as bleeding or perforation. Surgical options include severing the vagus nerve to eliminate stimulation of the gastric cells that produce the gastric acid. More involved

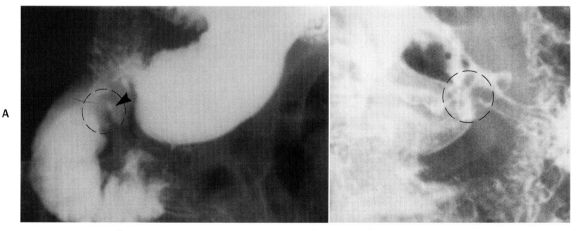

A

B

Fig. 4-27 A, Prone RAO projection of the duodenal bulb demonstrates a dense collection of barium in an ulcer crater, suggesting that it is on the anterior duodenal wall, **B,** persistent collection of barium in the middle portion of the duodenal bulb indicating a superficial ulcer crater, with radiating folds extending from the ulceration. An incisura (fold) along the lower bulb margin points toward the ulcer. (**A** and **B** Courtesy the American College of Radiology, Reston, Virginia.)

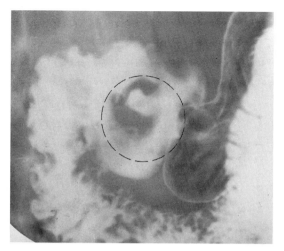

Fig. 4-28 A duodenal ulcer in a 25-year-old man, evidenced by an ulcer crater surrounded by edema represented by the radiolucent halo. (Courtesy the American College of Radiology, Reston, Virginia.)

procedures, including gastrectomy and variants of it, are used if additional complications arise from peptic ulceration. Thanks to better diagnosis and medical treatment, the need for surgery has continually decreased over the past 25 years.

The complications can include pneumoperitoneum or peritonitis if the ulcer perforates into the abdomen. Ulceration into an artery can produce life-threatening hemorrhage. Finally, the edema, spasm, and scarring produced by ulceration can result in bowel obstruction.

Gastroenteritis

A number of inflammatory disorders of the stomach and intestine fall into the general grouping of **gastroenteritis**, inflammation of the mucosal lining of the stomach and small bowel (Fig. 4-29). Erosive gastritis appears to

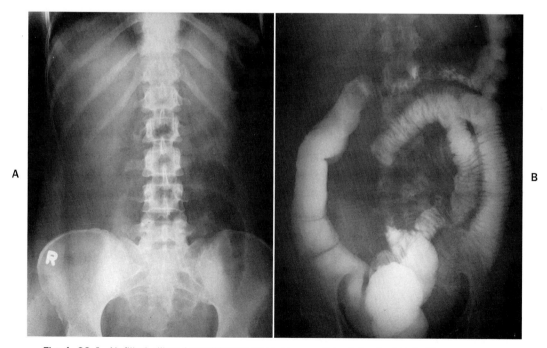

Fig. 4-29 A, Air-filled, dilated small-bowel loops seen on this abdominal plain film are suggestive of an obstruction in this 30-year-old patient with abdominal pain, nausea, and vomiting. **B,** Barium readily refluxes from a barium enema into the distal ileum, demonstrating dilatation without obstruction. The dilatation was due to inflammation caused by gastroenteritis. (**A** and **B** Courtesy the American College of Radiology, Reston, Virginia.)

be a precursor to gastric ulcer formation and results from a compromised mucosal barrier within the stomach. Causes of erosive gastritis include the ingestion of aspirin and other non-steroidal antiinflammatory drugs, alcohol, and steroids; physical stress, trauma; and viral or fungal infections. Acute gastric erosions heal rapidly once the cause is withdrawn. Gastric erosions may be identified on double-contrast examinations of the stomach. Complete erosion appears as slitlike collections of barium surrounded by radiolucent halos of swollen, elevated mucosa. In some cases, scalloped or nodular antral folds may also be visualized. Antral gastritis appears to result from alcohol, smoking, and *Helicobacter* infection. Radiographically, it is demonstrated by decreased distensibility of the antrum in combination with thickened mucosal folds within the antrum, which tend to be oriented on its longitudinal axis and result in a narrowed antrum.

Ingestion of foods contaminated with *Salmonella* and other types of bacteria—most commonly poultry, meat, dairy products, and eggs—may also result in gastroenteritis. Because of the methods used in the mass production of eggs, there was a dramatic increase in *Salmonella* infections in the 1980s. Diarrhea results from mild mucosal ulcerations within the small bowel and the ability of the *Salmonella* bacteria to produce a secretory factor. This is a threat to the normal electrolytic balance of the body, with the diarrhea lasting 3 to 4 days. A good patient history can often point out the offending agent, and treatment consists of proper fluid management and relief of nausea and vomiting.

Malabsorption Syndrome

Malabsorption syndrome is a group of diseases of various causes in which there is interference with normal digestion and absorption of food through the small bowel. Common symptoms of malabsorption syndrome include diarrhea, flatulence, weight loss, and abdominal distention. In addition, patients often present with nutritional deficiencies specific to the primary disease and the area of the gastrointestinal system affected by the disorder.

The best-known small-bowel malabsorption disorder is *celiac disease*, which occurs as a result of sensitivity to the gliadin fraction of gluten, an agent found in wheat and rye products such as bread. The gliadin acts as an antigen and combines with antibodies within the intestinal mucosa, which promotes the aggregation of K lymphocytes. These lymphocytes cause mucosal damage in combination with an increase in crypt cells within the mucosa. With such a condition, the bowel dilates, mucosal folds atrophy, and peristalsis slows or stops. Radiographic changes generally seen with malabsorption syndrome are segmentation of the barium column, flocculation (resembling tufts of cotton), and edematous mucosal changes (Fig. 4-30). Laboratory

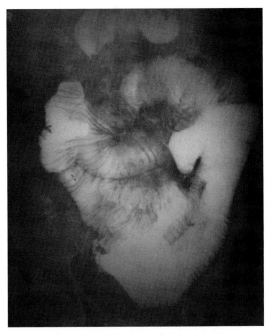

Fig. 4-30 Celiac disease in a 15-year-old patient with a history of diarrhea, indicated on this small bowel study by dilated bowel loops, thickened folds, a grayish appearance of the barium (due to excess fluid in the bowel), and a delayed transit time. (Courtesy the American College of Radiology, Reston, Virginia.)

tests demonstrate low albumin, calcium, potassium, and sodium levels in combination with elevated alkaline phosphatase and prothrombin time. Diagnosis is usually confirmed by biopsy of the small bowel. Treatment of celiac disease consists of avoidance of substances containing gluten and dietary substitution of other products. Vitamin therapy is also used to ensure adequate amounts of nutrients not available because of the malabsorption in the small bowel.

Lactose insufficiency is another form of the malabsorption syndrome, affecting about 60% of the nonwhite population and 20% to 30% of the white population. With this condition, the small bowel lacks enough of the enzyme lactase, which is used to digest lactose into simple sugars that can be absorbed. The result is that lactose stays in the bowel and acts as an osmotic agent, causing fluid to weep into the colon lumen from the wall and creating cramping and diarrhea. The diarrhea also leads to other nutri-

tional deficiencies because the nutrients are purged before they can be absorbed through the intestinal mucosa. Lactose mixed with barium shows the barium moving quickly through the bowel and becoming diluted in the distal ileum and colon (Fig. 4-31). Patients affected by this condition avoid symptoms through avoidance of dairy products.

Regional Enteritis

Regional enteritis, also known as *Crohn's disease* or *granulomatous colitis,* is a chronic inflammatory disease of unknown etiology. It is typically located in the lower ileum but may be seen anywhere throughout the bowel. Over half of all cases involve the colon. This disease typically affects young adults of both sexes in their twenties, with symptoms suggestive of appendicitis or acute bowel obstruction. Family history of Crohn's disease and emotional stress are

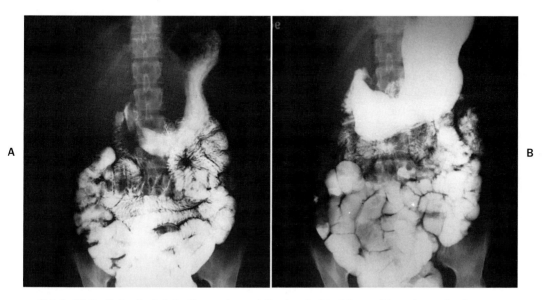

Fig. 4-31 A, Abdominal distention, pain, and diarrhea led to this small-bowel examination, diagnosed as normal for this 35-year-old patient. **B,** Mixing of lactose with barium on a repeat study led to mild bowel dilatation, rapid transit time, and dilution of barium in the distal small bowel, indicative of lactase insufficiency. (**A** and **B** Courtesy the American College of Radiology, Reston, Virginia.)

thought to be important causative factors of bowel dysfunction.

Regional enteritis starts as mucosal inflammation with ulceration of the bowel wall. It eventually affects all layers of the bowel wall. The bowel wall thickens in response to the inflammation and may form fistulas to adjacent loops of bowel, skin, or other abdominal viscera. Subsequent fibrotic scarring may give rise to mechanical obstruction of the bowel. The combination of mucosal edema and crisscrossing fine ulcerations gives the bowel a "cobblestone" radiographic appearance. The string sign (Fig. 4-32) is demonstrated where the terminal ileum is so diseased and stenotic that the barium mixture can only trickle through a small opening that looks like a string. Presentation of the disease in two or more areas with normal intervening bowel between is identified as "skip areas" (Fig. 4-33). Regional enteritis is a chronic disease characterized by periods of exacerbation interspersed with periods of inactivity. In addition, these patients tend to have an increased chance of developing carcinoma of the bowel with a very poor prognosis. Crohn's disease is classified as early stage, intermediate stage, or advanced stage, and the progression of the disease can be demonstrated radiographically, especially via enteroclysis.

Treatment of regional enteritis centers on decreasing inflammation, relief of diarrhea, and treatment of infection. Occasionally, bowel resection is used to remove the involved section of the intestine, particularly if perforation or hemorrhage is present. Recurrence of the disease in other areas of the bowel, however, is common.

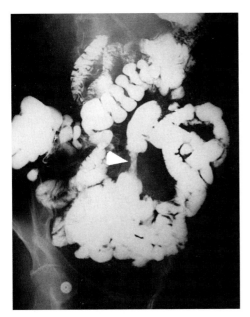

Fig. 4-32 The string sign, demonstrating a diseased, stenotic terminal ileum. (Courtesy Riverside Methodist Hospitals, Columbus, Ohio.)

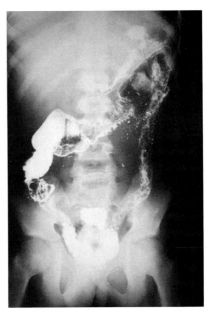

Fig. 4-33 Regional enteritis in an 11-year-old patient demonstrated by the "cobblestone" appearance of the cecum and left colon, with "skip" areas of normal bowel between. (Courtesy the American College of Radiology, Reston, Virginia.)

Appendicitis

Appendicitis is an inflammation of the vermiform appendix, resulting from an obstruction caused usually by a fecalith (Fig. 4-34) or rarely by a neoplasm. Most common abdominal surgical emergency in the United States, it affects approximately 250,000 individuals annually. Appendicitis is most frequent in the late teens and twenties and has a fairly equal distribution between males and females. Complications, usually resulting from gangrenous or perforated appendicitis, occur in about 3 to 5% of all cases. Delayed diagnosis and treatment of appendicitis account for much of the morbidity and mortality associated with this disease.

The obstruction leads to inflammation and distention and affects the blood supply to this portion of the bowel. Venous blood return is decreased, which in turn results in deoxygenation of the tissue. All of these factors leave the appendix susceptible to infection from bacteria, such as *Escherichia coli,* which is normally found within the intestinal tract. Poor blood supply can also lead to gangrene, perforation, and possible rupture. Once the vermiform appendix ruptures, the infection spreads to the peritoneum, leading to general peritonitis that could result in death.

The signs and symptoms of appendicitis include initial pain in the epigastrium that moves to the right-lower quadrant and becomes persistent. Nausea and vomiting may occur as a reflex symptom because the vagus nerve supplies both the stomach and appendix. Individuals also carry a low-grade fever, have a sudden onset of constipation, and present with an elevated white blood cell count. The elevation of white blood cells helps to distinguish appendicitis from other colicky abdominal disorders.

Surgical removal of the appendix is the most common treatment, and, in cases of early surgical intervention, the mortality is low. However, complications such as abscess formation or perforation and peritonitis place the individual at a greater risk and greatly increase the recovery period.

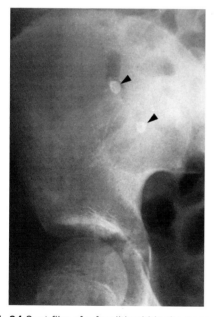

Fig. 4-34 Spot film of a fecalith within the appendix, a common cause of appendicitis. (Courtesy the American College of Radiology, Reston, Virginia.)

Ulcerative Colitis

Ulcerative colitis is an inflammatory lesion of the colon mucosa. Its etiology is unknown, but it is thought to be an autoimmune disease. It is 4 times more common in whites than in nonwhites, especially Jewish persons. Typically, it affects 15- to 25-year-olds. They present with symptoms of excessive diarrhea, with blood, pus, and mucus in the stools. The disease generally starts in the rectum and spreads to the sigmoid, sometimes involving the entire colon. Its clinical course is highly variable in severity and prognosis.

Inflammation of the mucosa and submucosa causes abscesses to form, separating them from their blood supply and leading to ulceration. Gradually, the mucosa is replaced by fibrous tissue whose crevices give a rough, cobblestone appearance to the involved colon.

Colon strictures are a rare complication of ulcerative colitis. Another complication of ulcerative colitis is *toxic megacolon,* an acute dilatation of the colon from colonic paralytic ileus (Fig. 4-35). The dilated bowel is particularly susceptible to rupture; a barium enema is absolutely contraindicated. People with ulcerative colitis have a greatly increased incidence of carcinoma.

Sigmoidoscopy and colonoscopy are the usual means of diagnosing ulcerative colitis in that 90% to 95% of the cases involve the distal colon or rectum. Barium enemas are used to support the clinical diagnosis and to assess the progression of the disease and its complications. When filled with barium, the normally smooth colon outline becomes irregular because of the ulceration present. *Pseudopolyps* are islands of unaffected mucosa that become visible when surrounded by affected mucosa. Another radiographic indication of ulcerative colitis is an easily recognized loss of colon haustration.

Certain characteristics of ulcerative colitis distinguish it from regional enteritis (Crohn's disease). Ulcerative colitis is a disease of the mucosa of the colon, whereas regional enteritis affects all layers of the bowel wall. Also, ulcerative colitis typically begins at the anus and ascends, often results in megacolon and bowel perforations, and frequently progresses to cancer; by contrast, regional enteritis usually begins in the terminal ileum and cecum and descends through the bowel, often with skip areas. It rarely produces megacolon or bowel perforations.

Treatment of ulcerative colitis is initially medical in nature and often involves steroid therapy. Development of an obstruction or neoplasm may require surgical intervention. This involves removal of the colon from cecum to sigmoid with establishment of an ileostomy or ileorectal or ileoanal anastomosis.

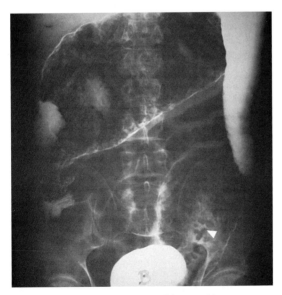

Fig. 4-35 Barium enema on a 61-year-old man demonstrates toxic megacolon secondary to ulcerative colitis. Pseudopolyps are seen in the descending colon. (Courtesy the American College of Radiology, Reston, Virginia.)

ESOPHAGEAL VARICES

Varicose veins are abnormally lengthened, dilated, and superficial veins; those in the esophagus are referred to as **esophageal varices.** They occur in the esophagus because of portal hypertension. Conditions that cause resistance to the normal blood flow through the liver (such as cirrhosis) cause a bypass of the normal venous drainage mechanism. Instead, the blood is directed through the esophageal and gastric collateral veins. The increase in blood flow through these channels results in venous dilatation.

Esophageal varices are best demonstrated in a recumbent position because gravity causes poor visualization in an erect position. A thin barium mixture radiographically demonstrates the varices as wormlike defects within the column of barium (Fig. 4-36). Use of thick barium may be counterproductive because it can cover the varices. Esophageal varices may also occasionally be visualized as a retrocardiac posterior mediastinal mass on a plain chest film obtained with the patient in a recumbent position.

Patients with esophageal varices are subject to their rupture and hemorrhage, which may be massive and often is fatal. Statistics show that ruptured varices have accounted for approximately one third of all death from cirrhosis. An erect film taken for this situation should be done with great caution as the patient's blood loss may be significant. The resultant reduced blood pressure along with the elevation may cause the patient to faint.

Treatment for esophageal varices may consist of endoscopic sclerotherapy, banding ligation, or infusion of vasopressin, a natural hormone useful in stopping hemorrhage. Compression of the varices through balloon tamponading may be occasionally used. Shunts such as transjugular untrahepatic portosystemic shunts (TIPS), applied via interventional radiology or in surgery may be used to help redirect liver blood flow, thus reducing portal hypertension and easing venous pressure in the esophageal and gastric collateral circulation.

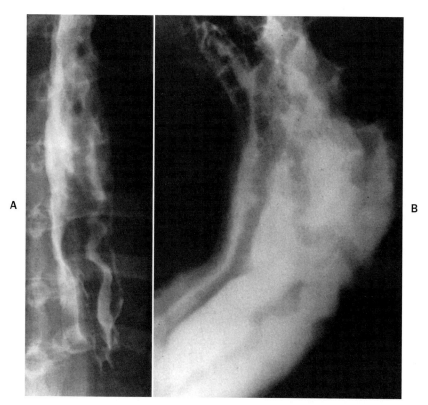

Fig. 4–36 **A,** Long, serpentine filling defects in the esophagus of a 41-year-old with chronic alcoholism, indicative of esophageal varices; **B,** similar filling defects seen in the cardia of the stomach of the same patient, indicative of gastric varices. (**A** and **B** Courtesy the American College of Radiology, Reston, Virginia.)

DEGENERATIVE DISEASES

Herniation

A **hernia** is a protrusion of a loop of bowel through a small opening, usually in the abdominal wall. Popularly referred to as a *rupture*, it occurs because of an anatomic weakness. As the bowel loop herniates, it pushes the peritoneum ahead of it. An *inguinal hernia*, which is common in men, occurs when a bowel loop protrudes through a weakness in the inguinal ring (Fig. 4-37) and may descend downward into the scrotum. Femoral and umbilical herniation (Fig. 4-38) occur in both sexes.

If a herniated loop of bowel can be pushed back into the abdominal cavity, it is said to be reducible. If it becomes stuck and cannot be reduced, it is an *incarcerated hernia*. As described previously, this can result in a bowel obstruction (Fig. 4-39). If the constriction through which the bowel loop has passed is tight enough to cut off blood supply to the bowel, it is called a *strangulated hernia*. Prompt surgical intervention is required in this case to avoid necrosis of that portion of the bowel. Bowel that has already necrosed can generally be surgically resected.

Hiatal Hernia

A **hiatal hernia** is a weakness of the esophageal hiatus, which permits some portions of the stomach to herniate into the thoracic cavity. Hiatal hernias occur in about half of the population over age 50. In its early stages, a hiatal hernia is reducible. Chronic herniation may be associated with reflux esophagitis.

A direct, or sliding, hiatal hernia occurs when a portion of the stomach and gastroesophageal junction are both situated above the diaphragm (Fig. 4-40). This type of hernia comprises the outstanding majority (about 99%) of all hiatal hernias. A *Schatzki's ring* is

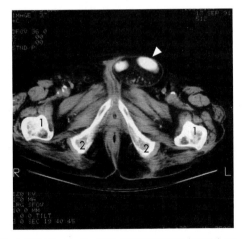

Fig. 4-37 Moderate left inguinal hernia (*arrow*) on this CT image of a 96-year-old man. Also well defined are *(1)* the femurs, showing the lesser trochanters projecting posteriorly, and *(2)* the ischial tuberosities. (Courtesy Riverside Methodist Hospitals, Columbus, Ohio.)

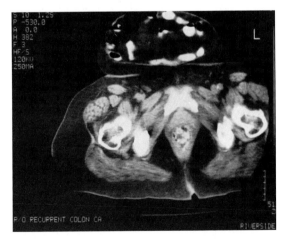

Fig. 4-38 CT demonstration of a large anterior abdominal hernia containing multiple loops of small bowel and possibly some large bowel, without evidence of obstruction in this 70-year-old man. (Courtesy Riverside Methodist Hospitals, Columbus, Ohio.)

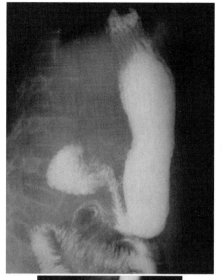

A

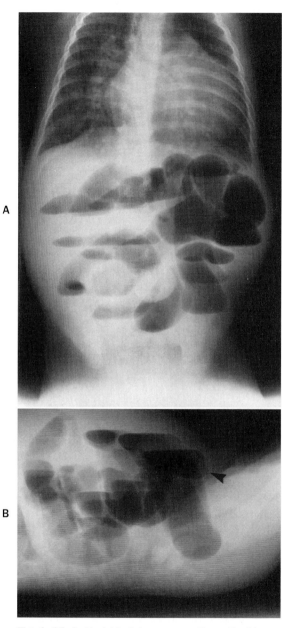

A

B

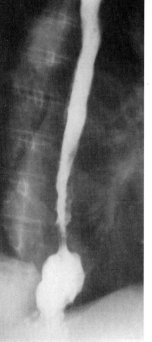

B

Fig. 4-39, A, Upright abdomen on a 3-month-old indicates multiple dilated loops of bowel with air-fluid levels present, suggesting a mechanical bowel obstruction; **B,** a prone cross-table lateral view shows the small bowel forming a beaklike projection at the point of obstruction at the internal inguinal ring in this incarcerated hernia. (**A** and **B** Courtesy the American College of Radiology, Reston, Virginia.)

Fig. 4-40 A, Demonstration of contrast material above the hemidiaphragm on an upper GI series of this 51-year-old woman; **B,** the esophagus narrows to the stomach, which is seen to empty passively, above the hemidiaphragm in this sliding hiatal hernia. (**A** and **B** Courtesy the American College of Radiology, Reston, Virginia.).

often visible with this condition (Fig. 4-41) and consists of a mucosal ring that protrudes into the lumen. Such a ring has traditionally been thought to be congenital but may be related to gastric reflux. It is, however, generally of no clinical significance unless it produces narrowing sufficient to cause dysphagia, usually less than 13 mm in diameter.

A far less common type of hiatal hernia is the rolling, or paraesophageal, hiatal hernia. This occurs when a portion of the stomach or adjacent viscera herniates above the diaphragm, while the gastroesophageal junction remains

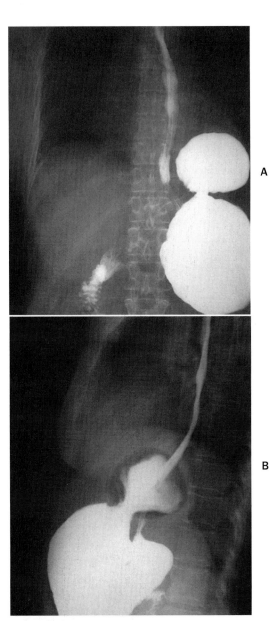

A

B

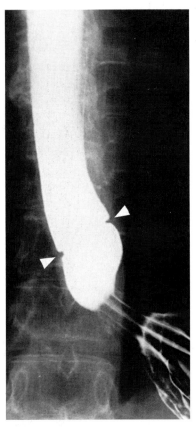

Fig. 4-41 Schatzki's ring as demonstrated in the case of a sliding hiatal hernia. (Courtesy Riverside Methodist Hospitals, Columbus, Ohio.)

Fig. 4-42 A, Paraesophageal hiatal hernia, demonstrating narrowing in the fundus; **B,** a lateral view of the same patient demonstrates the cardioesophageal junction in its normal place below the hemidiaphragm. The fundus is highlighted by the radiolucency of the lung.

(**A** and **B** Courtesy the American College of Radiology, Reston, Virginia.)

below the diaphragm (Fig. 4-42). If all of the stomach slides above the diaphragm, an *intrathoracic stomach* (Fig. 4-43) results. Unlike the sliding hiatal hernia, a paraesophageal hernia is potentially life-threatening because of the risk of volvulus, incarceration, or strangulation of the hernia.

Most hiatal hernias are asymptomatic, but some are accompanied by reflux. Most patients experiencing reflux complain of a full feeling in the chest, particularly after meals. Some reflux of gastric contents leads to complaints of heartburn. An upper GI examination can pinpoint the herniation and distinguish the cause of reflux esophagitis. Treatment of hiatal herniation is generally conservative and centered on efforts to reduce reflux esophagitis and minimize dis-

comfort. This includes modification of eating habits, weight loss, avoidance of smoking, medication to decrease acid, and elevation of the head of the bed.

BOWEL OBSTRUCTIONS

Both the small and large bowels of the normal patient are nearly always active in peristalsis. Many lesions of various types (e.g., inflammatory, degenerative) can interfere with this action and cause an obstruction of either small or large bowels. The resultant obstruction can be either a **mechanical bowel obstruction,** as occurs from a blockage of the bowel lumen, or a **paralytic ileus,** which results from a failure of peristalsis. There are gradations of each, and both may be present at the same time. Initial diagnosis of a small bowel obstruction by use of a plain abdominal radiograph may be difficult because of to the frequency of vomiting and the use of nasogastric decompression.

General signs and symptoms of a bowel obstruction include vomiting, abdominal distention, and abdominal pain. Sequential radiographs over 12 to 24 hours help to determine the diagnosis and to locate the level of the obstruction in individuals with mechanical obstructions. Most commonly, gas confined to the small bowel with multiple air-fluid levels visible on an erect abdominal radiograph indicates a mechanical obstruction, whereas gas distributed throughout both the large and small bowel is indicative of paralytic ileus. The small bowel tends to be more distended in cases of mechanical obstruction. Physical signs are also helpful in distinguishing the type of obstruction present. *Bowel sounds,* the normal sounds of a bowel in motion as heard on auscultation, are absent with an ileus; they are present with a mechanical obstruction and are often hyperactive and high- pitched. Emesis containing bile may also indicate a mechanical obstruction.

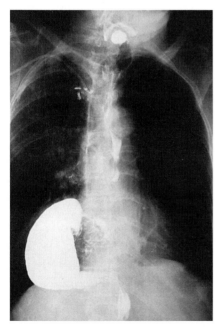

Fig. 4–43 Intrathoracic stomach indicated by the presence of the entire stomach above the diaphragm, also with malrotation of the stomach. (Courtesy Riverside Methodist Hospitals, Columbus, Ohio.

Mechanical Bowel Obstruction

A mechanical bowel obstruction (Fig. 4-44) is one in which the lumen of the bowel becomes occluded, as might occur for a variety of reasons, most often postoperatively from adhesions. Generally, these require surgical intervention to correct. Nearly half of all mechanical bowel obstructions are caused by an incarcerated (i.e., trapped) hernia, a condition discussed earlier in this chapter as a degenerative disease. Entrapment of a hernia, usually involving the small bowel, causes impairment of blood flow and swelling of the affected tissues. The resultant edema affects the arterial blood flow to the bowel and may lead to ischemic necrosis, perforation, and peritonitis. Prompt surgical intervention and reduction are required to relieve an incarcerated hernia.

Gallstone ileus is another cause for a mechanical bowel obstruction. This condition, a gallstone can erode from the gallbladder and create a fistula to the small bowel. This leads to an obstruction, usually when the gallstone reaches the ileocecal valve. Radiographic signs of this include air-fluid levels or air in the biliary tree (Fig. 4-45). The gallstone itself may also be visible, often in the terminal ileum where it causes the obstruction.

A **volvulus** is a twisting of a bowel loop about its mesenteric base, usually at either the sigmoid or ileocecal junction (Fig. 4-46). This most commonly occurs in the elderly and is identifiable on a plain abdomen radiograph as a collection of air conforming to the shape of the affected, dilated bowel. Some twists resolve spontaneously; however, bowel that is

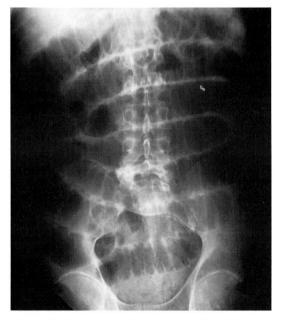

Fig. 4-44 Abdominal radiograph demonstrating a mechanical bowel obstruction, with numerous loops of dilated bowel seen within the midabdomen. The patient had an acute onset of abdominal pain, nausea, and vomiting. (Courtesy the American College of Radiology, Reston, Virginia.)

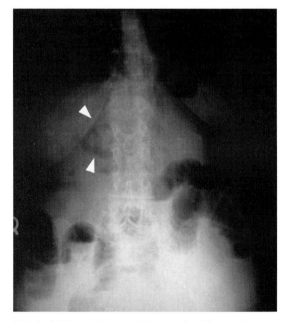

Fig. 4-45 Abdominal radiograph of a 43-year-old woman demonstrating air within the biliary ductal system and an overall density (gallstone) in the right lower abdomen. (Courtesy the American College of Radiology, Reston, Virginia.)

twisted more than 360 degrees requires surgical intervention. Surgical untwisting and resection is necessary to prevent necrosis and perforation of the bowel caused by a lack of blood supply.

An **intussusception** occurs when a segment of bowel, constricted by peristalsis, telescopes into a distal segment and is driven further into the distal bowel by peristalsis. Recall that the bowel is connected to the mesentery, so as the bowel telescopes into itself, the mesentery (with its rich blood supply) is also involved. Intussusception is responsible for approximately 5% of all mechanical obstructions and most frequently affects the ileocecal valve (Fig. 4-47). It is more common in children and infants than in adults. Its presence in an adult generally signifies an accompanying intraluminal mass and is generally reduced surgically so that the physician can search for the cause of the intussusception and correct the condition. In children and infants, an intussusception can often be reduced by an enema, sparing a surgical intervention.

Other causes of small bowel obstruction include adhesions, tumors, Crohn's disease, and appendicitis.

Paralytic Ileus

Paralytic ileus or adynamic ileus is a failure of normal peristalsis that may result from a variety of factors. The most common causes are following surgery, especially that requiring manipulation of the bowel (postoperative ileus), and intraperitoneal or retroperitoneal infection. It may

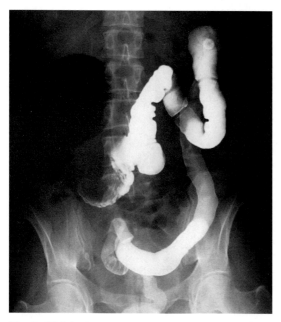

Fig. 4–46 A barium enema radiograph depicting a cecal volvulus. Note how the column of barium stops at the level of the volvulus. (Courtesy the American College of Radiology, Reston, Virginia.)

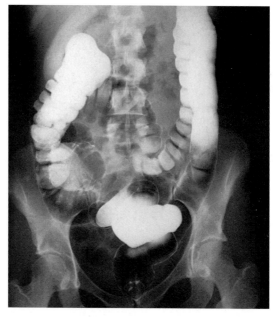

Fig. 4–47 Pediatric barium enema demonstrating intussusception at the ileocecal junction. (Courtesy the American College of Radiology, Reston, Virginia.)

also be associated with bowel ischemia, certain drugs, electrolyte imbalance, pancreatitis, or simply as a reaction to any stressful medical illness. Paralytic ileus generally lasts no longer than 3 days with proper medical treatment. The absence of peristalsis causes the lumen of both the small and large intestines to fill with gas and fluid, with the resultant dilatation extending to the rectum (Fig. 4-48). Treatment for paralytic ileus generally consists of medical stimulation of the bowel to restore peristalsis.

NEUROGENIC DISEASES

Achalasia

Achalasia is a neuromuscular abnormality of the esophagus that results in failure of the lower esophageal sphincter of the distal esophagus to relax, leading to dysphagia. It occurs equally in males and females and most commonly af-fects individuals between the ages of 40 and 50. Clini-

cally, these patients present with a slowly progressive dysphagia in swallowing both solids and liquids. Patients may also experience regurgitation.

Radiographically, the condition demonstrates as a dilated esophagus with little or no peristalsis. The distal esophagus itself is often described as having a "beaked" appearance (Fig. 4-49). Because the distal esophagus opens only intermittently, when the pressure is high enough, food residue may be seen in the distal esophagus or even on a chest radiograph. Because the esophageal contents act as a water seal, the normal gastric gas bubble may be absent.

Initial treatment of achalasia is conservative. Affected patients have sometimes learned on their own what induces pain and what prevents it, and they have modified their eating habits accordingly. Most patients, however, require other interventions for treatment, including medication, a pneumatic dilation done endoscopically, and surgical myotomy.

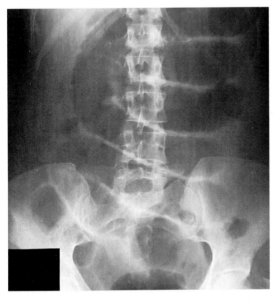

Fig. 4-48 Abdominal radiograph on a postoperative patient demonstrating paralytic ileus. Note the dilated bowel loops extending through the large intestine. (Courtesy Riverside Methodist Hospitals, Columbus, Ohio.)

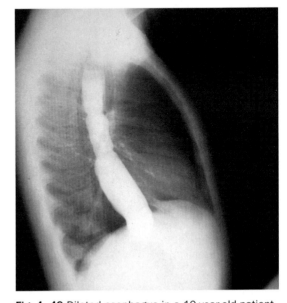

Fig. 4-49 Dilated esophagus in a 10-year-old patient that demonstrated no normal peristalsis on filling, indicating achalasia. The distal esophagus terminates into a beaked appearance. (Courtesy the American College of Radiology, Reston, Virginia.)

Hirschsprung's Disease

Hirschsprung's disease is an absence of neurons in the bowel wall, typically in the sigmoid colon, and is also known as *congenital megacolon*. Occurring in approximately 1 in 5000 births, this defect is a familial disease, primarily affecting males. The absence of neurons in the bowel wall prevents the normal relaxation of the colon and subsequent peristalsis, which results in gross dilatation to the point of narrowing and constriction.

This generally becomes apparent shortly after birth, when the affected infant passes little meconium and the abdomen becomes distended. As the patient ages, the continued effects are severe constipation and recurrent fecal impactions. Barium enemas demonstrate a transition from the narrow, distal rectum to a dilated proximal colon (Fig. 4-50). Initial treatment in an infant may consist of a temporary colostomy until surgical resection is possible later.

DIVERTICULAR DISEASES

Esophageal Diverticula

A **diverticulum** is a pouch or sac of variable size that occurs normally or is created by herniation of a mucous membrane through a defect in its muscular coat. Esophageal diverticula occur when mucosal outpouchings penetrate through the muscular layer of the esophagus. The two primary types of esophageal diverticula are pulsion and traction.

A *pulsion diverticulum* involves the mucosa only and results from a motility disorder of the esophagus, which allows the mucosa to herniate outward. This type of diverticulum appears radiographically as a rounded projection with a narrow neck and occurs more frequently in the upper and lower thirds of the esophagus. A *Zenker's diverticulum* is a pulsion type found at the pharyngoesophageal junction at the upper end of the esophagus (Fig. 4-51). An *epiphrenic diverticulum* is another pulsion type, but it is

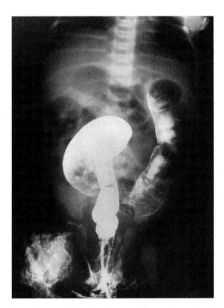

Fig. 4-50 Barium enema on a 6-day-old infant demonstrates a normal rectosigmoid leading to a distended large bowel consistent with Hirschsprung's disease. (Courtesy the American College of Radiology, Reston, Virginia.)

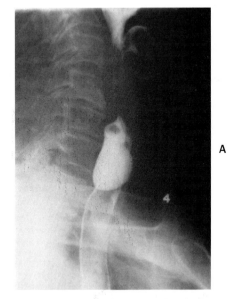

A

Fig. 4-51 **A,** Large Zenker's diverticulum in the esophagus of a 67-year-old man with complaints of difficulty in swallowing over the past 6 months. (**A** and **B,** Courtesy the American College of Radiology, Reston, Virginia.) *Continued*

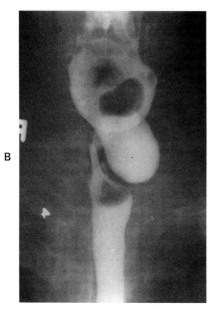

B

Fig. 4–51 cont'd **B,** Zenker's diverticulum in the same patient on a magnified view.

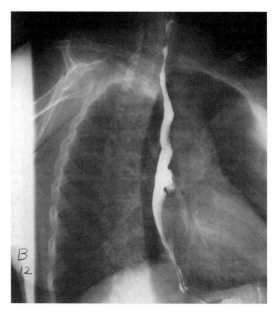

Fig. 4–53 Traction diverticulum indicated by the outpouching of the esophagus at the level of the carina seen in an esophagram of a 47-year-old woman with a history of ulcer disease. (Courtesy the American College of Radiology, Reston, Virginia.)

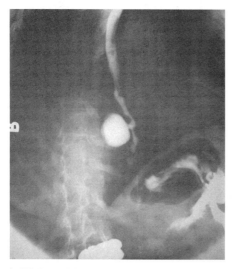

Fig. 4–52 An epiphrenic diverticulum shown as a large collection of barium connected and adjacent to the lower esophagus. (Courtesy the American College of Radiology, Reston, Virginia.)

found in the distal esophagus just above the hemidiaphragm (Fig. 4-52).

A *traction diverticulum* involves all layers of the esophagus and results from adjacent scar tissue that pulls the esophagus toward the area of involvement (Fig. 4-53). Such a diverticulum occurs more frequently in the middle third of the esophagus at the carina and appears radiographically as a triangle whose apex points toward the disease.

Usually, diverticula are asymptomatic until they reach a relatively large size, at which time complications may occur. For example, food and secretions can collect in the diverticulum and cause a mechanical obstruction of the esophagus. Such contents can also be aspirated by a recumbent patient, resulting in a chemical pneumonia. Failure to control the effects of diverticula through diet modifications may result in the need for surgical removal, dependent on the amount of food retention in the diverticulum.

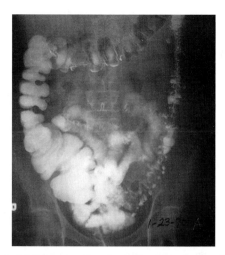

Fig. 4-54 Extensive diverticulosis of the descending and sigmoid colon in the barium enema of a 69-year-old woman. (Courtesy the American College of Radiology, Reston, Virginia.)

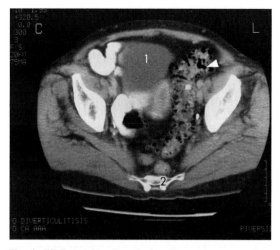

Fig. 4-55 Extensive diverticular disease seen as air-filled translucencies in the sigmoid colon on this CT film of an 87-year-old woman. Also well-defined are the *(1)* bladder, and *(2)* sacrum. (Courtesy Riverside Methodist Hospitals, Columbus, Ohio.)

Colonic Diverticula

Diverticulosis, the presence of diverticula without inflammation, is seen in all parts of the colon, most frequently in the sigmoid colon, and particularly among the elderly (Figs. 4-54 and 4-55). This anomaly is the most common colonic disease in the Western world. Diverticula are associated with hypertrophy of the muscular layer of the bowel and are thought to be caused by a refined diet with little dietary bulk. They generally occur where the terminal branches of the mesenteric vessels pierce the bowel wall and are present in 35 to 50% of patients over age 50. Factors contributing to the development of diverticula include a pressure gradient between the lumen and serosa of the bowel and areas of weakness within the bowel wall. The most common site for diverticula (95%) is the sigmoid colon, the narrowest portion of the colon, which generates the highest intrasegmental (between haustra) pressures.

Inflammation of a diverticulum, termed **diverticulitis** occurs in approximately 10% to 20% of patients with known diverticulosis. The inflammation is exacerbated by feces lodging in the diverticulum. Signs and symptoms include lower-left quadrant pain and tenderness, fever, and an increased white blood cell count. Because of these symptoms, sigmoid diverticulitis has been termed *left-sided appendicitis.* This condition can lead to bowel obstruction, perforation, and fistula formation. A barium enema examination may be indicated to demonstrate the affected diverticulum, most commonly in the distal colon. Radiographic signs of diverticulitis on barium enema include extraluminal or intraluminal contrast. Spasm may be seen as well, and the underlying colonic mucosa appears intact.

Treatment of diverticulitis centers on reduction of inflammation and infection. Mild cases are treated with antibiotic therapy. Complications such as peritonitis can result if perforation of a diverticulum occurs, and these, of course, must be treated. Surgical resection of the bowel may be used to remove the diseased portion in more severe cases.

NEOPLASTIC DISEASES

Tumors of the Esophagus

While benign and malignant tumors can occur anywhere in the esophagus, tumors of the lower third are the most common. Benign tumors are almost always a **leiomyoma,** which is a smooth muscle tumor, although these have an incidence of less than 10% that of malignant tumors of the esophagus. Many are discovered on x-ray examination for complaints not related to esophageal problems. These benign lesions demonstrate as an intramural defect in the barium-outlined esophageal wall (Fig. 4-56). The exact location of a leiomyoma, which appears as a homogeneous soft tissue mass, may be determined on CT. Treatment of a leiomyoma consists of surgi-

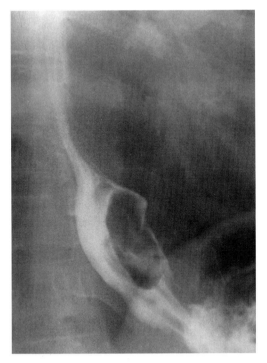

Fig. 4–56 Sharply defined filling defect in the distal esophagus indicative of a benign, esophageal leiomyoma. (Courtesy the American College of Radiology, Reston, Virginia.)

cal removal through a thoracic or abdominal incision that spares esophageal resection.

Cancers of the esophagus constitute approximately 7% of cancers of the GI system but carry a poor prognosis with an overall 5-year survival rate of less than 10%. Squamous cell carcinomas most commonly arise in the body of the esophagus; those at the gastroesophageal junction are typically adenocarcinomas. These two types of esophageal cancers have different clinical and radiographic features. Regardless of the type of esophageal cancer, however, CT is helpful to stage the spread of the disease by demonstrating tumor size, lymph node involvement, and metastases. Endoscopic ultrasonography is very accurate in detecting disease but less available in many medical institutions.

Chronic irritation of the esophagus is thought to be a predisposing factor to squamous cell carcinomas, with such irritation caused by particular agents, including reflux, alcohol, and smoking, and disorders such as achalasia and esophageal diverticula. The primary symptom of esophageal cancer is dysphagia. However, dysphagia may not become significant until the tumor has narrowed the lumen to 50% to 75% of its normal circumference, allowing metastatic spread to the adjacent lymph nodes and mediastinal structures prior to diagnosis. Surgery is used as a treatment, with the goal to excise the tumor and regional metastasis. The rapid spread of esophageal cancer, however, requires the goal to be palliation in many cases. The radiographic appearance of a malignant squamous cell tumor may include mucosal destruction, ulceration, narrowing, and a sharp demarcation between normal tissue and the malignant tumor.

As mentioned earlier, adenocarcinomas usually occur in the lower esophagus around the gastroesophageal junction. Many believe these begin as primary gastric carcinomas, which invade the lower esophagus. Others believe there is a direct link between a disorder termed Barrett's esophagus and the development of adenocarcinoma of the esophagus. Barrett's esophagus involves progressive columnar metaplasia of the distal esophagus due to chronic gastro-esophageal reflux. More than 90% of adenocarcinomas of the esophagus have been found to arise from Barrett's mucosa. Similar to squamous carcinomas, adenocarcinomas spread via the lymph nodes; however, unlike squamous carcinomas, they also spread below the diaphragm. Metastasis to mediastinal structures and hematogenous spread to the liver, lung, and bone occur readily (Fig. 4-57). Radiographically, early adenocarcinomas appear as plaquelike lesions or as sessile polyps, and advanced tumors appear as infiltrating lesions with irregular narrowing of the lumen with abrupt, asymmetric borders.

Tumors of the Stomach

Benign tumors account for fewer than 10% of all stomach tumors. Those that are clinically significant are quite rare. Most stomach tumors are malignant, and the outstanding preponderance

(about 95%) of these are **adenocarcinomas.** The incidence of gastric cancer varies strikingly by geographic area, race, diet, heredity, and sex. For example, the rate is nearly 5 times greater in Japan than in the United States. Factors that predispose an individual to gastric carcinoma include being male; being part of a fish-eating population; a salty, spicy, or high-cabbage diet; being black; and having type A blood. Like esophageal cancers, gastric carcinoma has a poor prognosis, with overall 5-year survival rates less than 20%.

Most gastric carcinomas develop in the pyloric and antrum regions, particularly along the lesser curvature, although they can be present anywhere (Fig. 4-58). Gastric ulcers are particularly suspect, as they may represent a carcinoma. Gastric carcinomas may also be polypoid with a plaquelike, lobulated appearance. Most gastric carcinomas are diagnosed at an advanced stage and invade other structures by a variety of routes. These tumors metastasize fairly readily

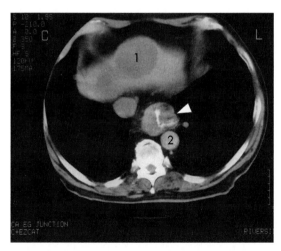

Fig. 4-57 A CT scan with contrast demonstrates an increased thickening of the esophageal wall and distortion of the lumen (*arrow*), compatible with a gastroesophageal junction malignancy. Also seen are (*1*) a large metastatic lesion in the superior portion of the liver and (*2*) the aorta. (Courtesy Riverside Methodist Hospitals, Columbus, Ohio.)

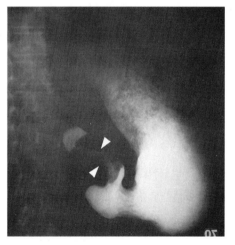

Fig. 4-58 Adenocarcinoma of the stomach in a 66-year-old woman, resulting in gastric outlet obstruction. Note the area of narrowing and the abrupt transition between normal stomach and the acutely narrowed area. (Courtesy the American College of Radiology, Reston, Virginia.)

outside the stomach to involve the omentum, liver, pancreas, and colon. Liver involvement creates the possibility of discharge into the bloodstream and dispersal throughout the body. Because of the abundance of lymphatics in the stomach, approximately 75% to 85% of these patients also demonstrate metastases via the lymphatic system.

Patients who complain of persistent GI pain should have a thorough workup, with the primary diagnostic study upper endoscopy, often followed by a GI series. Symptoms of gastric tumors are often vague but include bleeding, vomiting, loss of appetite, weight loss, and early satiety. Tumors are radiographically indicated by a relative rigidity of peristalsis and filling defects on compression. Filling defects demonstrate as areas of total or relative radiolucency within the barium column. Polypoid tumors are clearly visible on CT examination; however, ulcerated carcinomas are difficult to image with CT. By identifying lymphatic involvement and extragastric spread of the cancer, CT is also useful in the staging of gastric cancers.

Surgical removal of gastric cancer has been the only successful treatment; a subtotal gastrectomy is the usual procedure. Resection of the stomach to attach to the jejunum via a gastrojejunostomy usually accompanies this procedure. Radiation therapy and chemotherapy treatments for stomach carcinoma have been less effective.

Small-Bowel Neoplasms

Small-bowel tumors represent less than 2% of all benign and malignant GI neoplasms. The incidence of malignancy for this small amount is about 50%. The low overall incidence is surprising, considering that the small bowel composes 75% of the entire GI tract, with an enormous mucosal surface. Also, it is in constant contact with enteric carcinogenic substances. Reasons for this low incidence of tumors are not entirely known or understood. Most small-bowel cancers occur in the duodenum and proximal jejunum.

One predisposing factor for small-bowel neoplasms seems to be the degree of polyposis in other areas of the GI tract, a condition frequently determined by heredity. Intermittent abdominal pain sometimes described as cramps is the most common symptom. Small-bowel barium studies are the primary means of diagnosis. Surgical resection is the primary means of treating small-bowel neoplasms, both benign and malignant.

Colonic Polyps

Colonic polyps are small masses of tissue arising from the bowel wall to project inward into the lumen (Fig. 4-59). Polyps can be adenomatous or hyperplastic. An *adenomatous polyp* is a tumor of benign neoplastic epithelium. It consists of saccular projection into the bowel lumen and is either *sessile,* that is, attached directly to the bowel wall with a wide base—or *pedunculated,* that is, attached by a narrow stalk (Fig. 4-60). Polyps are more frequently noted in the left colon, and particularly in the rectosigmoid areas. It is the adenomatous polyp that has

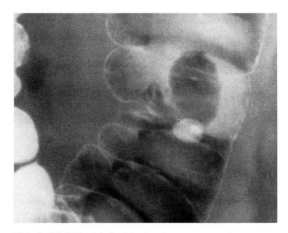

Fig. 4–59 Filling defect in the transverse colon near the splenic flexure indicates a polyp projecting into the lumen. A barium-filled diverticulum is seen immediately above it in this patient, who presented with blood in his stools. (Courtesy the American College of Radiology, Reston, Virginia.)

neoplastic potential. Other types of polyps are inflammatory, hyperplastic, and juvenile.

Although most polyps are benign, the larger and more sessile a polyp, the greater the chance of malignancy. Those over 2 cm in size have a malignancy rate over 50%. Most never reach this size, however. The complications of polyps include ulceration from chronic irritation or bowel obstruction from inflammation. Most cancers of the colon and rectum arise from previously benign polyps. Patients with polyps may present with rectal bleeding, constipation, diarrhea, or flatulence, but most are asymptomatic. Radiographically, an air-contrast barium enema is the examination of choice, with the polyps demonstrating as rounded filling defects or contour defects in the barium shadow. Although pedunculated polyps are easily recognized and often considered benign, size is a better indication of malignancy versus benignancy, as noted.

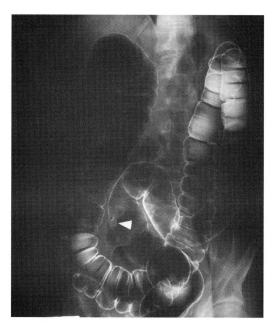

Fig. 4-60 Pedunculated polyp seen attached to the wall of the sigmoid colon by a long stalk on an air-contrast barium enema. (Courtesy the American College of Radiology, Reston, Virginia.)

At times, it is difficult to discriminate between fecal material and a polyp. In general, fecal material is mobile, while a polyp stays fixed to the stalk. Proctosigmoidoscopy and colonoscopy are critical in evaluation and removal of polyps. Patients with polyps are followed closely after discovery.

Colon Cancer

Carcinoma of the colon is one of the most common malignancies in the United States and the second most common cause of cancer mortality. The incidence of colon cancer rises significantly after age 40 and doubles with each decade, reaching a peak at about age 75. American adults have a 1 in 20 chance of developing colorectal cancer in their lifetime and a 1 in 40 chance of dying from this disease. Predisposing factors include a family history of familial polyposis and ulcerative colitis. Environmental factors also seem to correlate with colorectal cancer, as countries with higher intakes of sugar and animal fats (e.g., the United States) have a higher incidence than countries with a higher fiber intake.

Adenocarcinoma is the most common type of colorectal cancer and is derived from the glandular epithelium of the colon. It begins as a benign adenoma that which undergoes a slow, malignant transformation. Although the transformation may take up to 7 years to complete, all polypoid lesions larger than 1 cm should be removed from the colon. Adenocarcinoma is characterized by infiltration of the colon wall, as opposed to being a bulky, intraluminal mass.

Although the incidence of proximal colon cancers is increasing, nearly 50% still occur below the mid-descending colon. Most of these occur in the rectosigmoid area and are detectable by flexible sigmoidoscopy. Right colon lesions differ considerably from left colon lesions in terms of symptoms produced. Lesions in the right colon, on the one hand, may produce no early symptoms, often becoming quite large, ulcerating, and even bleeding without significant symptoms. They also tend to penetrate and extend into surrounding tissues without causing obstruction. Such patients often present initially with anemia and blood in their stools. Left colon lesions, on the other hand, present more often with obstruction and bleeding, largely because of a smaller lumen and an annular (ringlike) growth pattern.

The evaluation of colon cancer includes fecal blood testing, proctosigmoidoscopy, colonoscopy, and the barium enema. An air-contrast enema has been noted to produce more accurate diagnoses than the traditional single-contrast study. The radiographic appearance of adenocarcinoma has led to its designation as the "napkin-ring" carcinoma or the "apple-core" lesion, as the edges of the lesion tend to overhang and form acute angles with the bowel wall (Fig. 4-61).

Although it may be difficult to distinguish between carcinoma and an inflammatory lesion (e.g., regional enteritis or ulcerative colitis), a carcinoma generally has a more clear-cut transition between malignant and normal mucosa. In addition, the length of involved bowel is usually shorter with carcinoma than with an inflammatory lesion.

Without treatment, invasion of local tissue spreads the cancer via the lymphatics to the mesenteric nodes and on to the liver (Fig. 4-62) and lungs. Fortunately, the lesion does not metastasize early, leading to a good prognosis. The primary means of treatment are surgical excision of the primary tumor and its margins and resection of the bowel as possible. A colostomy may be required, depending on the site of the tumor. Radiation therapy is generally given before and after surgery for rectal cancers. For inoperable tumors, the radiation therapy is given to reduce the tumor size and its resultant complications (e.g., obstruction) and also to provide pain relief. Chemotherapy is given when the cancer has metastasized.

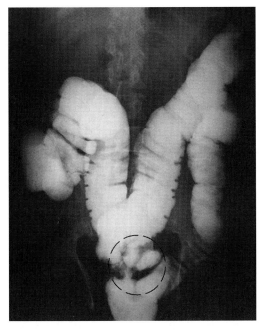

Fig. 4-61 The "apple core lesion" of the rectosigmoid colon consistent with adenocarcinoma, with characteristic appearance of abrupt change from normal to abnormal colon and shelflike appearance of overhanging edges caused by the mass. (Courtesy of the American College of Radiology, Reston, Virginia.)

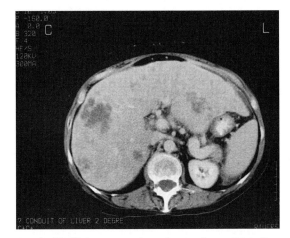

Fig. 4-62 CT demonstration of extensive metastatic disease from the colon to both lobes of the liver, ranging from punctate to up to 5 cm in this 50-year-old woman. (Courtesy Riverside Methodist Hospitals, Columbus, Ohio.)

QUESTIONS

1. Esophageal atresia is classified as a(n) _____ condition of the GI system.
   a. congenital
   b. degenerative
   c. inflammatory
   d. neurologic

2. An outpouching of the bowel wall caused by a weakening in its muscular layer is a(n):
   a. atresia
   b. carcinoma
   c. diverticulum
   d. polyp

3. The radiographic string sign is associated with which disease?
   a. achalasia
   b. adenocarcinoma
   c. regional enteritis
   d. ulcerative colitis

4. Celiac disease is a type of:
   a. atresia
   b. herniation
   c. malabsorption syndrome
   d. ulcerative colitis

5. The appearance of a Schatzki's ring is associated with a(n) _____ hernia.
   a. inguinal
   b. rolling
   c. sliding
   d. umbilical

6. A neurogenic disease of the GI system characterized by an absence of neurons in the bowel wall is:
   a. achalasia
   b. diverticulosis
   c. Hirschprung's disease
   d. toxic megacolon

7. The least number of all GI tumors, both benign and malignant, occur in the:
   a. colon
   b. esophagus
   c. large bowel
   d. small bowel

8. Which of the following statements are true of colon cancer?
   1. The majority of adenocarcinoma of the colon occur in the rectosigmoid area.
   2. The appearance of the "apple core" lesion is indicative of colon cancer.
   3. The prognosis with colon cancer is generally poor because of its early metastasis.
   a. 1 and 2
   b. 1 and 3
   c. 2 and 3
   d. 1, 2, and 3

9. A twisting of bowel about its mesenteric base best refers to a(n):
   a. ascites
   b. intussusception
   c. incarcerated hernia
   d. volvulus

10. The condition in which a gallstone erodes from the gallbladder and creates a fistula to the small bowel is:
    a. gallstone ileus
    b. intussusception
    c. incarcerated hernia
    d. volvulus

11. Describe the differences both clinically and radiographically between a mechanical bowel obstruction and paralytic ileus.

12. Explain the connection between colonic polyps and the development of colorectal cancer.

13. Describe the role of CT in the staging of various gastrointestinal cancers.

14. Explain the physiologic alteration that causes esophageal varices, and describe the radiographic appearance of this disorder.

15. Compare and contrast the various gastric tubes in terms of their uses and radiographic appearance.

Chapter 5

The Hepatobiliary System

Anatomy and Physiology Review
  The liver
  The biliary tree
  The gallbladder
  The pancreas
Imaging Considerations
  Plain films
  Contrast studies
    Oral cholecystogram
    Percutaneous transhepatic cholangiography
    Endoscopic retrograde cholangiopancre-
      atogram
    Operative cholangiography
    T-tube cholangiography
  Other studies
    Diagnostic medical sonography
    Computed tomography
    Hepatobiliary scans

Inflammatory Diseases
  Cirrhosis
  Viral hepatitis
  Cholelithiasis
  Pancreatitis
Metabolic Diseases
  Jaundice
Neoplastic Diseases
  Hemangioma
  Hepatoma
  Carcinoma of the gallbladder
  Carcinoma of the pancreas

Upon completion of Chapter 5, the reader should be able to:

■ Describe the anatomic components of the hepatobiliary system and how they are visualized radiographically.

■ Discuss the role of other imaging modalities in imaging of the hepatobiliary system, particularly ultrasound and CT.

■ Characterize a given condition as inflammatory, metabolic, or neoplastic.

■ Identify the pathogenesis of the pathologies cited and the typical treatments for them.

■ Describe, in general, the radiographic appearance of each of the given pathologies.

KEY TERMS

Milk of calcium
Cirrhosis
Ascites
Hepatitis
Hepatomegaly

Cholelithiasis
Cholecystitis
Gallstone ileus
Pancreatitis
Pseudocyst

Medical jaundice
Surgical jaundice
Hemangioma
Hepatoma
Carcinoma of the gallbladder

ANATOMY AND PHYSIOLOGY REVIEW

The hepatobiliary system is composed of the liver, gallbladder, and biliary tree (Fig. 5-1). The pancreas is closely related and shares a portion of the biliary ductal system, hence its inclusion here.

The Liver

The liver is the largest organ in the body and is sheltered by the ribs in the right-upper quadrant of the abdomen. It is kept in position by peritoneal ligaments and intraabdominal pressure from muscles of the abdominal wall. The

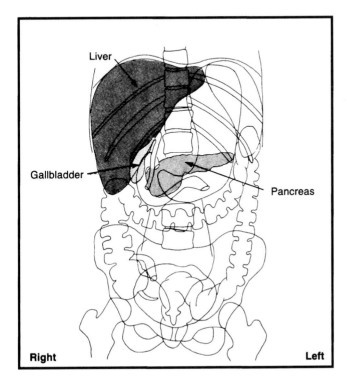

Fig. 5-1 The hepatobiliary system and the pancreas. (From Bontrager KL: *Textbook of radiographic anatomy and related positioning,* ed 3, St Louis, 1993, Mosby.)

functions of the liver are multiple, including metabolism of substances delivered via its portal circulation, synthesis of substances including those concerned with blood clotting, storage of vitamin B and other materials, and detoxification and excretion of various substances.

The liver has a double supply of blood, coming from the hepatic artery and the portal vein. The hepatic artery usually originates from the celiac axis and takes oxygenated blood to the liver. The portal vein is formed by the union of the superior mesenteric and splenic veins. It is located within the liver and serves to return venous blood from the abdominal viscera to the inferior vena cava. Any interference with blood flow, such as might occur with liver disease, results in consequences elsewhere in the abdominal viscera and spleen.

The Biliary Tree

A system of ducts acts to drain bile produced in the liver into the duodenum (Fig. 5-2). Bile from the liver's two main lobes is drained by the right and left hepatic ducts. These unite to form the common hepatic duct, which is joined usu-ally in its midportion by the cystic duct from the gallbladder. Together, the cystic duct and the common hepatic duct form the common bile duct.

The common bile duct descends posterior to the descending duodenum to enter at its posteromedial aspect. Before its entrance into the duodenum, the common bile duct may be joined by the pancreatic duct from the head of the pancreas. The short part of the common bile duct, after joining the pancreatic duct, is known as the hepatopancreatic ampulla or, more commonly, the ampulla of Vater.

The flow of both bile and pancreatic juice into the duodenum is regulated by the hepatopancreatic sphincter, more commonly known as the sphincter of Oddi. The release of bile into the duodenum is triggered by cholecystokinin, a hormone released by the presence of fatty foods in the stomach. The purpose of bile is to emulsify fats so that they may be absorbed.

The Gallbladder

The gallbladder is a pear-shaped sac located on the undersurface on the right lobe of the liver.

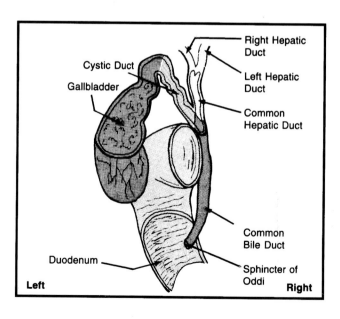

Fig. 5-2 The biliary system. (From Bontrager KL: *Textbook of radiographic anatomy and related positioning,* ed 3, St Louis, 1993, Mosby.)

Normally, the walls are quite thin, but they often thicken in the presence of inflammation. The sole function of the gallbladder is to store and concentrate bile that has been produced in the liver.

The Pancreas

The pancreas is an elongated, flat organ that obliquely crosses the left side of the abdomen behind the stomach; it is a powerful digestive organ. Its functions are both exocrine and endocrine. Exocrine function is concerned with production of digestive enzymes. These are discharged through the pancreatic duct into the duodenum. The endocrine portion of the pancreas consists of multiple clusters of specialized cells, the islets of Langerhans. Their function is to produce insulin and glucagon, which are discharged directly into the blood from the pancreas. Insulin and glucagon regulate carbohydrate metabolism.

IMAGING CONSIDERATIONS

Plain Films

A conventional abdominal radiograph may contain information about the hepatobiliary system through the demonstration of faint calcifications that might otherwise be obscured by contrast media. A plain radiograph of the gallbladder may demonstrate **milk of calcium** as a semiliquid sludge (Fig. 5-3) composed of calcium carbonate mixed with bile in the gallbladder. The hazy radiopacity is due to a settling of bile as a result of an obstruction at the neck of the gallbladder.

Gas may occasionally be seen in the wall or lumen of the gallbladder because of the presence of gas-forming organisms in the gallbladder walls. This is most generally seen in patients with poorly controlled diabetes. Gas visualized in the biliary tree may also be a result of a spontaneous fistula, as might be seen in gallstone ileus, or postoperative biliary anastomosis (Fig. 5-4).

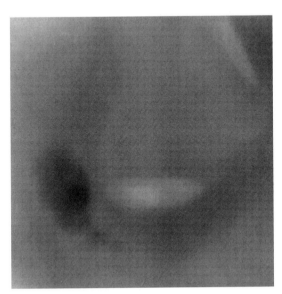

Fig. 5-3 Milk of calcium bile as seen in the bottom of this gallbladder in an erect spot film. (Courtesy Riverside Methodist Hospitals, Columbus, Ohio.)

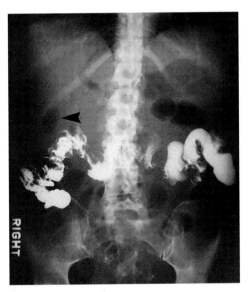

Fig. 5-4 Gas in the lumen of the gallbladder as a result of postsurgical fistula development to the bowel as seen on plain film. (Courtesy the American College of Radiology, Reston, Virginia.)

Contrast Studies

ORAL CHOLECYSTOGRAM

An examination formerly widely used to study the biliary system is an oral cholecystogram (OCG), although it has been largely replaced by ultrasound. It still has use in certain clinical situations. In this examination, the contrast media is absorbed in the small bowel and passes through the portal vein to the liver. The contrast agent is excreted from the liver with bile and is stored in the gallbladder (Fig. 5-5). About 25% of all patients' gallbladders fail to visualize on the first attempt at oral cholecystography. The most common causes of nonvisualization are an obstruction of the cystic duct secondary to a stone and chronic cholecystitis, with poor concentration of the contrast agent.

PERCUTANEOUS TRANSHEPATIC CHOLANGIOGRAPHY

A percutaneous transhepatic cholangiogram (PTC) is used to visualize the biliary tree and involves insertion of a needle into the biliary tree by puncture directly through the wall of the abdomen. With the use of a flexible, 22-gauge, skinny needle (Chiba), this procedure is safe and fairly easy to perform. The subsequent injection of contrast media (Fig. 5-6) is useful in distinguishing medical jaundice, caused by hepatocellular dysfunction, from surgical jaundice, which results from biliary obstruction. Also, the examination is useful for detecting the presence of calculi or a tumor in the distal common bile duct. It has a high success rate in imaging the biliary ductal system, is less expensive than ERCP, and has a low complication rate of approximately 3.5%. It also may be immediately followed by a therapeutic procedure such as a

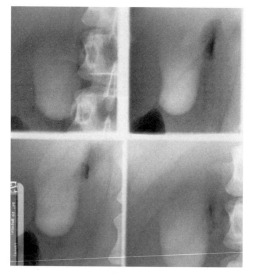

Fig. 5-5 A normal oral cholecystogram, with no evidence of stones as demonstrated on this standard 4-on-1 spot film in various projections. (Courtesy Riverside Methodist Hospitals, Columbus, Ohio.)

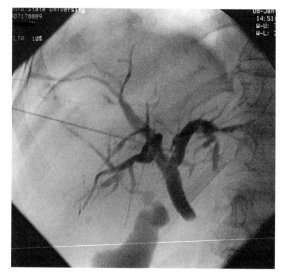

Fig. 5-6 Demonstration of the biliary system via a percutaneous transhepatic cholangiogram (PTC). (Courtesy the Ohio State University Medical Center, Columbus, Ohio.)

biliary drainage, stone removal or crushing via contact lithotripsy or laser fragmentation, stent placement, or biopsy. This procedure is preferred in the evaluation of proximal obstructions involving the hepatic duct bifurcation, which is difficult to image with the retrograde approach via an ERCP.

ENDOSCOPIC RETROGRADE CHOLANGIOPANCREATOGRAM

The endoscopic retrograde cholangiopancreatogram (ERCP), an imaging procedure performed by a gastroenterologist, is a means of visualizing the biliary system and main pancreatic duct, which provides drainage for the pancreatic enzymes into both the digestive tract and the common bile duct. A fiberoptic endoscope is passed through the duodenal C-loop to visualize the ampulla of Vater. A thin catheter is then directed into the orifice of the common bile duct or pancreatic duct, followed by an injection of contrast media (Fig. 5-7). In many cases, the ERCP is preferred over the transhepatic cholangiogram and is often preceded with an ultrasonic examination or CT investigation of the pancreas. Although an ERCP is more expensive than a PTC, it is often used to visualize nondilated ducts, distal obstructions, patients with bleeding disorders, and the pancreas. The complication rate (2% to 3%) is similar to PTC and also offers the ability to perform therapeutic procedures such as sphincterotomy, stone extractions, stent placement, and biliary dilatation. Cytology and biopsy may also be performed.

OPERATIVE CHOLANGIOGRAPHY

Operative cholangiography is performed during surgery at the time of a cholecystectomy to detect biliary calculi and the need for common bile duct exploration (Fig. 5-8). A needle is placed directly into the cystic duct or common bile duct by the surgeon, and a small volume (5 ml) of contrast material is injected, followed by a radiograph. A second injection of 5 ml is made, followed by a second radiograph. The resulting images are reviewed for possible areas of concern prior to completing the surgery. It is imperative that no air bubbles be injected into the ductal system with the contrast agent during this procedure because they can mimic stones.

T-TUBE CHOLANGIOGRAPHY

T-tube cholangiography is used after a cholecystectomy to demonstrate patency of the common bile duct and to check for calculi. With a

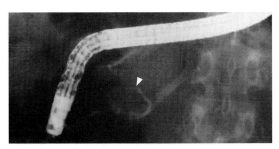

Fig. 5-7 An ERCP showing abrupt termination of the pancreatic duct about 4 cm from its opening. (Courtesy Riverside Methodist Hospitals, Columbus, Ohio.)

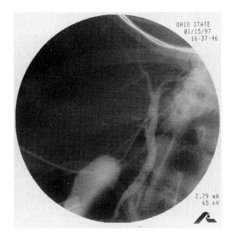

Fig. 5-8 A digital image of an operative cholangiogram taken during surgery. (Courtesy the Ohio State University Medical Center, Columbus, Ohio.)

T-shaped tube already inserted surgically into the common bile duct, contrast media are injected to verify removal of all calculi. The radiologist must take care not to inject air bubbles because they may give the radiographic appearance of radiolucent calculi.

Other Studies

DIAGNOSTIC MEDICAL SONOGRAPHY

Real-time diagnostic medical sonography is now the modality of choice for evaluating the gallbladder (Fig. 5-9). This procedure is noninvasive, and the gallbladder can be satisfactorily imaged in almost all fasting patients regardless of the body habitus or clinical condition of the patient. Sonography has proven to be 95% accurate in detecting gallstones. It is also an excellent tool for determining the presence of common bile duct obstruction, evaluation of the intrahepatic biliary ductal system, and abscesses. The liver may also be evaluated by sonography because of its ideal location in the right-upper quadrant and broad contact with the abdominal wall. Advances in Doppler flow technology have greatly enhanced the diagnostic capabilities of ultrasound to allow for clear

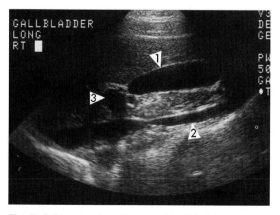

Fig. 5–9 Sonography of a normal gallbladder readily demonstrates *(1)* the gallbladder, *(2)* inferior vena cava, and *(3)* the portal vein. (Courtesy Riverside Methodist Hospitals, Columbus, Ohio.)

analysis of the circulatory dynamics, including portal blood flow. Doppler sonography can also differentiate between vessels and biliary ducts based on flow characteristics. In addition, ultrasound is increasingly used for needle-directed biopsies of the hepatobiliary systems, and, in cases where respiratory motion is a problem, it is preferred to CT-directed biopsy.

COMPUTED TOMOGRAPHY

The role of computed tomography (CT) in the hepatobiliary system is similar to its role in the GI tract. It is the accepted modality for following malignancies and assessing masses, particularly of the gallbladder, liver, and pancreas. It is also helpful in evaluating complications of cholecystitis, such as perforations and abcess formations. As mentioned in the last chapter, spiral or helical CT ensures that the entire liver is imaged in one breath and that anatomy is not lost due to respiratory artifact. In addition, the use of large-bolus IV injections during dynamic CT examination has also improved CT evaluations of the liver and biliary ductal system. If a biliary obstruction is not visible on sonographic examination, CT can generally identfy the location and extent of the obstruction. In addition, CT can often differentiate between benign and malignant obstructions. Lacerations of the liver and resultant abdominal bleeding are readily detected on CT (Fig. 5-10), and CT-guided biopsy procedures for the liver (Fig. 5-11), pancreas, and kidney allow for analysis and drainage and offer significant advantages over conventional surgical biopsy and drainage.

HEPATOBILIARY SCANS

With improvements in real-time sonography and CT, the use of conventional nuclear medicine liver and spleen scans with Tc 99m sulfur colloid has decreased because their limited spatial resolution produces poorer quality images. However, single-photon emission computed tomography (SPECT) examinations provide much better detection of lesions, especially those located deep within the liver parenchyma. It provides a noninvasive method of evaluating hepatic function and hepatic and splenic perfusion. Beacuse nuclear medicine imaging can provide information regarding physiologic function, these scans can often provide information prior to the onset of the anatomic changes that are visible with CT. White cells labeled with radioactive indium are useful in locating sites of infection for treatment. Cholescintography scans performed in nuclear medicine are very useful to confirm cholecystitis, and they may be useful for distinguishing acute from chronic cholecystitis (Fig. 5-12). In addition, it is a noninvasive method of evaluating biliary drainage and segmental obstruction.

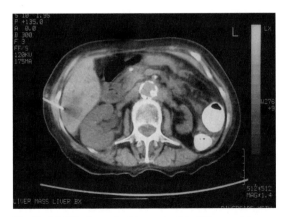

Fig. 5-10 CT of this 39-year-old woman after a car accident reveals large lacerations to the liver. (Courtesy Riverside Methodist Hospitals, Columbus, Ohio.)

Fig. 5-11 CT of needle biopsy in this 87-year-old woman clearly demonstrates the needle in the liver. (Courtesy Riverside Methodist Hospitals, Columbus, Ohio.)

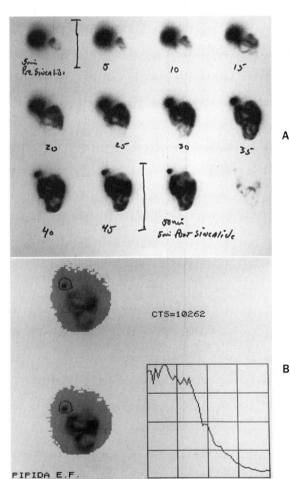

Fig. 5-12 A, Nuclear medicine hepatobiliary scan demonstrates ready ejection of the radionuclide from the gallbladder (large in upper-left image) through sequential images into the duodenum (large in lower-right image) in this 44-year-old woman. **B,** Computer analysis of the accompanying data generates a graph showing 95% ejection of the agent. Above 50% is considered acceptable. (**A** and **B** Courtesy Riverside Methodist Hospitals, Columbus, Ohio.)

INFLAMMATORY DISEASES

Cirrhosis

Cirrhosis is a chronic liver condition in which the liver parenchyma and architecture are destroyed, fibrous tissue is laid down, and regenerative nodules are formed. In its early stages, it is usually asymptomatic, as it can take months or even years before damage becomes apparent. Cirrhosis is considered an end-stage condition resulting from liver damage by chronic alcohol abuse, drugs, autoimmune disorders, metabolic and genetic disease, chronic viral infections, cardiac problems, and chronic biliary tract obstruction. It is the sixth leading cause of death in the United States, with one third of the deaths secondary to hemorrhage from esophageal varices.

The scarring and formation of regenerative nodules associated with cirrhosis can have serious complications for the afflicted individual. The two functional impairments caused by cirrhosis are impaired liver function resulting from hepatocyte damage, generally resulting in jaundice, and portal hypertension. Because of interference of portal blood flow through the liver, portal hypertension may lead to development of collateral venous connections to the venae cavae. Most commonly, such connections involve the esophageal veins, which dilate to become esophageal varices, as described in the preceding chapter. These are best evaluated with endoscopy but may be seen on an esophagram. Also, the patient with cirrhosis has a tendency to bleed because the liver is unable to make the necessary clotting factors found in plasma or as a result of an esophageal variceal rupture. Such hemorrhaging may be, in fact, the first indication of portal hypertension.

Ascites, the accumulation of fluid within the peritoneal cavity (Fig. 5-13), is also seen as a result of portal hypertension and the leakage of excessive fluids from the portal capillaries. Much of this excess fluid is composed of hepatic lymph weeping from the liver surface. It is associated with approximately 50% of deaths due to cirrhosis. Ascites may also result from chronic hepatitis, congestive heart failure, renal failure, and certain cancers. When the cause of ascites is uncertain, diagnostic paracentesis may be conducted with sonographic guidance. This involves removal of 50 to 100 ml of peritoneal fluid for analysis. Patients with ascites generally

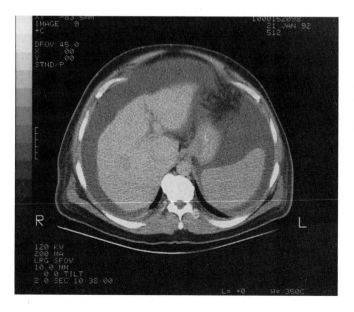

Fig. 5-13 Cirrhosis of the liver as indicated on this CT scan showing a shrunken liver with significant ascites around it within the abdomen. (Courtesy Riverside Methodist Hospitals, Columbus, Ohio.)

complain of nonspecific abdominal pain and dyspnea. Medical treatment of ascites includes bed rest, dietary restrictions of sodium, use of diuretics to avoid excess fluid accumulation, and treatment of the underlying cause.

It is important for the technologist to be aware of the clinical diagnosis of ascites because the fluid accumulation can make it difficult to adequately penetrate the abdomen. An increase in exposure factors is necessary to obtain a diagnostic-quality radiograph. Radiographically, large amounts of ascitic fluid give the abdomen a dense, gray, ground-glass appearance. With the patient in a supine position, the fluid accumulates in the pelvis and ascends to either side of the bladder to give it a dog-eared appearance. Gradually, the margins of the liver, spleen, kidneys, and psoas muscles become indistinct as the volume of fluid increases. Loops of bowel filled with gas float centrally, and a lateral decubitus radiograph demonstrates the fluid descending and the gas-filled loops of bowel floating on top.

Although sonography is helpful in determining the presence of liver cirrhosis, the diagnosis is generally accomplished through a biopsy of liver tissue. Conventional radiographic signs of cirrhosis are few and not specific. Morphologic changes in the liver due to cirrhosis may cause displacement of other abdominal organs such as the stomach, duodenum, colon, gallbladder, and kidney. The primary means of evaluating the complications arising from cirrhosis is CT. Fatty infiltration of the liver, an initial feature in alcoholic liver disease, is well visualized by computed tomography. The most characteristic finding in cirrhosis is an increase in the ratio of the caudate lobe and the right lobe because with cirrhosis the right lobe and medial segment of the left lobe atrophy while the caudate lobe and the lateral segment of the left lobe hypertrophy. Because of its dual arterial blood supply, the caudate lobe of the liver is usually spared in cirrhosis. Studies show that individuals with cirrhosis have an increased risk of developing hepatic carcinoma, so CT is also of value in assessing the presence of complications

of cirrhosis, such as ascites and hepatocellular carcinoma.

Diagnostic medical sonography is utilized to detect portal hypertension and evaluate portosystemic collateral circulation. Ultrasound is used to measure the vessel size of the portal vein, which ranges from 0.64 to 1 cm in a normal adult. A portal vein larger than 1.3 cm in diameter is indicative of portal hypertension. In addition, the portal vein should distend with deep inspiration, but in patients with portal hypertension, the vein lacks distensibility. Sonographic evaluation of the other venous structures such as the superior mesenteric and splenic veins adds additional information to the clinician.

Treatment of cirrhosis depends on the extent of liver damage and the involvement of other organs (e.g., the esophagus and stomach). The primary goal of treatment is to eliminate the underlying causes of the disease and to treat its complications. Surgical treatment of portal hypertension may be achieved by diverting blood from the portocollateral system into the lower-pressure systemic circulation. This is accomplished by placing a shunt, eliminating the chance of variceal bleeding. A distal splenorenal shunt in which the splenic vein is divided, with the distal portion anastomosed to the left renal vein, is most commonly used. If the patient is not a candidate for this type of shunt, a total shunt, either portocaval or mesocaval, must be placed. However, these shunts have a tendency to thrombose, requiring patency to be assessed by angiography, CT, or ultrasound.

Viral Hepatitis

Hepatitis is a relatively common liver condition, with an estimated 70,000 cases reported annually. A virus causes acute inflammation of the liver and interferes with the liver's impaired ability to excrete bilirubin, the orange or yellowish pigment in bile. Evidence of the disease is seen clinically by nausea, vomiting, discomfort, and tenderness over the liver area, and laboratory results indicate a disturbance in liver function. Additional signs and symptoms include fatigue, anorexia, photophobia, and general malaise. Jaundice may also develop within 1 or 2 weeks because of the disturbance of bilirubin excretion. If the liver inflammation lasts 6 months or more, the condition is classified as chronic. Different viruses give rise to the three types of viral hepatitis, with their names describing the usual methods of transmission.

Hepatitis A, infectious hepatitis, is excreted in the GI tract in fecal material and is spread by contact with an infected individual, normally through ingestion of contaminated food or water. It is the most common form and highly contagious. The incubation period of the disease is relatively short (15 to 50 days), and its course is usually mild.

Hepatitis B, serum hepatitis, is transmitted parenterally in infected serum or blood products. Its incubation period is much longer (50 to 160 days) and its effects more severe than those of hepatitis A. Hepatitis type B can result in an asymptomatic carrier state, acute hepatitis, chronic hepatitis, cirrhosis, and hepatocellular carcinoma.

A third type of viral hepatitis, hepatitis C, is non-A, non-B, and is caused by a parenterally transmitted RNA virus. Type C accounts for 90% of the cases of hepatitis that develop after blood transfusions. Recently, a routine test for anti–hepatitis C antibody has been developed, so transmission via transfused blood has been significantly decreased. Hepatitis C can cause either acute or chronic hepatitis, with 10% to 20% of these patients eventually developing cirrhosis of the liver.

The diagnosis of viral hepatitis is usually made through laboratory testing because the disease is carried in the bloodstream during the acute phase. Evidence of hepatitis may be seen radiographically on a plain film of the abdomen that demonstrates **hepatomegaly,** or enlargement of the liver, although this is a nonspecific finding. Cellular necrosis can be confirmed through nuclear medicine scanning of the liver, CT, or a liver biopsy. Ultrasound is also useful in distinguishing the characteristics of the liver.

Viral hepatitis is usually mild; the majority of patients recover without complications. Treatment generally consists of bed rest and medication to fight nausea and vomiting. In a healthy individual, the liver regenerates after hepatitis damage, and complete recovery is gained. Approximately 10% of patients with type B and 60% with type C progress into chronic hepatitis. In some, the disease may become progressive and lead to liver failure.

Cholelithiasis

The incidence of **cholelithiasis** (gallstones) is fairly common, with at least 10% of all persons developing them at some point. Females are more likely than males to have them. Their occurrence is also greater in diabetics, the obese, and in parous women. Heredity plays a role in their development. Although most commonly found in the gallbladder, they can be located anywhere in the biliary tree. Symptoms associated with cholelithiasis may be vague, including bloating, nausea, and pain in the right-upper quadrant.

The characteristics of gallstones are quite varied. They may occur as a single stone or as multiple stones. About 80% of all stones comprise a mixture of cholesterol, bile pigment (bilirubin), and calcium salts. The remaining 20% are composed of pure cholesterol or a calcium-bilirubin mixture. Most stones are radiolucent because only about 10% of all stones contain enough calcium to be radiopaque. Those that are radiopaque may be difficult to distinguish from renal stones, but oblique radiographs help separate the two structures (kidney and gallbladder) from each other, demonstrating the gallbladder anterior to the kidney. As noted before, sonography readily demonstrates the presence of cholelithiasis (Fig. 5-14). The best image is obtained when the gallbladder is distended and filled with bile; therefore, patients should fast 8 hours prior to

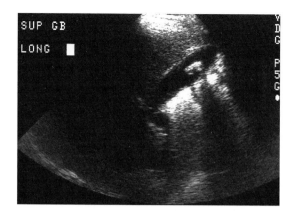

Fig. 5-14 Cholelithiasis with ready visibility of a single stone as seen in this sonogram of the gallbladder in this young woman. (Courtesy Riverside Methodist Hospitals, Columbus, Ohio.)

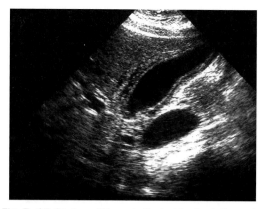

Fig. 5-15 Cholecystitis as indicated by the inflamed, thickened gallbladder walls in this 23-year-old woman. (Courtesy Riverside Methodist Hospitals, Columbus, Ohio.)

sonographic examination. The three major sonographic criteria for gallstones include (1) an echogenic focus, (2) acoustic shadowing below the stone, and (3) gravitational dependence. Gallstones can be the size of a pinhead to the size of a large marble. The small stones, commonly referred to as *gravel,* tend to travel into the biliary tree and may result in obstruction. Obstruction of the bile duct causes pain and jaundice and may result in cholangitis.

Surgical removal of the gallbladder (cholecystectomy) is usually the treatment of choice, although laparoscopic cholecystectomy has replaced many traditional open cholecystectomies. The newer technique allows a less traumatic entry, excision, and removal of the gallbladder, with a shortened hospitalization and reduced costs. Radiographers are commonly called to the operating environment to film injections of contrast media into the exposed biliary duct to determine if all stones have been removed. If additional stones are suspected but not visualized, a T-tube may be inserted to allow for later study, as noted earlier. An alternative treatment method, shock wave lithotripsy of gallstones, has not proven as successful in the gallbladder as it has in the kidneys for kidney stones. Investigation of it as an alternative in the United States

continues, although it is used to some extent elsewhere in the world.

Cholecystitis is an acute inflammation of the gallbladder. It is characterized clinically by a sudden onset of pain, fever, nausea, and vomiting in individuals with chronically symptomatic cholelithiasis. Its diagnosis is clinically suspected and supported through an ultrasound examination or radionuclide cholescintography. A radiopharmaceutical comprised of Tc 99m in combination with disopropyliminodiacetic acid (DISIDA) allows visualization of the biliary ductal system and results in a highly sensitive examination with consistently reliable results. Non visualization of the gallbladder is a good indicator of acute cholecystitis. Repeated attacks of acute cholecystitis cause damage to the gallbladder, thickening of the walls, (Fig. 5-15) and decreased function.

Complications of untreated gallbladder disease include infarction and a possible gangrenous state, prompting a rupture of the walls. Perforation of the gallbladder occurs in approximately 5% to 15% of all patients with acute cholecystitis and can be diagnosed in several ways. Cholescintography provides the best images of perforation; however, stones may be visible outside the gallbladder on plain abdominal films, CT images, or sonographic images. Ultrasound and CT often also demonstrate a nonspecific pericholecystic fluid collection. If a rupture does occur, bile peritonitis may result and require immediate treatment.

Occasionally, a stone can erode through the wall of the gallbladder in cases of chronic cholecystitis and create a fistula to the bowel, most frequently the duodenum. If the stone becomes impacted in the small bowel and causes an obstruction, the condition is referred to as **gallstone ileus** (Fig. 5-16). Gallstone ileus is characterized by air in the biliary ductal system, clearly visible on a conventional abdominal radiograph. The radiopaque gallstone may also be visible within the bowel surrounded by intestinal gas. Surgical removal of the stone is necessary to relieve the obstruction.

Pancreatitis

An acute or chronic inflammation of the pancreatic tissue is known as **pancreatitis**. It is one of the most complex and clinically challenging disorders of the abdomen and is classified as acute or chronic pancreatitis according to clinical, morphologic, and histologic criteria. Its causes include excessive and chronic alcohol consumption and obstruction of the ampulla of Vater by a gallstone or tumor, and even the injection of contrast media during an ERCP has been known to cause pancreatitis. Once activated by any of these causes, trypsin, the pancreatic enzyme that is normally excreted through the ducts into the duodenum, begins to autodigest the organ itself. This can be quite serious and carries a high mortality rate. Hemorrhagic pancreatitis is a complication of pancreatitis and consists of erosion into local tissues and blood vessels, with subsequent hemorrhaging into the retroperitoneal space. A **pseudocyst** is a fluid collection caused by pancreatitis. It is readily visualized by sonographic or CT examination (Fig. 5-17).

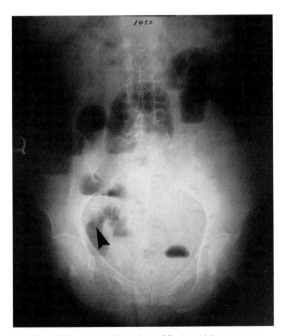

Fig. 5-16 Gallstone ileus in a 43-year-old woman as a result of cholecystitis. The gallstone is in the lower-right abdomen (*arrow*) with the small-bowel air pattern because of the resultant bowel obstruction. (Courtesy the American College of Radiology, Reston, Virginia.)

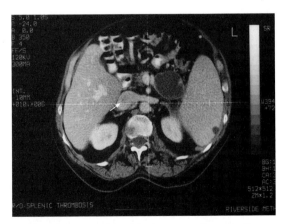

Fig. 5-17 Pancreatitis with demonstration of a 5-cm pseudocyst in the tail as seen on CT. (Courtesy Riverside Methodist Hospitals, Columbus, Ohio.)

Symptoms of pancreatitis vary from mild abdominal pain, nausea, and vomiting to severe pain and shock. Radiographic indications of pancreatitis are subtle and previously centered on displacement of the duodenal C-loop or the stomach by the diseased pancreas. However, CT has made a major contribution to the diagnosis and staging of acute pancreatitis. It adequately demonstrates not only the pancreas itself but also the retroperitoneum, the ligaments, the mesenteries, and the omenta. The infected pancreas is usually enlarged, with a shaggy and irregular contour. In advanced cases, fluid collections are demonstrated within the pancreas, as well as within the retroperitoneum. An ERCP is of value in determining the reasons for acute recurrent pancreatitis, chronic pancreatitis, or the complications associated with pancreatitis. Ultrasound examination is also of significant value in assessing pancreatic disease and most frequently demonstrates a diffusely enlarged hypoechoic pancreas. Laboratory testing is the most common way to diagnose pancreatitis, through evaluation of serum, and occasionally the urine amylase level.

Management of patients with pancreatitis consists of a pain-relieving drug in mild cases and maintaining proper fluid levels to prevent shock, a frequent occurrence in acute pancreatitis. Proper dietary restrictions (e.g., abstinence from alcohol) are also important. The role of surgery in chronic pancreatitis remains controversial in regard to the effectiveness of results.

METABOLIC DISEASES

Jaundice

Jaundice, the yellowish discoloration of the skin and whites of the eyes, is not a disease itself but rather a sign of disease. The accumulation of excess bile pigments (i.e., bilirubin) in the body tissues "stains" the skin and eyes this yellowish color. Normally, bile and its pigments are secreted into the bowel and eliminated. Bilirubin is a type of bile pigment that is produced when

hemoglobin breaks down. Normal serum bilirubin levels are equal to or less than 1 mg per 100 ml but must exceed 3 mg per 100 ml to be visible to the observer.

Medical (nonobstructive) **jaundice** occurs because of hemolytic disease in which too many red blood cells are destroyed or because of liver damage from cirrhosis or hepatitis. Its most common appearance is transient in the first few days after birth, when more bile pigments are released than can be handled. A liver that is damaged from disease simply cannot excrete the bilirubin in a normal fashion, and it enters the bloodstream.

Surgical (obstructive) **jaundice** occurs when the biliary system is obstructed and prevents bile from entering the duodenum. A common cause of this obstruction is blockage of the common bile duct caused by stones or masses. The longer the obstruction persists, the more likely it is that complications (e.g., liver injury, infection, or bleeding) will arise.

The jaundiced patient often undergoes an ultrasound examination of the liver, biliary tree, and pancreas to determine if the jaundice is obstructive or nonobstructive. The common bile duct is readily identified, and, generally speaking, a normal size implies nonobstructive jaundice and a dilated common bile duct suggests an obstruction. A variety of other methods may be used to diagnose the cause of jaundice, including ERCP and CT. An ultrasound or CT-directed needle biopsy may be used if an intrahepatic cause of the hepatitis is suspected. Treatment of jaundice centers on diagnosis and treatment of its underlying cause. In the case of obstructive jaundice, surgical excision of the obstructing body may be necessary. Endoscopic removal of common duct stones is frequently done, and endoscopy also offers the opportunity to stent or bypass a tumor.

NEOPLASTIC DISEASES

Hemangioma

A **hemangioma** is the most common tumor of the liver. It is a benign neoplasm composed of newly formed blood vessels, and these neoplasms can form in other places within the body. For instance, a port-wine stain on the face (a superficial purplish red birthmark) is an example of a hemangioma elsewhere in the body. Hemangiomas are generally well circumscribed, solitary tumors. They can range in size from microscopic to 20 cm. They are more common in females than in males, especially postmenopausal women.

A hemangioma does not become malignant and is generally insignificant. It can, however, present symptoms such as right-upper quadrant pain as a result of tissue displacement or bleeding. Diagnosis can be complicated when it occurs with a known malignancy because its characteristics may be difficult to distinguish from metastasis. Nuclear medicine scans using labeled red blood cells that are attracted to the highly vascular tumor are virtually diagnositic in assessing the presence of a hemangioma. These scans demonstrate the tumor as a defect in early phases and display prolonged and persistent uptake on delayed scans. A CT of the liver following an injection of IV contrast demonstrates the hemangioma with peripheral enhancement. Magnetic resonance imaging

demonstrates marked hyperintensity on T_2 weighted images, which corresponds with fibrosis within the tumor. Following an IV injection of a gadolinium contrast agent, peripheral enhancement of the hemangioma occurs in early scans, followed by filling in of the tumor (Fig. 5-18), similar to the appearance on an enhanced CT examination.

Hepatoma

Hepatoma (hepatocarcinoma), a primary carcinoma of the liver, is uncommon in the United States, accounting for less than 2% of all cancers. An association between cirrhosis and hepatoma exists, with alcoholism and poor nutrition associated with each. Most primary hepatomas originate in liver parenchyma, creating a large central mass with smaller satellite nodules. Although vascular invasion is common, death occurs from liver failure, often without extension of the cancer outside the liver.

The liver is also a common site for metastasis from other primary sites, which makes sense, given the liver's role in filtering blood that has traveled from these sites. Primary cancers located in the abdomen, especially those drained

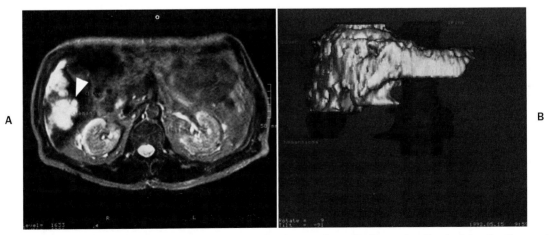

Fig. 5-18 A, An axial MRI slice through the liver reveals a hemangioma. **B,** Reconstruction isolates the liver and the hemangioma in this lateral view of the liver. (**A** and **B** Courtesy Riverside Methodist Hospitals, Columbus, Ohio.)

by the portal venous system, often metastasize to the liver (Fig. 5-19).

Patients with cirrhosis and unexpected deterioration are suspect for hepatoma. Other symptoms include increased jaundice, abdominal pain, weight loss, ascites, and a rapid increase in liver size. Plain abdominal radiographs of patients with hepatoma may demonstrate hepatomegaly. Ultrasound and CT are often used to reveal the extent of the tumor (Fig. 5-20). Arteriography may demonstrate the increased vascularity associated with a carcinoma.

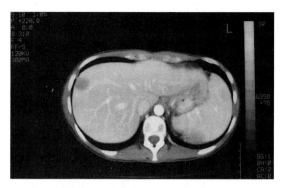

Fig. 5–19 CT scan after duodenal cancer resection in a 21-year-old woman demonstrates local recurrence and metastases to the liver on its lateral border in this slice. (Courtesy Riverside Methodist Hospitals, Columbus, Ohio.)

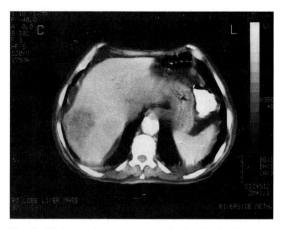

Fig. 5–20 Large, heterogeneous lesion in the liver as consistent with hepatoma. (Courtesy Riverside Methodist Hospitals, Columbus, Ohio.)

Surgical resection of the hepatoma represents the only possibility for cure. Those hepatomas that are diffuse or have multiple nodules generally preclude surgery. The general lack of radiosensitivity of these tumors makes radiotherapy ineffective. Patients treated with chemotherapy demonstrate tumor shrinkage and an addition of a few months to their lives. The disease, however, is generally fatal except for those who have had successful resection of a single liver mass.

Carcinoma of the Gallbladder

Carcinoma of the gallbladder occurs infrequently, but most neoplasms within the gallbladder are malignant. Most primary carcinomas of the gallbladder, approximately 85%, are adenocarcinomas, with the remaining 15% being anaplastic or squamous cell cancers. Carcinoma of the gallbladder is more common in women and the elderly, with gallstones present in about 75% of all cases. The symptoms are nonspecific, right-upper quadrant including pain, jaundice, and weight loss. Another risk factor associated with the development of gallbladder carcinoma is a "porcelain" gallbladder, which results from chronic cholecystitis (Fig. 5-21).

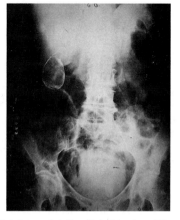

Fig. 5–21 A "porcelain" gallbladder in a 70-year-old man with a history of recurrent indigestion. (Courtesy the American College of Radiology, Reston, Virginia.)

Approximately 22% of patients with porcelain gallbladders develop carcinoma.

The best methods of imaging gallbladder carcinoma include CT and ultrasound. Radiographically, the appearance of the carcinoma may vary. It may appear as a mass replacing the gallbladder or a polypoid mass within the gallbladder, or the appearance may be as subtle as focal thickening of the gallbladder wall. Clinically and radiographically, this cancer may be difficult to differentiate from cholecystitis with pericholecystic fluid accumulation or an abscess. Unfortunately, the prognosis with gallbladder carcinoma is often poor because metastases to the liver usually occur before the primary disease is diagnosed (Fig. 5-22). It may spread via direct invasion of the liver, via intraductal tumor extension, or via the lymphatic system to regional lymph nodes. Approximately 88% of these patients die within 1 year of diagnosis, and only 4% survive 5 years following diagnosis.

Carcinoma of the Pancreas

Pancreatic cancer is usually rapidly fatal and is the fifth most common cause of cancer death within the United States. Its diagnosis is difficult because of the location of the pancreas and lack of symptoms before extensive local spread. Even with advances in CT and ultrasound, the prognosis is poor. In most cases, the tumor is well advanced before the diagnosis is made. Its incidence is greater in men than in women and in blacks than in whites. A clear-cut association with cigarette smoking has been demonstrated, and other risk factors include alcoholism, chronic pancreatitis, diabetes mellitus, and a family history of adenocarcinoma. Most tumors (approximately 90%) arise as epithelial tumors of the duct (adenocarcinoma) and cause pancreatic obstruction (Fig. 5-23). In addition, the majority (60 to 70%) of these neoplasms arise in the head of the pancreas, followed by the body (10% to 15%), and then the tail (5% tp 10%). The rich supply of nerves to the pancreas results in pain as a prominent feature of this carcinoma. The tumor infiltrates and replaces normal tissue without significant hemmorhage, necrosis, or calcification. Symptoms are nonspecific, including pain, weight loss, jaundice, fatigue, nausea, vomiting, and diabetes. Carcinomas of the pancreatic head may be visible on barium studies of the stomach and small bowel because the head of the pancreas lies within the duodenal C-loop. Carcinomas of the body and

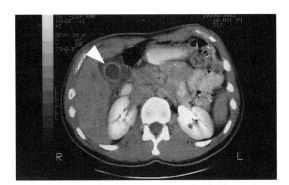

Fig. 5-22 Gallbladder carcinoma, resulting in metastasis to surrounding structures, as seen on this CT of a 23-year-old man. The gallbladder (*arrow*) is surrounded by metastasis, with significant metastasis into the pancreas area and right kidney. (Courtesy Riverside Methodist Hospitals, Columbus, Ohio.)

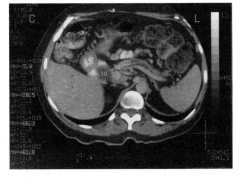

Fig. 5-23 Pancreatic carcinoma in the head of the pancreas, as indicated by atrophy of the pancreatic body and tail on this CT scan of the same patient shown in Fig. 6-6. Numbers shown are for density sampling, with *1, 2,* and *3* in the pancreas. (Courtesy Riverside Methodist Hospitals, Columbus, Ohio.)

tail may affect the duodenojejunal junction and cause distortion on a barium-filled small-bowel study. Computed tomography is the best method of imaging the pancreas, with the most common finding a mass deforming the pancreas. However, in most cases, the tumor is unresectable because of its size by the time the mass is visible on the CT image. Radical surgery as a treatment mode is about the only hope for cure, but it carries a high mortality rate. Radiation therapy is difficult because of the proximity to very radiosensitive structures such as the spinal cord, and chemotherapy also produces poor results. The prognosis with pancreatic carcinoma is very poor, demonstrating only a 2% survival rate for 5 years.

QUESTIONS

1. Bile drains from the liver's right and left hepatic ducts directly into the:
   a. common bile duct
   b. common hepatic duct
   c. cystic duct sample
   d. duodenum

2. The modality of choice for visualization of gallbladder disease is:
   a. CT
   b. diagnostic medical sonography
   c. MRI
   d. nuclear medicine

3. Impairment of normal liver function might result in:
   a. cirrhosis
   b. jaundice
   c. milk of calcium
   d. viral hepatitis

4. Patients with liver cirrhosis have a tendency to develop:
   1. ascites
   2. esophageal varices
   3. jaundice
      a. 1 and 2
      b. 1 and 3
      c. 2 and 3
      d. 1, 2, and 3

5. Which of the following is more characteristic of hepatitis A than of hepatitis B?
   a. effects generally more severe
   b. excreted through blood products
   c. has a longer incubation period
   d. more common form of the two

6. The radiographic appearance of a porcelain gallbladder may be an indication of:
   a. biliary obstruction
   b. carcinoma of the gallbladder
   c. cirrhosis
   d. cholelithiasis

7. The yellowish discoloration of the skin associated with jaundice is due to:
   a. an accumulation of milk of calcium
   b. infected fecal material transmission
   c. paralysis of the small-bowel wall
   d. presence of bilirubin in the blood
   e. none of the above

8. Gallstone ileus refers to impaction of a gallstone in the:
   a. biliary tree
   b. gallbladder
   c. liver
   d. small bowel

9. The diagnostic imaging modality of choice for following the progress of a liver malignancy is:
   a. CT
   b. MRI
   c. radiography
   d. ultrasonography

10. The most common liver tumor is a(n):
    a. hepatitis
    b. hemangioma
    c. hepatoma
    d. jaundice

11. Compare and contrast medical versus surgical jaundice.

12. Explain why cholelithiasis in a nonfunctioning gallbladder can be imaged with sonography and an oral cholangiogram would be ineffective in assisting a diagnosis.

13. What are the advantages of imaging the biliary ductal system antegrade with a PTC versus retrograde with an ERCP? What are the disadvantages with PTC?

14. Explain why cancers of the gallbladder and pancreas carry a poor prognosis.

15. Describe the physiologic cause of esophageal varices in conjunction with cirrhosis of the liver.

Chapter 6

The Urinary System

Anatomy and Physiology Review
Imaging Considerations
    Intravenous urography
    Other studies
    Urinary tubes and catheters
Congenital and Hereditary Diseases
    Number and size anomalies of the kidney
    Fusion anomalies of the kidney
    Position anomalies of the kidney
    Renal pelvis and ureter anomalies
    Lower tract anomalies
    Polycystic kidney disease
    Medullary sponge kidney

Inflammatory Diseases
    Urinary tract infection
    Pyelonephritis
    Acute glomerulonephritis
    Cystitis
Degenerative and Metabolic Disease
    Nephrosclerosis
    Nephrocalcinosis
    Renal failure
    Calcifications
Neoplastic Diseases
    Renal cysts
    Renal carcinoma
    Nephroblastoma (Wilms' Tumor)
    Bladder carcinoma

Upon completion of Chapter 6, the reader should be able to:

- Describe the anatomic components of the urinary system and their functions.

- Discuss the role of other modalities in imaging the urinary system, particularly ultrasound and computed tomography.

- Discuss common congenital anomalies of the urinary system.

- Characterize a given condition as inflammatory, metabolic, or neoplastic.

- Identify the pathogenesis of the pathologies cited and the typical treatments for them.

- Describe, in general, the radiographic appearance of each of the given pathologies.

KEY TERMS

Nephrostomy tube
Ureteral stent
Foley catheter
Renal agenesis
Supernumerary kidney
Hypoplasia
Hyperplasia
Horseshoe kidney
Crossed ectopy
Malrotation
Ectopic kidney
Nephroptosis
Ureterocele

Ureteral diverticula
Bladder diverticula
Urethral valve
Polycystic kidney disease
Medullary sponge kidney
Urinary tract infection
Pyelonephritis
Pyuria
Acute glomerulonephritis
Bright's disease
Cystitis
Vesicoureteral reflux
Neurogenic bladder

Bladder trabeculae
Nephrosclerosis
Nephrocalcinosis
Renal failure
Uremia
Renal calculi
Staghorn calculus
Renal colic
Hydronephrosis
Renal cyst
Adenocarcinoma
Nephroblastoma
Bladder carcinoma

ANATOMY AND PHYSIOLOGY REVIEW

The urinary system consists of two kidneys, two ureters, a urinary bladder, and a urethra (Fig. 6-1). The urinary system forms urine to remove waste from the bloodstream for excretion. The kidneys are the site where urine is formed and excreted through remarkable processes of filtration and reabsorption, involving up to 180 L of blood per day. Urine formed in this process amounts to about 1 to 1.5 L per day and passes from the kidneys to the bladder through the ureters. Stored in the bladder, it is eventually excreted through the urethra.

The kidneys are retroperitoneal, normally located between the twelfth thoracic vertebra and the third lumbar vertebra. The right kidney lies slightly lower because of the presence of the liver superiorly. The notch located on the medial surface of each kidney is the hilus, the area where structures enter and leave the kidney. These structures include the renal artery and vein, lymphatics, and a nerve plexus. Microscopically, the

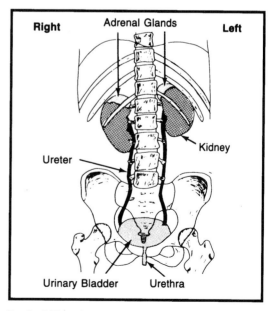

Fig. 6-1 The urinary system. (From Bontrager KL: *Textbook of radiographic positioning and related anatomy,* ed 3, St Louis, 1993, Mosby.)

nephron is the functional unit of the kidney responsible for forming and excreting urine (Fig. 6-2). The nephron unit terminates into a collecting tubule, which helps to form a tube opening at the renal papilla into a minor calix. Minor calices terminate in the major calices, which, in turn, terminate at the renal pelvis (Fig. 6-3).

The ureters extend from the kidneys to the urinary bladder and are approximately 10 inches in length (Fig. 6-4). They normally enter the bladder obliquely in the posterolateral portion of the bladder, equidistant from the urethral orifice in a triangular fashion. A number of variations of this can exist. The function of the ureters is to drain the urine from the kidneys to the bladder.

The bladder is located posterior to the symphysis pubis. It serves as a reservoir for urine before it is expelled from the body. The bladder is very muscular and capable of distention. Valves located at the junction of the ureters and bladder prevent the backflow of urine.

The urethra is a tube leading from the urinary bladder to the exterior of the body. In the male, it also serves as a part of the reproductive system by receiving watery fluid via prostatic ducts that open into the urethra from the prostate.

IMAGING CONSIDERATIONS

Intravenous Urography

Many different examinations exist to study the various aspects of the urinary system. The most common of these is the intravenous urogram (intravenous pyelogram or IVP), which remains the usual starting point for the diagnosis of urinary tract dysfunction. The indications for performing an intravenous urogram include suspected urinary tract obstruction, abnormal urinary sediment (especially hematuria), systemic

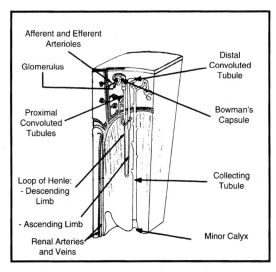

Fig. 6-2 The microscopic structure of a nephron. (From Bontrager KL: *Textbook of radiographic positioning and related anatomy,* ed 3, St Louis, 1993, Mosby.)

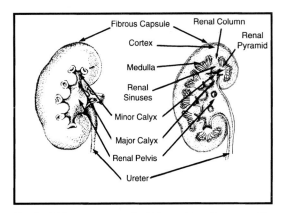

Fig. 6-3 The structure of a kidney. (From Bontrager KL: *Textbook of radiographic positioning and related anatomy,* ed 3, St Louis, 1993, Mosby.)

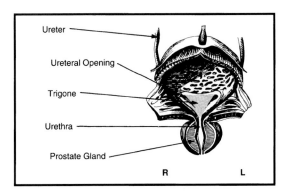

Fig. 6-4 An anterior, cut-away view of the bladder. (From Bontrager KL: *Textbook of radiographic positioning and related anatomy,* ed 3, St Louis, 1993, Mosby.)

hypertension, or, frequently in men, symptoms of prostatism. While few or no serious adverse effects typically accompany the injection of urographic contrast agents, about 1 of 40,000 patients dies as a result of an allergic reaction to the contrast agents. The use of nonionic, low osmolar contrast agents significantly reduces minor and moderate reactions, although reduction of the mortality figure associated with ionic agents has not been proven.

A plain abdominal radiograph, often termed a *scout* or *preliminary* film, is the usual beginning for most intravenous urograms (Fig. 6-5, *A*). Its primary purposes are to determine if adequate bowel preparation has been accomplished and to visualize radiopaque calculi of the kidneys, ureters, and bladder that may otherwise be hidden by the presence of contrast media. The radiologist also examines areas unrelated to the urinary tract, as they may hold clues to the diagnosis. The kidneys are frequently radiographically visible on this film because of the perirenal fat capsule that surrounds them. The kidneys are generally well fixed to the abdominal wall and are seen to move with respiratory effort. In addition, a male's kidneys are generally larger than those of the female.

Many intravenous urogram routines allow for a radiograph to be taken within 1 minute after contrast media injection. This is termed a *nephrogram* (phase) radiograph and may be used to demonstrate the contrast agent in the nephrons before it reaches the renal calices. Ready visualization of the renal parenchyma allows for an inspection of the renal outline. Indentations or bulges may indicate the presence of disease. The nephrogram radiograph is also used to check for normal kidney position, which may be altered by congenital malposition, ptosis, or the presence of a retroperitoneal mass.

Although the number and type of radiographs taken may vary from one institution to another, a series of collecting system sequence films are the final part of an intravenous urogram (Fig. 6-5, *B*). The renal pelvis, calices, ureters, and bladder are examined for any abnormalities. The calices should be evenly distributed and

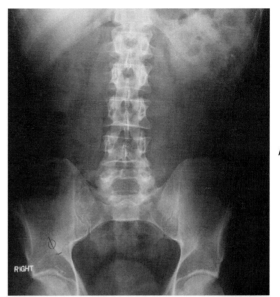

A

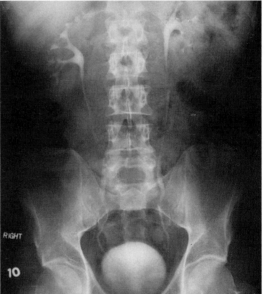

B

Fig. 6-5 A, Scout film of the abdomen taken in preparation for an intravenous urogram readily demonstrates renal and psoas shadows in this 39-year-old man. **B,** With other films interspersed, this 10-minute follow-up IVP film demonstrates good renal function with normal renal contours and collecting system. (**A** and **B** Courtesy Riverside Methodist Hospitals, Columbus, Ohio.)

Continued

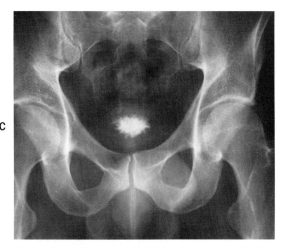

C

Fig. 6–5 cont'd C, Postvoid film taken as part of this IVP series demonstrates good bladder function, evidenced by the expulsion of nearly all of the contrast agent. This completes a normal intravenous urogram. (C Courtesy Riverside Methodist Hospitals, Columbus, Ohio.)

reasonably symmetrical. Usually, they present as buttercup-shaped projections surrounding the renal papillae. Caliceal dilatation may be demonstrated as a result of acute or chronic urinary tract obstruction, postobstructive uropathy, or reflux. Dilatation secondary to destruction of the renal pyramids is less common.

Because of the peristaltic activity of ureters, only part of their length in a collecting system sequence may be demonstrated. Sometimes nonopaque ureteral calculi cause filling defects and an obstructive dilatation of the ureter. The majority of all urinary tract calculi are found at the vesicoureteral junction. Any pronounced deviation of the ureter suggests the presence of a retroperitoneal mass. Various filling defects may be demonstrated in the contrast agent–filled ureter during an intravenous pyelogram, including tumors, blood clots, and nonopaque calculi. Common bladder defects visualized during an intravenous urogram include urinary catheter balloons, normal uterus and colon, and extrinsic deformities such as uterine or sigmoid colon tumors. A "postvoid" film usually com-

pletes an intravenous urogram procedure and allows assessment of the bladder function (Fig. 6-5, C).

Other Studies

In addition to the intravenous urogram, the physician may order one of several additional tests designed to look at a select aspect of the urinary tract. Nephrotomography, for example, may be used as a primary study in lieu of the standard intravenous urogram or as an adjunct study, using tomograms of the kidneys taken at suitable intervals. Tomographic views obtained before intravenous contrast are used to look for calculi, whereas those after contrast administration are used for closer examination of the renal parenchyma and collecting systems.

With retrograde pyelography, a catheter is placed into the ureteric orifice, usually by a urologist, at cystoscopy to allow injection of contrast medium to outline the renal collecting system. Indications for this study may include hematuria of unknown cause, hydronephrosis, and, in cases of a nonfunctioning kidney, where further information about possible obstruction is desired. A percutaneous nephrostogram involves posterolateral insertion of a needle or catheter into the renal pelvis using medical sonography, fluoroscopy, or sometimes a combination of both modalities. The nephrostomy tube may be left in place to provide drainage of an obstructed kidney or to allow retrieval of the calculus with a basket catheter. Sometimes the procedure is used to relieve obstruction in patients for whom immediate surgery is not possible.

Extracorporeal shock wave lithotripsy (ESWL) is a method used to locate and treat renal calculi. After location of the stone is attained radiographically, fluoroscopy aids in alignment of a high-frequency shock wave directed at the stone of a patient. If the treatment is successful, the stone disintegrates into fragments that can be voided by the patient, often sparing a surgical procedure and a much lengthier recovery period (Fig. 6-6).

A

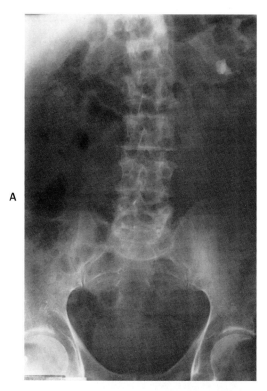

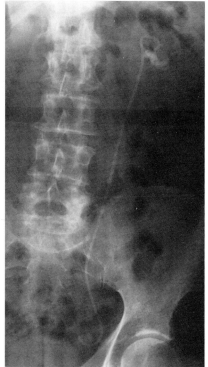

B

C

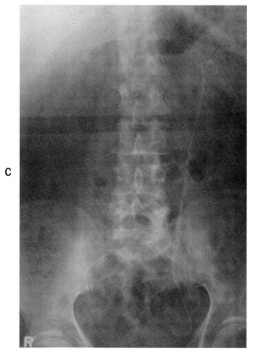

Fig. 6-6 A, Scout film taken before lithotripsy demonstrates a large, solid renal stone in the right kidney. **B,** Two months after lithotripsy, the stone is clearly seen to be fragmented and beginning to descend the right ureter. A stent has been placed in the right ureter to aid in draining urine. **C,** A film taken 2 months later demonstrates further movement of stone fragments down the ureter. The stent is still in place. (A, B, and C Courtesy the Ohio Kidney Stone Center, Columbus, Ohio.)

Renal angiography is usually indicated to further evaluate a renal mass suspected of being malignant, but it also allows an assessment of renal artery stenosis, a cause of hypertension, as well as other vascular disease (e.g., fibromuscular hyperplasia). In renal angiography, a catheter is introduced into the femoral artery, with injection of contrast media into or above the renal arteries.

The most common examination for studying the lower urinary tract is the cystogram. This involves insertion of a catheter into the urethra and retrograde filling of the bladder with contrast material (Fig. 6-7). A frequent indication for this procedure is to identify vesicoureteral reflux. In the normal bladder, increased pressure as the bladder fills effectively shuts down any chance of reflux. Bladder infection, however, can render the ureteral "valve" incompetent, refluxing infection into the kidney. Cystography is also used to study congenital bladder anomalies, tumors, diverticula, calculi (Fig. 6-8), or neurogenic bladder.

Voiding (micturition) cystography is sometimes used as a follow-up to a cystogram to al-low study of the urethra upon voiding. Urethrography may be accomplished antegrade, as with a voiding cystourethrogram, or retrograde when a cystogram is not necessary. The antegrade approach is used to study the posterior urethra, and the retrograde approach is helpful in studying the anterior urethra. The usual intent of voiding cystography is to allow study of a urethral stricture (Figs. 6-9 and 6-10).

For imaging other than radiographic or fluoroscopic, both ultrasound and computed tomography (CT) play large roles. Ultrasound is useful in diagnosis of kidney stones, calcifications, hydronephrosis, abscesses, renal masses and cysts, and to assess renal atrophy; CT is particularly important in determining the nature of renal masses, either solid or cystic, and allowing for accurate biopsy. It is also useful in looking for sites of obstruction, assessing renal infection or trauma, and in staging of tumors of the lymph nodes or bladder. Nuclear medicine has a role in assessing the physiology associated with urine flow and in evaluating renal artery stenosis. As in the abdomen, the role of magnetic resonance imaging (MRI) is still being defined, as respiratory motion problems are present.

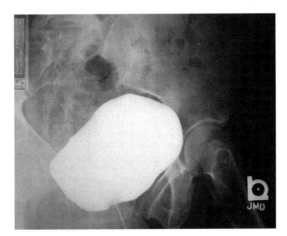

Fig. 6-7 Normal cystogram without reflux as seen in this oblique projection of the bladder in a 56-year-old woman. (Courtesy Riverside Methodist Hospitals, Columbus, Ohio.)

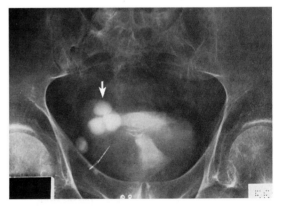

Fig. 6-8 Bladder diverticula in an 88-year-old man demonstrate the presence of numerous calculi within them. (Courtesy the American College of Radiology, Reston, Virginia).

Urinary Tubes and Catheters

When certain types of pathology, such as tumors or stone formation, inhibit the normal flow of urine through the urinary system, several types of tubes may be used to allow drainage of the urine. A **nephrostomy tube** connects the renal pelvis to the outside of the body (Fig. 6-11). It is inserted percutaneously through the renal cortex and medulla into the renal pelvis to allow the urine to drain outside of the body directly from the renal pelvis. Special care must be taken when dealing with this these patients, who are readily prone to infections because of the direct opening into the urinary system.

Ureteral stents may also be placed in cases of ureteral obstruction. Unlike nephrostomy tubes, ureteral stents do not connect the urinary system to the outside of the patient's body (see Fig. 6-6, *B*). Ureteral stents are placed surgically or via cystoscopy, with the upper portion of the stent in the renal pelvis and the lower portion within the urinary bladder. The stent allows patency of the diseased ureter and enables the urine to flow normally. These stents are

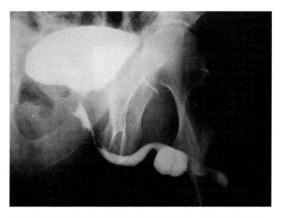

Fig. 6-10 A voiding cystourethrogram demonstrates a urethral diverticula. The mucosal margin of the prostatic urethra is ragged as a result of scarring after transurethral resection. (Courtesy the American College of Radiology, Reston, Virginia.)

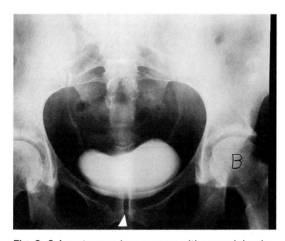

Fig. 6-9 A cystogram in a woman with unexplained recurrent urinary tract infections reveals an ovoid calculus superimposed on the symphysis pubis. A voiding cystourethrogram demonstrates the stone to be within a urethral diverticulum. (Courtesy the American College of Radiology, Reston, Virginia.)

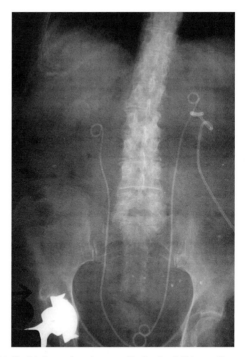

Fig. 6-11 A nephrostomy catheter is visible on the left, along with a stent catheter between the right and left renal pelves and urinary bladder in this abdominal view of a 68-year-old man. (Courtesy Riverside Methodist Hospitals, Columbus, Ohio.)

radiographically visible on plain abdominal radiographs.

Urinary catheterization is performed to obtain urine specimens, relieve urinary retention, monitor renal function, and manage urinary incontinence. A **Foley catheter** is the most common indwelling urinary catheter. It is placed within the urinary bladder using sterile technique. Once the catheter is placed through the urethra and urinary sphincter, a small balloon is inflated to help the catheter remain in place within the urinary bladder. This catheter is generally connected to a bag that collects the urine as it flows through the catheter to the outside of the body. Care must be taken to ensure the catheter is not displaced during a radiographic procedure, and the urine collection bag must remain lower than the patient's bladder at all times to prevent the reflux of urine back into the bladder, which could result in a urinary tract infection. A Foley catheter must be placed in an individual before performing cystography or cystourethrography to allow the installation of contrast material into the bladder. Again, the importance of proper sterile technique cannot be overemphasized.

CONGENITAL AND HEREDITARY DISEASES

Anomalies of the kidneys and ureters are caused by errors in development. They can be classified as anomalies of number, size and form, fusion, and position. About 10% of all persons have some sort of congenital malformation of the urinary system. At least half of those with kidney anomalies have malformations elsewhere in the urinary system or other systems, most commonly the reproductive system.

Number and Size Anomalies of the Kidney

Renal agenesis is a relatively rare anomaly that demonstrates as the absence of the kidney on one side and an unusually large kidney on the other side (Fig. 6-12), a condition known as *compensatory hypertrophy*. The left kidney is more frequently missing, and the condition is

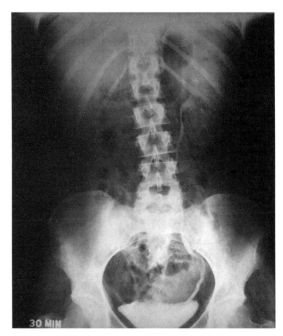

Fig. 6-12 No kidney is visible on the right side on this intravenous urogram. Angiography confirmed lack of a renal artery, and cystoscopy demonstrated no ureteric orifice; all are consistent with renal agenesis on the right. (Courtesy Riverside Methodist Hospitals, Columbus, Ohio.)

more common in males than in females. A single kidney occurs in approximately 1 in 1000 individuals. It is more subject to trauma because of its enlarged size. Protection against disease in an individual with only one kidney is very important.

A **supernumerary kidney** is also relatively rare and consists of the presence of a third, small, rudimentary kidney. It has no parenchymal attachment to a kidney, with about half of occurrences draining from an independent renal pelvis into the ureter on that side. It often becomes symptomatic as a result of infection.

Hypoplasia is a rare anomaly of size involving a kidney that is developed less than normal (Fig. 6-13). Usually hypoplasia is associated with hyperplasia of the other kidney. It requires renal arteriography to differentiate congenital

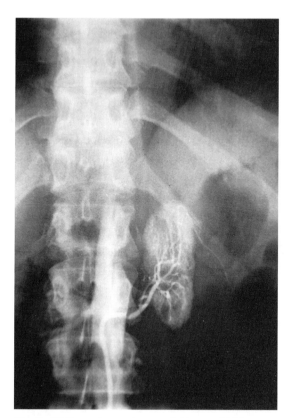

Fig. 6-13 Normal vasculature of this small kidney demonstrates renal hypoplasia. (Courtesy Riverside Methodist Hospitals, Columbus, Ohio.)

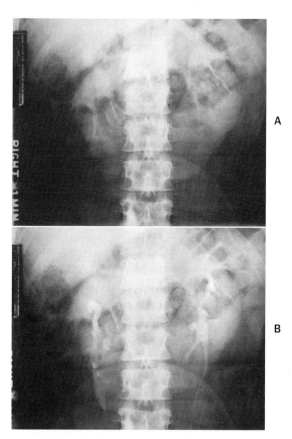

Fig. 6-14 A, Nephrogram phase of an intravenous urogram demonstrates fusing of the lower poles, as consistent with horseshoe kidney. **B,** Further excretion in the intravenous urogram demonstrates emptying of the malrotated kidneys via separate ureters. (**A** and **B** Courtesy Riverside Methodist Hospitals, Columbus, Ohio.)

hypoplasia from a kidney that is atrophic due to acquired vascular disease. The clinical significance of hypoplasia depends on the volume of functioning kidney. **Hyperplasia** is the opposite condition; it involves an overdeveloped kidney. Again, this is often associated with renal agenesis or hypoplasia of the other kidney.

Fusion Anomalies of the Kidney

Fusion anomalies of the kidneys are often distinguishable on plain radiographs. **Horseshoe kidney** describes a condition affecting about 0.25% of the population, with males affected twice as frequently as females. With it, the lower poles of the kidneys are joined across midline by a band of soft tissues, causing a rotation anomaly on one or both sides. The ureters exit the kidneys anteriorly instead of medially, and the lower pole calices point medially rather than laterally with this condition (Figs. 6-14 and 6-15). Kidney function is generally unimpaired with this condition. The lower bridge frequently lies on a sacral promontory where it is susceptible to trauma and may be palpated as an abdominal mass. **Crossed ectopy** exists when one kidney lies across the midline and is fused to the other kidney (Fig. 6-16). Both kidneys demonstrate various anomalies of position, shape, fusion, and rotation with crossed ectopy. The crossed kidney generally lies inferior to the uncrossed one.

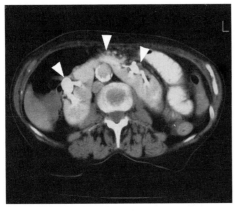

Fig. 6–15 Horseshoe kidney with apparent obstruction as seen on this CT of a 72-year-old woman. (Courtesy Riverside Methodist Hospitals, Columbus, Ohio.)

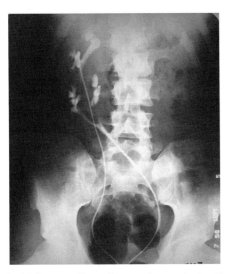

Fig. 6–16 Retrograde pyelogram demonstrates the left ureter crossing midline to connect with the lower pelvis of an anomalous right kidney, as consistent with crossed fused renal ectopy. (Courtesy Riverside Methodist Hospitals, Columbus, Ohio.)

Its drainage may be impaired by malposition of its ureter.

Position Anomalies of the Kidney

Anomalies of position are relatively common. **Malrotation** consists of incomplete or excessive rotation of the kidneys (Fig. 6-17) as they ascend from the pelvis in utero. This is generally of little clinical significance unless an obstruction is created. An **ectopic kidney** is one that is out of its normal position, a condition found in approximately 1 in 800 urologic examinations. Most are asymptomatic throughout life. Ectopic kidneys are usually lower than normal, often in a pelvic (Fig. 6-18) or sacral location. In rare cases, the ectopic kidney may be intrathoracic. In some lean and athletic persons, the kidney is mobile and may drop toward the pelvis in an

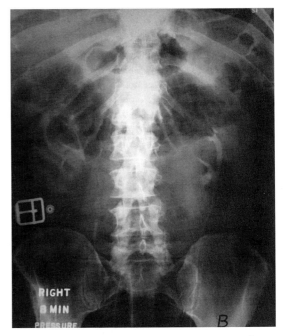

Fig. 6–17 Intravenous urography demonstrates that the left kidney's collecting system is along the lateral margin, consistent with malrotation. A restraining band is in place to slow renal excretion. (Courtesy Riverside Methodist Hospitals, Columbus, Ohio.)

erect position. **Nephroptosis** (prolapse) can be distinguished from a pelvic kidney by the length of the ureter; if the ureter is short, it is a congenital pelvic kidney.

Renal Pelvis and Ureter Anomalies

Renal pelvis and ureter anomalies are frequent. They may be unilateral or bilateral, and they have a tendency to be asymmetric. Such anomalies may occur as double renal pelvis, either isolated or in combination with a double ureter (Figs. 6-19 and 6-20). The problem with these and other upper tract anomalies is that they may impair renal drainage, predisposing the patient to infection and calculi formation.

Lower Tract Anomalies

A simple **ureterocele** is a cystlike dilatation of a ureter near its opening into the bladder (Fig.

6-21). These usually result from congenital stenosis of the ureteral orifice. Radiographically, a ureterocele presents as a filling defect in the bladder with a characteristic "cobra head" appearance. A ureterocele that appears with ureteral

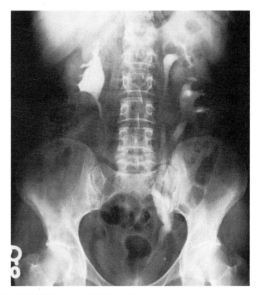

Fig. 6–19 Congenital double ureter is clearly seen on the left side. (Courtesy Riverside Methodist Hospitals, Columbus, Ohio.)

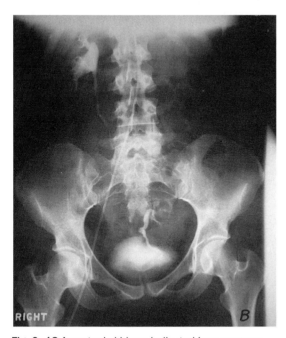

Fig. 6–18 An ectopic kidney, indicated by a urogram film taken at the end of an angiogram, demonstrates the left kidney with a shortened ureter in the left pelvis. (Courtesy Riverside Methodist Hospitals, Columbus, Ohio.)

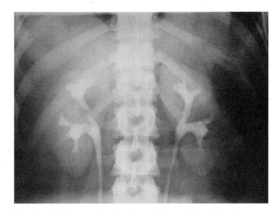

Fig. 6–20 Normal variation of the pelvicaliceal junction is seen in both kidneys. (Courtesy the American College of Radiology, Reston, Virginia.)

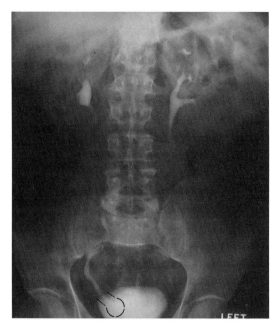

Fig. 6-21 A simple ureterocele seen as an opacified mass continuous with the terminal right ureter. (Courtesy the American College of Radiology, Reston, Virginia.)

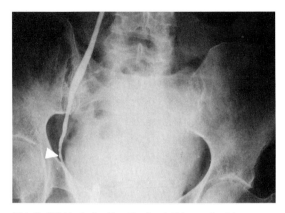

Fig. 6-22 Ureteric diverticula visible as double densities superimposed on the lower ureter just above the ischial spine in this retrograde pyelogram on a 62-year-old woman with recurrent urinary tract infection. (Courtesy the American College of Radiology, Reston, Virginia).

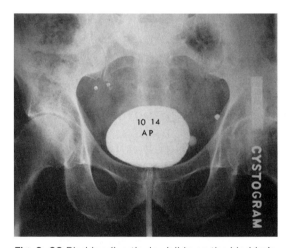

Fig. 6-23 Bladder diverticula visible on the bladder's left margin in this cystogram. (Courtesy Riverside Methodist Hospitals, Columbus, Ohio.)

duplication is an "ectopic" ureterocele; it often causes substantial obstruction, primarily of the upper pole, and kidney infection. Treatment in this situation involves surgical removal to allow for increased flow of urine into the bladder.

Ureteral diverticula are probably a congenital anomaly and may actually represent a dilated, branched ureteric remnant. The appearance of these is the same as that of any other diverticula and is best demonstrated by retrograde urography (Fig. 6-22). **Bladder diverticula** (Fig. 6-23) may occur as a congenital anomaly or be caused by chronic bladder obstruction and resultant infection. They usually occur in middle-aged men, with treatment aimed at eliminating the cause of obstruction and relief of infection.

Urethral valves are mucosal folds that protrude into the posterior urethra as a congenital condition. These can cause significant obstruction to urine flow (Fig. 6-24). Such "valves" oc-

cur in males and are usually discovered during infancy or early childhood.

Polycystic Kidney Disease

Polycystic kidney disease is a familial kidney disorder that, though congenital in origin, usually

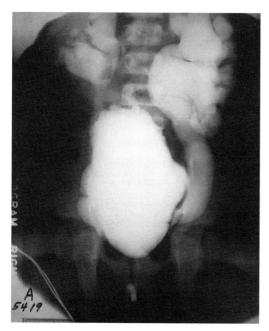

Fig. 6–24 Large, trabeculated bladder and large tortuous ureters and renal pelves seen on this cystogram of a 15-year-old boy, consistent with bladder outflow obstruction due to congenital posterior urethral valves. (Courtesy the American College of Radiology, Reston, Virginia.)

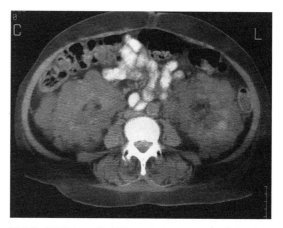

Fig. 6–25 Polycystic kidney disease as seen in both kidneys on this CT study of a 66- year-old man. (Courtesy Riverside Methodist Hospitals, Columbus, Ohio.)

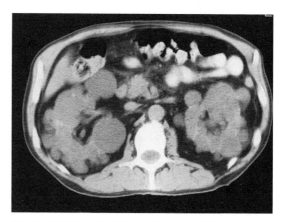

Fig. 6–26 Polycystic kidney disease visible as multiple masses in the kidneys in this CT of a 64-year-old man. (Courtesy Riverside Methodist Hospitals, Columbus, Ohio.)

presents in adults in their thirties. Innumerable tiny cysts that are present at birth gradually enlarge as the patient ages. This enlargement compresses and eventually destroys normal tissues. The late presentation of the condition occurs because the cysts are initially very small and do not cause problems until tissue destruction becomes significant. Radiographic indications of polycystic kidney disease show bilateral enlargement of the kidneys with poorly visualized outlines (from the presence of cysts) and caliceal stretching and distortion (Figs. 6-25 and 6-26). The diagnosis of multiple cysts is readily confirmed by ultrasound, which reveals multiple echo-free areas in both kidneys. Therapy for this condition consists of basic fluid and electrolyte management, avoidance of physical activities that could cause trauma to the abdomen, and management of pain caused by the occasional rupture of a cyst.

Medullary Sponge Kidney

Although the diagnosis is not usually made until the fourth or fifth decade, when infective complications emerge, **medullary sponge kidney** is considered by most as a congenital anomaly. The only visible abnormality is the dilatation of the medullary and papillary portions of the collecting ducts, usually bilaterally (Fig.

6-27). Calculi are contained in about 60% of symptomatic patients, with infection and intrarenal obstruction common. Intravenous urography reveals linear markings in the papillae or cystic collections of contrast media in the enlarged collecting ducts. Therapy for this condition consists of treatment of infection and, if possible, resolution of nephrolithiasis with lithotripsy.

INFLAMMATORY DISEASES

Urinary Tract Infection

Urinary tract infection (UTI) is the most common of all bacterial infections. Up to 35% of all women experience UTI at least once. A quantitative urine culture is essential in approaching UTI because its causes are broad. In most cases of UTI, the infecting organism is a gram-negative bacillus that invades the urinary system by an ascending route through the urethra to the bladder to the kidney. Some believe that the offending bacteria ascend during micturition, possibly related to a turbulent stream or reflux upon completion of voiding. The only clearly demonstrated mechanism, however, is by instrumentation of the urethra and bladder by cys-

toscopy, urologic surgery, or Foley catheter placement. Antibiotics are used to clear the infectious bacteria.

Pyelonephritis

Acute **pyelonephritis** is a bacterial infection of the calices and renal pelvis and thought to represent the most common renal disease. Any stagnation or obstruction to urine flow in any part of the urinary tract predisposes the patient to kidney infection. The bacteria involved likely reach the kidney via the bloodstream. The condition is more common among women than men because of their increased incidence of reflux from the bladder. Acute pyelonephritis can occur during pregnancy as the increased size of the uterus acts to compress the ureter and decrease urine clearance of bacteria.

Patients presenting with acute pyelonephritis have fever, flank pain, and general malaise. Urinalysis demonstrates **pyuria,** the presence of pus (white cells) created by the body's reaction to the infection. Abscesses may form in the kidneys and create the flow of pus into the collecting tubules. Diagnosis of the condition is usually

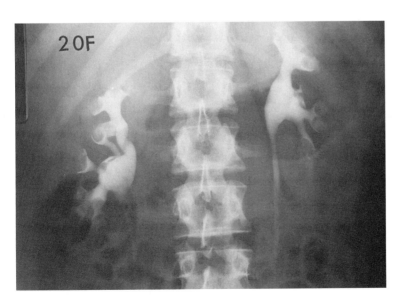

Fig. 6-27 Medullary sponge kidney demonstrated by large bilateral papillae and dilated tubules visible within the papillae in this 20-year-old woman with recurrent cystitis. (Courtesy the American College of Radiology, Reston, Virginia.)

made by laboratory results, as radiographic findings are often nonspecific. In most cases, an intravenous urogram is normal even during an acute attack. The calices may be blunted and collecting structures may be less well visualized because of interstitial edema. Treatment consists of administering antibiotics to eliminate the infectious bacteria.

Recurrent or persistent infection of the kidneys, such as caused by chronic reflux of infected urine from the bladder into the renal pelvis, can result in chronic pyelonephritis. It generally has no relation to acute pyelonephritis and is sometimes seen in patients with a major anatomic abnormality (e.g., an obstruction) or, most commonly, in vesicoureteral reflux in children. Chronic pyelonephritis is often bilateral

and leads to destruction and scarring of the renal tissue, with marked dilatation of the calices. The eventual result is an overall reduction in kidney size, readily seen on intravenous urography (Fig. 6-28, *A*). The renal pyramids atrophy, giving the calices a clubbed appearance. Scars may also be seen and appear as indentations of the renal cortex on the kidney outline in the nephrogram phase (Fig. 6-28, *B*). In addition to being caused by a congenital duplication of ureters that allows a chronic reflux of urine, it may also occur with obstruction or neurogenic bladder. Hypertension may result from chronic pyelonephritis. Treatment of pyelonephritis in a chronic stage centers on control of hypertension, removal of any cause for obstruction, and use of antibiotics to control infection.

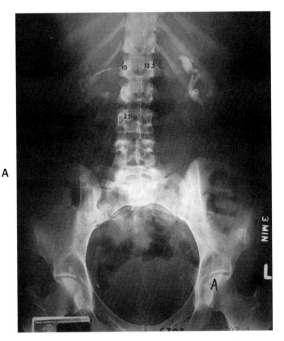

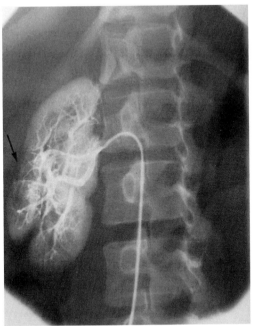

Fig. 6-28 A, Right kidney is small and has a scarred surface as seen on this intravenous urogram on a 25-year-old woman with recurrent urinary tract infections. **B,** Selective renal angiography demonstrates a thinned cortex caused by scarring and bunching of the renal vessels, as consistent with chronic pyelonephritis. (**A** and **B** Courtesy the American College of Radiology, Reston, Virginia.)

Acute Glomerulonephritis

An antigen-antibody reaction in the glomeruli causes an inflammatory reaction of the renal parenchyma known as **acute glomerulonephritis** or **Bright's disease.** Often this immunologic reaction occurs following streptococcal infection of the upper respiratory tract or the middle ear. It differs from acute pyelonephritis, which primarily affects the interstitial tissue rather than the nephrons. The condition occurs mainly in children following streptococcal infection, with most patients recovering completely. The diagnosis is again best made with laboratory results. Radiographically, the kidneys appear larger, particularly during the nephrogram phase of an intravenous urogram, because of edematous accumulation. Treatment may include diuretic therapy to lessen edema and its resultant pressure on the glomeruli. Also, antibiotic therapy and bed rest may be used. Renal dialysis may be used for severe, chronic cases (Fig. 6-29).

Cystitis

Cystitis, inflammation of the bladder, is a fairly common infection, generally caused by bacteria, that may be either acute or chronic. Cystitis is more prevalent in women than in men because their short urethra permits bacteria easier access into the bladder. The bladder lining's natural resistance to inflammation, however, serves as a protective mechanism. Inflammation and congestion of the bladder mucosa cause the patient to experience burning pain on urination or the desire to urinate frequently. Although cystitis is not serious, the infection can cause further problems by spreading into the upper urinary passages, including the renal pelvis and kidney.

Vesicoureteral reflux (VUR), the backward flow of urine out of the bladder and into the ureters, may be seen in cases of cystitis. In the normal urinary tract, vesicoureteral reflux is prevented by compression of the bladder musculature on the ureters during micturition. Failure of this valve mechanism usually is due to a shortening of the intravesical portion of the ureter caused by abnormal embryologic development, resulting in ureteric orifices that are displaced laterally. As this portion of the ureter lengthens with growth, this type of vesicoureteral reflux may disappear completely with age. Congenital VUR is also seen in duplication of collecting systems and ureters with reflux into an ectopically placed ureter serving the upper pole of the kidney. Vesicoureteral reflux can also result from a **neurogenic bladder,** a bladder dysfunction caused by interference with the nerve impulses concerned with urination. Cystography may demonstrate the presence of reflux and grade its severity. It may show a roughening of the normally smooth bladder wall, a radiographic appearance referred to as **bladder trabeculae** (Fig. 6-30). Treatment of cystitis includes antibiotic ther-

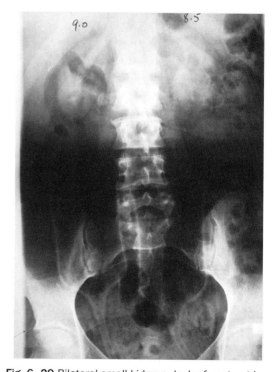

Fig. 6-29 Bilateral small kidneys, lack of contrast in the bladder, and a patient history of attacks of acute glomerulonephritis indicate chronic glomerulonephritis in this 28-year-old patient. (Courtesy the American College of Radiology, Reston, Virginia.)

apy and an abundance of fluids. Prevention of pyelonephritis is paramount.

DEGENERATIVE AND METABOLIC DISEASE

Nephrosclerosis

Nephrosclerosis is intimal thickening of predominantly the small vessels of the kidney. It may occur as part of the normal aging process as well as in younger patients in association with hypertension and diabetes. Reduced blood flow caused by arteriosclerosis of the renal vasculature causes atrophy of the renal parenchyma. Local infarction may occur, demonstrating as an irregularity of the cortical margin, usually an indentation. The collecting system of the affected kidney is usually normal, but the kidney itself is decreased in size. Other conditions that cause the kidneys to appear smaller than normal include hypoplasia, atrophy following obstruction, and ischemia from large vessel obstruction. Treatment of nephrosclerosis consists of managing the associated hypertension and administration of diuretic agents and proper dietary restrictions (e.g., low-sodium diet).

Nephrocalcinosis

Disturbances of calcium metabolism (e.g., hyperparathyroidism) may result in **nephrocalcinosis,** a condition characterized by tiny deposits of calcium dispersed throughout the renal parenchyma (Fig. 6-31). These deposits are readily seen on an intravenous urogram and even on plain films of the abdomen. Calcium may also be deposited throughout the parenchyma as a result of tissue damaged by some other disease process or injury. In the case of a metabolic cause, treatment of the specific metabolic condition indirectly treats nephrocalcinosis. Treatment designed to lower serum calcium levels is also important.

Renal Failure

Although it can arise acutely, **renal failure** usually represents the end result of a chronic process such as chronic glomerulonephritis or polycystic kidney disease that gradually results in

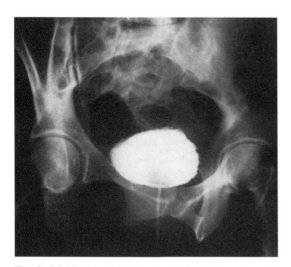

Fig. 6-30 Mildly trabeculated bladder as seen in this 34-year-old woman with a small capacity bladder. (Courtesy Riverside Methodist Hospitals, Columbus, Ohio.)

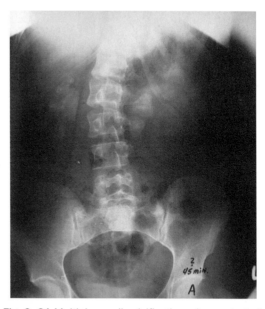

Fig. 6-31 Multiple small calcifications demonstrated in the renal pyramids of both kidneys caused by nephrocalcinosis secondary to hyperparathyroidism. (Courtesy the American College of Radiology, Reston, Virginia.)

diminished kidney function. The kidney's normal regulatory and excretory functions become impaired because of loss of glomerular filtration and subsequent deterioration of the renal parenchyma (Fig. 6-32). **Uremia** which is characteristic of renal failure, consists of retention of urea in the blood. Although not toxic in itself, urea is normally excreted by the kidneys. Its blood level correlates with retention of other waste products and is thus a measure of the severity of renal failure.

The gradual deterioration of renal function brings with it a host of changes in other body systems. The affected patient experiences moderate anemia, hypertension, heart arrhythmia, congestive heart failure, and other problems related to the body's severe electrolyte and acid-base imbalances. Treatment consists of dialysis and possible transplantation.

Calcifications

With the exception of the gallbladder, more calculi are found in the urinary tract than anywhere else in the body. **Renal calculi** are stones that develop from urine, which can precipitate crystalline materials, especially calcium and its salts. If the body's normal equilibrium is upset, these products may precipitate out of the solution. Factors that can cause this precipitation include metabolic disorders such as hyperparathyroidism, excessive intake of calcium, and a metabolic rate that causes high urine concentration. Chronic urinary tract infections are also related to stone formation.

Males develop calculi more often than females, especially after age 30. Nearly all urinary tract calculi are calcified to some extent, appearing partially or totally opaque (Fig. 6-33). About 5% of stones do not calcify (Fig. 6-34).

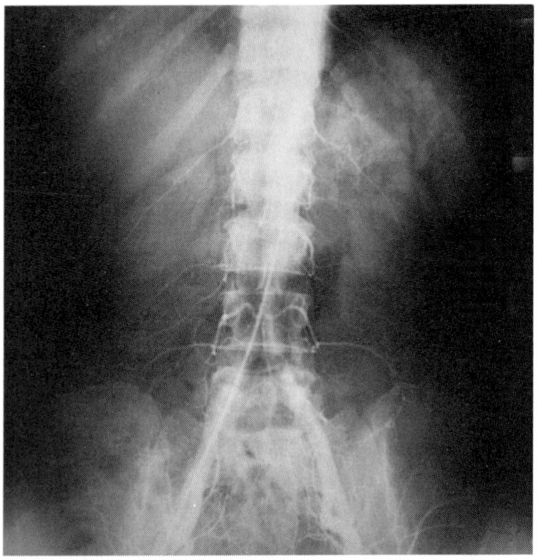

Fig. 6-32 Renal failure caused by chronic glomerulonephritis, indicated by bilaterally small kidneys with small outlines, no evidence of obstruction, and arterial changes associated with end-stage kidneys. (Courtesy the American College of Radiology, Reston, Virginia.)

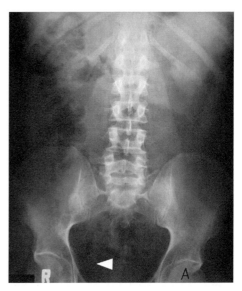

Fig. 6-33 A 3-mm, slightly calcified density is seen at the level of the right ischial spine on this plain film for an intravenous urogram. Subsequent films show distention of the collecting system to this point, as consistent with an opaque calculus at the ureterovesicular junction. (Courtesy the American College of Radiology, Reston, Virginia.)

These are generally made of pure uric acid and present a more difficult diagnosis to the physician because they are one of several filling defects, including blood clots and tumors. Most stones are formed in the calices or renal pelvis. A **staghorn calculus** is a large calculus that assumes the shape of the pelvicaliceal junction (Fig. 6-35). Beside intravenous urography, ultrasound can demonstrate stones (Fig. 6-36).

Stones tend to be asymptomatic until they begin to descend or cause an obstruction. The most common site for a calculus to lodge and create an obstruction is the ureterovesical junction (Fig. 6-37). Obstructions can also occur at the junction of the ureter and bladder and in the ureter at the pelvic brim. Movement of stones or acute obstruction results in severe pain known as **renal colic.** It refers along the course of the ureter toward the flank or genital regions and

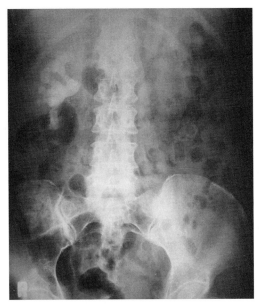

Fig. 6-35 Staghorn calculus of the right kidney as seen in a patient with a history of chronic pyuria. (Courtesy the American College of Radiology, Reston, Virginia.)

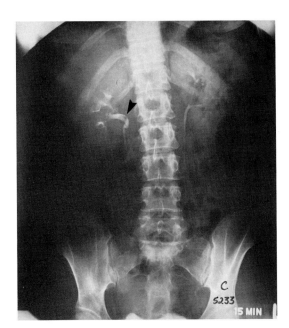

Fig. 6-34 Smooth, oval, noncalcified filling defect is seen in the right renal pelvis, as suggestive of a radiolucent uric acid stone in this 40-year-old woman with hematuria. (Courtesy the American College of Radiology, Reston, Virginia.)

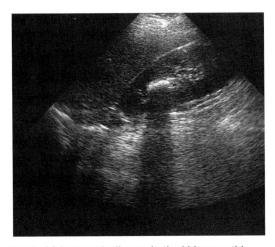

Fig. 6-36 Large calculi seen in the kidney on this ultrasound of a young female. Note the absence of sound transmission beyond the stone as indicated by the dark pathway beneath it. (Courtesy Riverside Methodist Hospitals, Columbus, Ohio.)

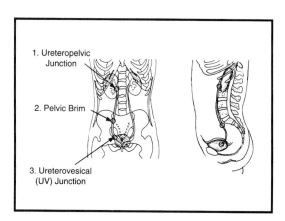

Fig. 6–37 The three usual points where kidney stones become lodged. (From Bontrager KL: *Textbook of radiographic positioning and related anatomy,* ed 3, St Louis, 1993, Mosby.)

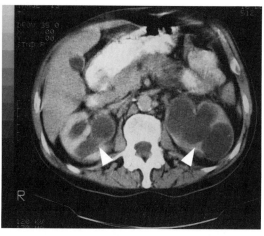

Fig. 6–38 Gross bilateral hydronephrosis as caused by pyelonephritis in this 64-year-old man. (Courtesy Riverside Methodist Hospitals, Columbus, Ohio.)

is highlighted by paroxysmal attacks, between which a constant low-grade pain is felt. The physician is generally able to distinguish between biliary and renal colic because biliary colic usually causes referred pain to the subscapular area or epigastrium, and renal colic causes referred pain as described.

Hydronephrosis is an obstructive disease of the urinary system that causes a dilatation of the renal pelvis and calices with urine (Fig. 6-38). If long-standing, the resultant increase in intrarenal pressure causes ischemia, parenchymal atrophy, and loss of renal function. Although the most common cause of hydronephrosis is a calculus, it can also occur as a congenital defect or blockage of the system by a tumor, stricture, blood clot, or inflammation. Patients with hydronephrosis often complain of pain in their flanks, and their urine may demonstrate blood or pus. The long-term changes of hydronephrosis are reversible if the cause of obstruction is relieved early in the process. A CT scan (Fig. 6-39), an intravenous urogram, or ultrasound readily demonstrates the marked dilatation characteristic of the condition. Treatment

of obstructive disease includes antibiotics for the presence of any infection, and either lithotripsy of the stone or surgical excision of the cause of obstruction, or waiting until the stone passes.

In addition to the kidneys, other sites of calcification in the urinary tract include the wall of the bladder and the prostate gland in the male. Calcification of the bladder wall is very rare and is usually due to calcium deposition in a tumor extrinsic to the bladder, such as from the ovary or rectum. Rarely, it may also be on the surface of a bladder tumor. Prostatic calcification appears as numerous flecks of calcium of varying size below the bladder. It does not, however, correlate with either prostatic hypertrophy or carcinoma and usually is of no real significance.

Urinary tract calcifications are sometimes difficult to distinguish from other abnormal calcifications, such as gallstones, vascular calcifications, and calcified costal cartilages. To be in the kidney, the calcification must remain within the outline of the kidney on both frontal and oblique projections or be confirmed with plain

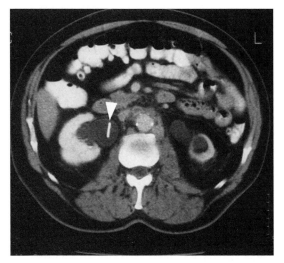

Fig. 6–39 Hydronephrosis of both kidneys as seen on this CT film, particularly in the right kidney where a stent is placed (*arrow*) to drain excess fluid to the bladder. (Courtesy Riverside Methodist Hospitals, Columbus, Ohio.)

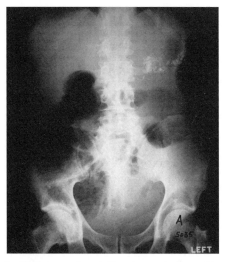

Fig. 6–40 Pancreatic calcification as indicated by the masses of calcium in the left-upper quadrant that conform neatly to the shape of the pancreas. (Courtesy the American College of Radiology, Reston, Virginia.)

tomography. In the case of gallstones, oblique projections of the abdomen help demonstrate whether the calculus in question is anterior to the kidney. The pancreas may also demonstrate calcification that usually conforms to its shape (Fig. 6-40).

NEOPLASTIC DISEASES

Masses can cause filling defects in the urinary tract, becoming visible when they stretch and displace the collecting system or form an evident mass. Almost all solitary masses are either malignant tumors or simple cysts.

Profuse hematuria resulting from a blood clot also causes a filling defect. The diagnosis of such depends on the radiologist's awareness of the history of hematuria. The distinction between a blood clot and a tumor is difficult for the physician. However, blood clots tend to have a smooth outline and show change on repeat examinations following treatment.

Renal Cysts

Renal cysts are an acquired abnormality common in adults. It is estimated that more than half of people at age 50 have renal cysts. Simple cysts may be solitary or multiple and bilateral. They are usually asymptomatic and not an impairment to renal function, but they may cause symptoms from rupture, hemorrhage, infection, or obstruction. Their pathogenesis is unknown, but obstruction of nephrons by an acquired disease may have a relationship. They are commonly found in a lower pole of the kidney (Fig. 6-41) and are readily demonstrated by CT (Fig. 6-42) and ultrasound.

Radiographically, cysts have sharply defined margins and show caliceal spreading, but they can be distinguished from tumors by nephrotomography, in which a cyst shows an absence of a nephrogram phase after contrast media injection. By contrast, tumors, the majority of which have vascularity, may show irregular opacification during the nephrogram phase. Treatment,

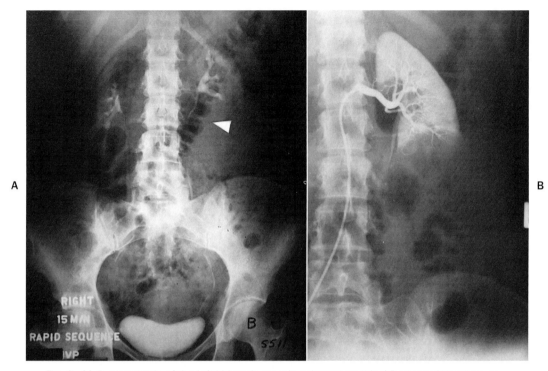

A   B

Fig. 6-41 A, Lower pole of the left kidney is grossly enlarged on this 15-minute film taken as part of an intravenous urogram, suggestive of a space-occupying lesion. **B,** Selective arteriography of the left kidney demonstrates an avascular mass, with vessels near it normal except for displacement. The diagnosis was simple renal cyst. (**A** and **B** Courtesy the American College of Radiology, Reston, Virginia.)

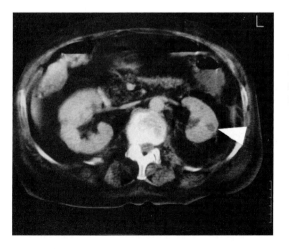

Fig. 6-42 Small renal cysts are visible on the relatively atrophic left kidney in this abdominal CT scan of a 73-year-old woman. (Courtesy Riverside Methodist Hospitals, Columbus, Ohio.)

if needed, consists of aspiration of the cyst contents (Fig. 6-43). Most cysts are asymptomatic, and no treatment is needed.

Renal Carcinoma

The most common malignant tumor of the kidney is **adenocarcinoma** (hypernephroma), arising from the proximal convoluted tubule. It occurs 2 to 3 times as frequently in males as in females, with an increased incidence after age 40. Its etiology is unknown, but chronic inflammation as from obstruction, cigarette smoking, and other agents is thought to contribute to the development of renal carcinoma. The affected patient often first presents for an intravenous urogram with hematuria.

Radiographically, the space-occupying lesion may be evident and can distort, stretch, and displace the kidney's collecting system (Fig. 6-44, *A*). Computed tomography is also useful in demonstrating renal carcinoma and its metastases. Abnormal vascularity is readily seen on angiography (Fig. 6-44, *B*), sometimes

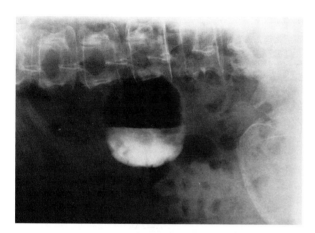

Fig. 6-43 An air-fluid level reveals removal of much of the contents of a renal cyst via a needle aspiration. (Courtesy Riverside Methodist Hospitals, Columbus, Ohio.)

A 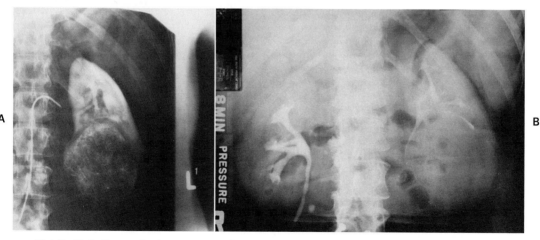 B

Fig. 6-44 **A,** Urography demonstrates displacement of the left lower pole calices in this 54-year-old woman with hematuria. **B,** Arteriography of the same patient demonstrates a large vascularized mass of the left lower pole, with grossly abnormal vasculature, indicative of renal cell carcinoma. (**A** and **B** Courtesy of Riverside Methodist Hospitals, Columbus, Ohio.)

surrounding an avascular necrotic center. Computed tomography provides a good method to follow the progress of renal carcinoma (Fig. 6-45).

If caught early, surgical excision of the kidney provides a good cure rate, as renal carcinoma is relatively insensitive to chemotherapy. The tendency of adenocarcinoma to metastasize early from the kidneys, however, poses a serious threat. The most common sites of metastasis are the lungs, brain, liver, and bone.

Nephroblastoma (Wilms' tumor)

Nephroblastoma is a malignant renal tumor found in approximately 1 child in every 13,500 live births. It almost invariably develops before 5 years of age, with equal incidence between sexes. Children with nephroblastoma often have no symptoms but may have the tumor discovered by a parent or physician who feel a large, palpable abdominal mass. The relative firmness and immobility help distinguish Wilms' tumor from hydronephrosis and renal cysts. On urography, the kidneys appear quite enlarged with marked caliceal spreading—an indication nearly diagnostic of the condition when seen in children (Fig. 6-46). Left untreated, the tumor shows widespread metastases to the lungs, liver, adrenal glands, and bone. Early surgical excision combined with radiation therapy and

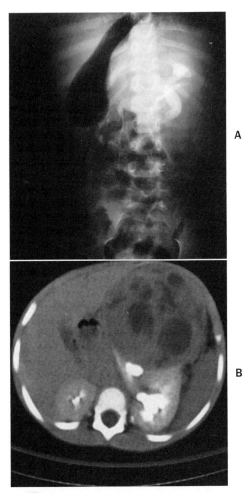

Fig. 6-46 **A,** An intravenous urogram on a 4-year-old girl demonstrates an enlarged left kidney with distortion of the collecting system and significant displacement of the stomach by the large mass. **B,** A CT image demonstrates a huge, noncalcified mass arising from the left kidney, as seen in nephroblastoma. (A and B Courtesy the American College of Radiology, Reston, Virginia.)

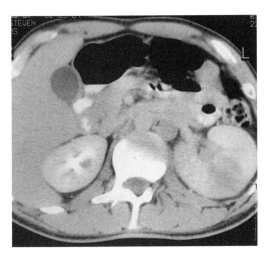

Fig. 6-45 CT demonstration of a large metastatic lesion in the left kidney of this 25-year-old man with renal adenocarcinoma. (Courtesy Riverside Methodist Hospitals, Columbus, Ohio.)

chemotherapy, results in a cure rate of approximately 80%.

Bladder Carcinoma

<u>Bladder carcinoma</u> is usually seen 3 times more often in men than in women, particularly after age 50. Its etiology is clearly related to cigarette smoking and certain industrial chemicals, and a link to excessive coffee drinking is being investigated. Painless hematuria is the chief symptom. Tumors are generally small and located in the area of the trigone. An intravenous urogram may reveal a filling defect in the bladder (Figs. 6-47 and 6-48), but it is often difficult to distinguish among tumor, stone, and blood clot. Therefore, cystoscopy is the method of choice for investigation of bladder carcinoma.

Treatment consists of resection or a total cystectomy, depending on the amount of involvement and extent of metastasis, if any. Radiation therapy of the region follows. In the case of total cystectomy, the distal ureters are generally attached into a loop of the ileum. Distant metastases are usually late developing with bladder carcinoma.

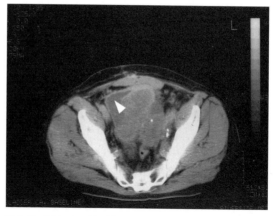

Fig. 6-48 Large bladder carcinoma in this 65-year-old man as seen on CT. (Courtesy Riverside Methodist Hospitals, Columbus, Ohio.)

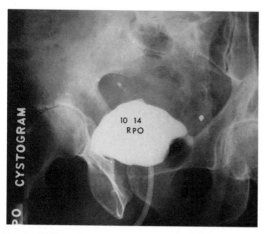

Fig. 6-47 Transitional cell carcinoma of the bladder, seen as a space-occupying lesion on this right posterior oblique view of the bladder on a cystogram of a 67-year-old man. (Courtesy the American College of Radiology, Reston, Virginia.)

QUESTIONS

1. A malignant tumor of the kidney in young children is:
   a. adenocarcinoma   c. fibroadenoma
   b. hypernephroma   d. nephroblastoma

2. Which of the following statements are true about the anatomy and function of the urinary system?
   1. The amount of urine formed in a typical day is about 1 to 1.5 L.
   2. Urine is formed and excreted in the nephron, the microscopic unit of the kidney.
   3. The left kidney lies lower than the right because of the spleen's presence above it.
      a. 1 and 2   c. 2 and 3
      b. 1 and 3   d. 1, 2 and 3

3. Which of the following statements are true of intravenous urography?
   1. Demonstration of contrast filling of only a partial ureter is always pathologic.

2. Low osmolar contrast agents reduce the rate of mild and moderate reactions.
3. Presence of renal colic is an indication for performing intravenous urography.
   a. 1 and 2   c. 2 and 3
   b. 1 and 3   d. 1, 2 and 3

4. Horseshoe kidney is an anomaly of:
   a. fusion   c. position
   b. number   d. size

5. Which of the following statements are true of urinary system anomalies?
   1. Crossed ectopy exists when one kidney lies across midline, fused to the other.
   2. Nephroptosis and a pelvic kidney are identical conditions.
   3. Ureteroceles are ureteral dilatations near the ureter's termination.
      a. 1 and 2   c. 2 and 3
      b. 1 and 3   d. 1, 2 and 3

6. Vesicoureteral reflux refers to the backward flow of urine into the:
   a. bladder   d. urethra
   b. major calix   e. any of the above
   c. ureters

7. The "cobra head" is a radiographic appearance associated with:
   a. cystitis   c. pyelonephritis
   b. nephrosclerosis   d. ureteroceles

8. Which of the following conditions can make the kidneys appear smaller than normal?
   a. atrophy following obstruction
   b. chronic pyelonephritis
   c. hypoplasia
   d. nephrocalcinosis
   e. all of the above
   f. all but one of a through d

9. The most common renal disease overall is:
   a. cystitis
   b. glomerulonephritis
   c. nephrocalcinosis
   d. pyelonephritis

10. Medical treatment designed to lower serum calcium levels is important in management of:
    a. cystitis
    b. nephrocalcinosis
    c. nephrosclerosis
    d. polycystic kidney disease

11. Gradual and chronic deterioration of the renal parenchyma eventually results in:
    a. glomerulonephritis
    b. polycystic kidney disease
    c. renal calculi
    d. renal failure

12. Renal failure is characterized by the abnormal retention of _____ in the blood.
    a. bilirubin   c. pus
    b. calcium   d. urea

13. Which of the following statements are true of renal calculi?
    1. Precipitation of solutes out of urine is the pathogenesis of renal calculi.
    2. Renal colic causes referred pain into the subscapular area or epigastrium.
    3. Stones tend to be asymptomatic until they move or cause an obstruction.
       a. 1 and 2   c. 2 and 3
       b. 1 and 3   d. 1, 2 and 3

14. Significant dilatation of the renal pelvis and calices as a result of an obstruction from a stone is characteristic of:
    a. hypernephrosis
    b. renal failure
    c. nephroblastoma
    d. vesicoureteral reflux

15. Which of the following statements are true of neoplastic diseases of the urinary system?
    1. Chronic inflammation from obstruction can result in adenocarcinoma.
    2. Wilms' tumor is generally associated with elderly patients in renal failure.
    3. Early excision of nephroblastoma has shown a very high cure rate.
       a. 1 and 2   c. 2 and 3
       b. 1 and 3   d. 1, 2 and 3

16. A film taken later in an intravenous urogram routine demonstrates only a portion of the ureters. Is this cause for concern? Why or why not?

17. How can one distinguish between nephroptosis and a pelvic kidney?

18. Identify at least three mechanisms through which bacteria can enter the urinary tract.

19. A 30-year-old pregnant woman demonstrates fever, flank pain, and general malaise. Although the intravenous urogram looks normal, urinalysis demonstrates pyuria. What might you suspect?

20. In renal failure, what causes the kidney to lose its normal regulatory and excretory function?

The Reproductive System

The Female Reproductive System
    Anatomy and physiology review
    Imaging considerations
    Congenital abnormalities
    Inflammatory disease
    Neoplastic diseases
    Uterine masses
    Breast masses
    Disorders during pregnancy

The Male Reproductive System
    Anatomy and physiology review
    Imaging considerations
    Neoplastic diseases

Upon completion of Chapter 7, the reader should be able to:

- Discuss the basic anatomic structures associated with the male and female reproductive systems.

- Describe the limitation of general radiography in the diagnosis and treatment of reproductive disorders.

- Briefly explain the role of diagnostic medical sonography in the diagnosis and treatment of reproductive system disorders.

- Compare and contrast breast imaging modalities, including diagnostic versus screening mammography, localization techniques, and sonography.

- Differentiate among the major congenital anomalies of the female reproductive system.

- Describe the various neoplastic diseases of both the female and male reproductive systems in terms of etiology, incidence, signs and symptoms, treatment, and prognosis.

- Differentiate among the common disorders during pregnancy, and explain the role of diagnostic medical sonography in the management of the gravid female.

KEY TERMS

Pessary
Hysterosalpingogram
Pelvimetry
Bicornuate uterus
Unicornuate uterus
Uterus didelphys
Pelvic inflammatory disease
Mastitis
Follicular ovarian cyst
Corpus luteum ovarian cyst
Endometriosis
Polycystic ovaries
Cystic teratoma
Dermoid cysts

Cystadenocarcinoma
Cervical carcinoma
Cervical dysplasia
Leiomyoma
Uterine fibroid
Fibroadenoma
Fibrocystic breasts
Breast carcinoma
Oligohydramnios
Polyhydramnios
Ectopic pregnancy
Placenta previa
Placental abruption
Placental accreta

Hydatiform mole
Prostatic hyperplasia
TURP
Prostatic calculi
Adenocarcinoma of the
  prostate
Epididymoorchitis
Hydrocele
Spermatocele
Testicular seminoma
Testicular embryonal
  carcinoma
Testicular teratoma
Testicular choriocarcinoma

THE FEMALE REPRODUCTIVE SYSTEM

Anatomy and Physiology Review

The female reproductive system comprises one pair of ovaries, which are the primary sex organs, and the secondary sex organs, which include one pair of uterine tubes, the uterus, the vagina, and two breasts (Fig. 7-1). This system functions in the production of the female reproductive cell (the ovum) and hormones and provides a cavity for the development of the zygote.

The external genitalia (the vulva) includes the mons pubis, the labia majora and minora, the clitoris, the openings of the urethra and vagina,

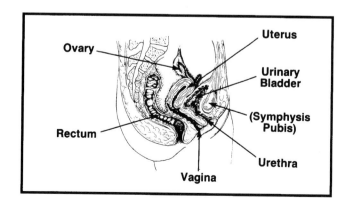

Fig. 7-1 Female pelvic organs. (From Bontrager KL: *Textbook of radiographic positioning and related anatomy,* ed 3, St Louis, 1993, Mosby.)

and the perineum. The vagina connects the external genitalia with the uterus and is the mode of exit of menstrual fluids and conception products.

The uterus is a pear-shaped organ whose purpose is to provide the environment for fetal growth and development. Located within the pelvic cavity, it can be divided into the upper portion, termed the *body* and the lower, neck portion, termed the *cervix*. The cervix connects the uterine cavity with the upper vagina. Anatomically, the uterus is flexed so that the cervix and lower portion of the body lie anterior to the rectum, posterior to the urinary bladder, and with the upper portion of the body normally lying superior to the bladder. The walls of the uterus include an inner, endometrial layer; a middle, muscular, myometrial layer; and an outer layer termed the *parietal peritoneum*. In actuality, the parietal peritoneum drapes over the upper three fourths of the body but does not enclose the lower fourth of the body or the cervix. The actual cavity within the uterus is fairly small and can be well visualized via hysterosalpingography. It is divided into the internal os leading to the cervical canal and into the external os, which opens into the vagina. The uterus is held in place within the pelvic cavity via eight ligaments. Occasionally, lack of proper uterine support is present, and a device known as a **pessary** (Fig. 7-2) is inserted into the vagina to provide proper support.

The uterine (fallopian) tubes extend from the upper, outer edges of the uterus and expand distally into the infundibulum located close to, but not attached to, the ovaries. Suspended in place by the broad ligament, they are 8 to 12 cm long and tend to fall behind the uterus. These tubes serve as a passageway for the mature ova and are the normal site of fertilization. In a normal pregnancy, the fertilized ovum continues to travel through the uterine tube and implants into the endometrium of the uterus.

The ovaries are the primary reproductive glands and are responsible for ovulation and secretion of estrogen and progesterone. Attached to the broad ligament and the posterior uterine wall, each ovary contains numerous graafian follicles enclosing ova. Following puberty, several graafian follicles and ova grow and develop each month. Normally only one follicle matures, migrates to the surface of the ovary, and degenerates, thus expelling a mature ovum. This is termed *ovulation*.

The breasts, like the uterine tubes, uterus, and vagina, are also secondary sex organs. Breast

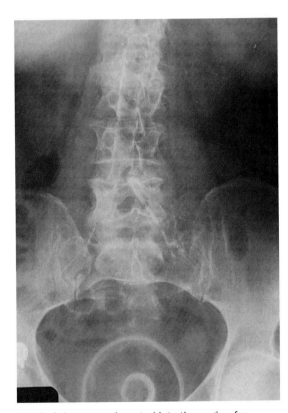

Fig. 7-2 A pessary, inserted into the vagina for uterine support, is readily visible on this abdomen radiography of an 88-year-old woman. (Courtesy Riverside Methodist Hospitals, Columbus, Ohio.)

parenchyma differs according to age and parity. Women in their twenties and thirties, especially nulliparous women, have dense, fi-broglandular parenchyma that may hide breast masses on both physical and mammographic examination. However, as age and parity increase, the breast typically becomes fattier, which enhances the radiographic visibility of possible masses.

Anatomically, the breasts are attached via connective tissue to the pectoral muscles and consist of about 12 lobes separated by connective tissue, much like the spokes of a wheel. The lobes are further divided into lobules clustered around small ducts. These small ducts join to form larger ducts, which terminate at the nipple (Fig. 7-3). The breasts function as an accessory reproductive gland to secrete milk for the newborn infant. During pregnancy, changes in the estrogen and progesterone levels prepare the breasts for lactation. Approximately 3 days after delivery, a lactogenic hormone stimulates the secretion of milk.

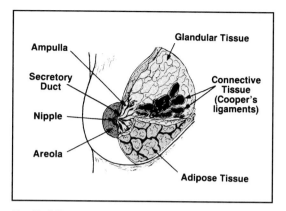

Fig. 7–3 Breast, anterior. (From Bontrager KL: *Textbook of radiographic positioning and related anatomy,* ed 3, St Louis, 1993, Mosby.)

Imaging Considerations

Radiographic studies of the female reproductive system include investigation of gravid and nongravid females. The **hysterosalpingogram** is a common examination for screening of the nongravid female. A common finding in cases of infertility is nonpatent uterine tubes. Additionally, although it does not define the extent of certain conditions such as endometriosis, it is useful in revealing the shape of the uterus and certain characteristics of the uterine tubes other than their patency. Hysterosalpingography is performed by injecting about 5 to 10 cc of an opaque medium into the uterine cavity. Spillage of the contrast media from the uterine tubes indicates their patency (Fig. 7-4). Typically, hysterosalpingography is for diagnostic purposes, but it can also be used therapeutically for restoring tubal patency or to dilate or stretch the uterine tubes.

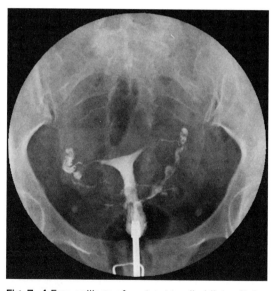

Fig. 7–4 Free spillage of contrast media bilaterally in this 38-year-old woman indicates uterine tubes are open in this hysterosalpingogram. (Courtesy Riverside Methodist Hospitals, Columbus, Ohio.)

Radiography may also be used to locate intrauterine devices (IUDs) used for contraception (Fig. 7-5).

Although uncommon today, **pelvimetry** is used to measure the dimensions of the bony pelvis in a gravid female. A fetal age study provides rough approximation of fetal age by visualizing ossification patterns of the fetal bones. However, much of this same information can be obtained with the use of diagnostic medical sonography.

Ultrasound has replaced radiographic examinations of the female reproductive system because of its excellent accuracy and because it presents no radiation hazards to the fetus or mother. Not only is ultrasound applicable in pregnancy but also it is useful in normal gynecologic examinations to visualize reproductive organs, to locate lost IUDs, or to follow the progress of a regimen of fertility medication.

Traditional pelvic sonography requires a distended urinary bladder to serve as an "acoustic window" for good visualization of the pelvic organs. In addition, the fluid within the urinary bladder helps to displace bowel gas away from the area of interest. Recent sonographic advance have led to the use of transvaginal transducers that also provide accurate clinical information. The most common indications for sonography in the nongravid female include evaluation of pelvic, uterine, and ovarian masses because ultrasound can give information about mass size, location, internal characteristics, and the effect on surrounding organs. Sonography is often used to locate and identify IUDs. Obstetrically, ultrasound is the method of choice in visualizing the position of the placenta, multiple gestations, and ectopic pregnancies and determining gestational age. It is used to assist and guide the physician during amniocentesis and is invaluable in assessing fetal abnormalities, such as anen-

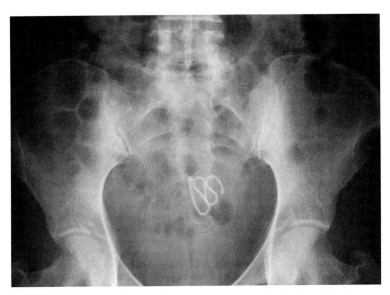

Fig. 7-5 Pelvic radiograph of a 47-year-old woman who presented with pelvic abscesses drained percutaneously. The IUD present had been in place for more than 20 years. (Courtesy Riverside Methodist Hospitals, Columbus, Ohio.)

cephaly, hydrocephaly, congenital heart defects, polycystic kidney disease, urinary tract obstructions, and GI tract obstructions, as well as determining fetal death.

The use of mammography as a diagnostic procedure for symptomatic patients is well documented. Mammography provides important information about specific clinical problems such as a breast mass, pain, nipple discharge, and abnormalities of the skin and lymph nodes. With modern mammographic equipment and techniques, radiation exposure is minimal. It is not known for certain if very low doses of radiation cause breast cancers; however, there is no evidence to suggest significant risk to women over 35 years of age. If a risk does exist, it is thought to be so minimal that it has never been observed, only inferred, scientifically. In the accuracy of detecting breast pathologies, clinical investigations have revealed no significant difference between film/screen mammography and xeromammography; however, the glandular radiation dose is higher with xeromammography. Xeromammography is seldom used in modern radiology applications.

Whether mammography is a safe method of screening asymptomatic women remains controversial. The use of mammography for screening purposes is based on its ability to detect nonpalpable breast lesions at an early stage when they are too small to be identified by physical examination. Current literature suggests that mammography can detect some cancers 2 years before they are palpable, and survival depends on tumor size and lymph node involvement. It is generally agreed that women 50 years of age and older should undergo regular mammographic screening because in this age range the breast tissue is less sensitive to radiation and the incidence of breast cancer increases with age. The benefits far outweigh associated risks from radiation exposure.

Mammography is also a valuable examination tool in the detection and evaluation of breast disease in individuals with augmentation prostheses. Although experience with augmentation mammoplasty patients is limited, current research indicates mammography can demonstrate both palpable and nonpalpable breast lesions. To demonstrate the underlying breast parenchyma in these individuals, technologists are encouraged to use manual exposure techniques, as well as additional "pinch" or axillary projections. Pinch projections require pushing the prosthesis posteriorly against the chest wall so the anterior breast tissue can be compressed and radiographed.

Needle or guidewire localization is a specialized procedure to identify nonpalpable, mammographically detected abnormalities of the breast. They help direct the surgeon to the lesion in question and allow excision of the suspect tissue for biopsy. Needle guidewire localizations cause minimal morbidity, with complications including hematoma formation, intraoperative wire dislodgement, and wire breakage. The development and refinement of localization techniques have greatly increased the percentage of positive findings upon surgical biopsy and allow more accurate diagnosis and treatment of early-stage carcinoma of the breast. Fine-needle and large-core biopsy techniques offer an alternative to surgical biopsy as an initial step in investigation of breast masses.

Ultrasound is an excellent modality for differentiating cystic masses from solid masses within the breast. However, sonography has major limitations in the diagnosis of malignant breast disease because of the solid nature of most breast cancers. It is not indicated as an established screening procedure for solid breast lesions and cannot differentiate between a solid benign mass and malignant disease.

Congenital Abnormalities

Congenital anomalies of the female reproductive system occur in approximately 1% to 2% of women. The most common anomaly is the **bicornuate uterus,** paired uterine horns that extend to the uterine tubes (Fig. 7-6). A **unicornuate uterus** occurs when the uterine cavity is elongated and has a single uterine tube emerging from it. Often, the kidney on the side of the missing uterine tube is also absent. **Uterus didelphys** is a rare congenital anomaly with complete duplication of the uterus, cervix, and vagina. The most serious complication of these anomalies is problems with reproduction, although various surgical corrections can be employed.

In the normal female, the fundus of the uterus lies anterior to the cervix as well as away from the rectum. Occasionally, the normal uterus may lie in an abnormal position. If the uterus is more vertical than normal, it is termed *retroflexed* and lies against the rectosigmoid region of the bowel. A uterus that lies more horizontal is termed *anteflexed,* and it lies on top of the urinary bladder. Although neither is normal, they are generally of little clinical significance.

Inflammatory Disease

Pelvic Inflammatory Disease

Pelvic inflammatory disease (PID) is a bacterial infection of the female genital system, specifically the uterine tubes, most often caused by gonococcus, *Staphylococcus,* or *Streptococcus* bacteria. It may result from an unsterile abortion, insertion of an IUD, or introduction of a pathogen from other sources. This inflammation is generally bilateral, and without treatment the infection spreads to the peritoneum, resulting in bacteremia. Tuboovarian abscess formation may also occur with PID, often resulting in sterility.

Common signs and symptoms of PID include pelvic and abdominal pain, dysmenorrhea, nausea and vomiting, elevated temperature, and leukocytosis. The most common treatment of PID is antibiotic therapy, but healing often results in scarring and obstruction of the uterine tubes, which predisposes the individual to ectopic pregnancy because of the narrowing of the

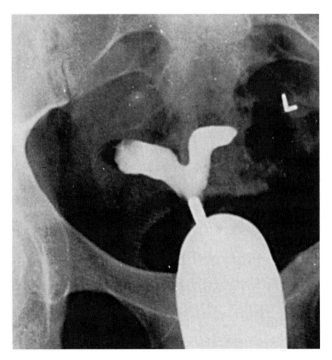

Fig. 7-6 Hysterosalpingogram demonstrates bicornuate uterus. (Courtesy Riverside Methodist Hospitals, Columbus, Ohio.)

uterine tubes. It is a common indication for sonographic evaluation in a nongravid female. Severe cases with abscess formation may also require surgical intervention.

MASTITIS

Inflammation of the breast or **mastitis** is most often caused by *staphylococcus aureus*. This bacterial infection usually occurs in the breasts of lactating females through cracks in the skin surrounding the nipple. Common signs and symptoms of mastitis include pain, redness, and swelling of the affected breast, elevated temperature, and, in severe cases, abscess formation. Mastitis is treated medically with antibiotic therapy and heat application to the affected breast. Mammography plays a very limited role in the diagnosis and treatment of mastitis.

Neoplastic Diseases

OVARIAN CYSTIC MASSES

Single cystic ovarian masses are fairly common in females within the reproductive age group. They include **follicular ovarian cysts** and **corpus luteum ovarian cysts.** The formation of follicular and corpus luteum cysts occurs as a part of the normal menstrual cycle. Follicular cysts result from faulty resorption of the fluid from incompletely developed follicles (Fig. 7-7). Corpus luteum cysts occur when resorption of any blood leaked into the cavity following ovulation leaves behind a small cyst. Changes in the size of follicular and corpus luteum cysts occur quickly and vary with the menstrual cycle. These cysts may occasionally increase in size and cause pelvic discomfort or abnormal pressure on the urinary bladder. These cysts are readily visible with ultrasound, and treatment is generally not necessary because they often disappear completely without medical intervention.

Multiple cystic masses may indicate **endometriosis,** a disease caused by the presence of endometrial tissue or glands outside the uterus, in abnormal locations within the pelvis. External endometriosis commonly involves the ovaries, uter-

ine ligaments, the rectovaginal septum, and the pelvic peritoneum; however, it may also attach to the rectal wall, the ureters, or the urinary bladder. The etiology of endometriosis is unknown, but it seems to respond to normal hormonal stimuli and is clinically significant in females between the ages of 20 and 40. The external endometrial tissue contains normal functioning endometrium. Responsive to hormonal changes, it continues to bleed cyclically. These blood-filled cysts are often visible upon ultrasonic examination. Long-standing endometriosis results in the development of fibrosis, adhesions, scarring, and eventually sterility. Common signs and symptoms include pelvic and low back pain, dysmenorrhea, and infertility. Although ultrasound is useful in the diagnosis of endometriosis, a positive diagnosis is generally made via laparoscopy. Mild cases of endometriosis may be treated with hormone therapy; severe cases generally require surgical intervention.

Polycystic ovaries consist of enlarged ovaries containing multiple small cysts. The ovaries are bilaterally enlarged and have a smooth exterior surface, with the multiple cysts lying just below the outer surface. Polycystic ovaries are often associated with Stein-Leventhal syndrome, a fairly

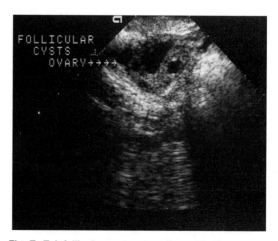

Fig. 7-7 A follicular cyst seen adjacent to the ovary on this transverse ultrasound view. (Courtesy Riverside Methodist Hospitals, Columbus, Ohio.)

rare disease. Women with Stein-Leventhal syndrome rarely ovulate because of an endocrine abnormality that inhibits maturation and release of the ovarian follicle. In addition, these individuals may experience amenorrhea and sterility. The primary treatment is use of drugs to induce ovulation.

Benign **cystic teratomas** of the ovary, often called **dermoid cysts,** account for approximately 20% to 25% of ovarian tumors and are the most common type of germ cell tumor containing mature tissue. These masses arise from an unfertilized ova that undergoes neoplastic change. Cystic teratomas are composed of tissue derived from the ectoderm, endoderm, and mesoderm, and they often contain hair, thyroid tissue, keratin, sebaceous secretions, and occasionally teeth (Fig. 7-8). The treatment for cystic teratomas is surgical removal of the mass.

CYSTADENOCARCINOMA

Cystadenocarcinoma is a malignant neoplasm of the ovary (Fig. 7-9), which occurs in women over age 40. Although it is less common than other female genital carcinomas, cystadenocarcinoma is the most lethal and has a very poor prognosis. The etiology of this neoplasm is unknown. Sonographic evaluation demonstrates a rough, irregular ovarian surface with the tumor often containing both cystic and solid areas. Serous tumors are frequently bilateral; mucinous tumors are more likely to be unilateral.

The signs and symptoms of cystadenocarcinoma are very vague, including urinary bladder or rectal pressure. In many cases, the disease is completely asymptomatic and discovered only on routine pelvic examination. This tends to delay diagnosis and treatment, thus reducing the chance for cure. These tumors often spread to other pelvic organs, the small intestines, the

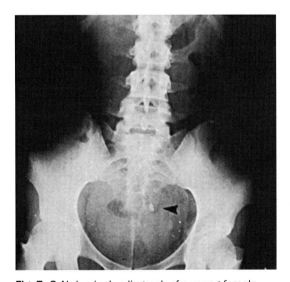

Fig. 7–8 Abdominal radiograph of a young female demonstrates a radiographically visible tooth within a cystic teratoma. (Courtesy Riverside Methodist Hospitals, Columbus, Ohio.)

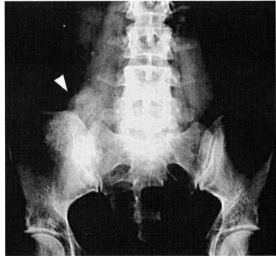

Fig. 7–9 Abdominal radiograph of a 47-year-old woman diagnosed with a cystadenocarcinoma. Note the calcifications within the lesion that make it radiographically visible. (Courtesy Riverside Methodist Hospitals, Columbus, Ohio.)

omentum, the stomach, and the liver, frequently presenting with associated ascites and pleural effusions. Common treatment of cystadenocarcinoma includes surgery in combination with chemotherapy or radiation therapy.

CARCINOMA OF THE CERVIX

Cervical carcinoma or **dysplasia** is a common malignancy of the female genital system caused by an abnormal growth pattern of epithelial cells around the neck of the uterus. Cervical intraepithelial neoplasias (CIN) are classified or staged as mild (I), moderate (II), or severe (III) and are generally diagnosed by a Pap smear and confirmed by surgical biopsy. Research indicates that a history of multiple sexual partners or prior sexually transmitted infections predisposes women to this disease. Symptoms commonly associated with cervical dysplasia include abnormal bleeding, especially postcoitally. Additionally, impaired renal function resulting from ureteral obstruction is often seen. The treatment of cervical dysplasia varies according to the classification. Pap smears allow early detection of this disease, thus improving the chance of cure and survival. The 5-year survival rate ranges from 90% for stage I dysplasias to less than 15% for advanced disease. The primary treatment is radiation therapy; however, surgical intervention may also be necessary.

Uterine Masses

LEIOMYOMAS (UTERINE FIBROIDS)

Leiomyomas are benign, solid masses of the uterus that develop from an overgrowth of the uterine smooth muscle tissue. They are present in approximately 25% of all women over age 30 and are the most common benign tumors of the female genital system. The etiology of this neoplasm is unknown; however, they tend to grow under the influence of estrogen, may enlarge during pregnancy, and stop growing at menopause. Following menopause, leiomyomas are replaced largely by fibrous scar tissue, leading to

the misnomer **uterine fibroids.** In addition, they often contain radiographically visible calcifications (Fig. 7-10). The tumors vary in size, number, and location; they are frequently asymptomatic until they grow large enough to place pressure on surrounding structures, and they are usually detected upon pelvic examination. Sonographically, they appear as sharply circumscribed, encapsulated lesions and may contain cystic areas. Malignant transformation is rare, and treatment depends on patient symptoms, ranging from no treatment to surgical removal of the uterus.

ADENOCARCINOMA OF THE ENDOMETRIUM

Adenocarcinoma of the endometrium is by far the most common malignancy of the uterus. It is often termed *carcinoma of the uterus.* It is histopathologically different from cervical carcinoma

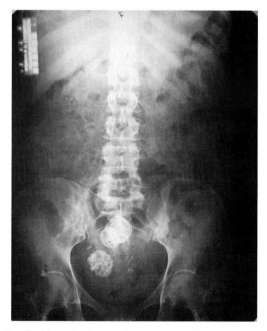

Fig. 7-10 Abdominal radiograph of a 50-year-old woman demonstrates leiomyomas of the uterus with radiographically visible calcifications. (Courtesy the American College of Radiology, Reston, Virginia.)

and is one of the most common cancers of the female reproductive system, second only to breast cancer. The incidence of adenocarcinoma of the endometrium has remained fairly static, occurring mainly in postmenopausal women and increasing in incidence with age. The development of this neoplasm has strong ties to hormonal changes within the female and is more common in nulliparous women. Adenocarcinoma of the endometrium is believed to be preceded by adenomatous hyperplasia. It then passes through an in situ stage before reaching its final invasive stage, often completely filling the uterine cavity. The cancer is graded according to cellular differentiation and staged according to the extent of the disease. The most frequent symptom is irregular or postmenopausal bleeding. Treatment varies with the stage of the disease. Stage 0 is curable via hysterectomy and stages I and II are usually treated with a combination of surgery and radiation therapy, with a 5-year survival rate of 80%.

Breast Masses

FIBROADENOMA

A **fibroadenoma** is a common benign breast tumor. It is usually unilateral and consists of a solid, well-defined mass that does not invade surrounding tissue. The neoplasm is formed by an overgrowth of fibrous and glandular tissue and is commonly located in the upper, outer quadrant of the breast. Fibroadenomas occur most frequently in women between the ages of 15 and 35, appear to be estrogen dependent, and may grow rapidly during pregnancy. These lesions are often painless and can usually be moved about within the breast. Mammography, in conjunction with physical breast examination and sometimes ultrasound, plays a vital role in the detection of fibroadenomas (Figs. 7-11 and 7-12) and is useful in distinguishing them from mammary dysplasia (fibrocystic breast disease) and breast carcinoma. Surgical removal of the lesion is curative.

FIBROCYSTIC BREASTS

An overgrowth of fibrous tissue or cystic hyperplasia results in **fibrocystic breasts.** This is the most common disorder of the female breast and occurs to some degree in approximately 50% of premenopausal women. This condition may be unilateral; however, it is most frequently bilateral, with variably sized cysts located throughout the breasts (Fig. 7-13). The severity of this disorder varies greatly, and it is believed to result from fluctuations in the hormone levels during the menstrual cycle. The most common sign or symptom associated with fibrocystic breasts is a mass or masses that increase in size and tenderness immediately preceding the onset of the menstrual period. Ultrasound is extremely useful as a follow-up to mammography in differentiating solid masses from cystic masses in women with fibrocystic breasts (Fig. 7-14). Large cysts are commonly aspirated for cytologic evaluation

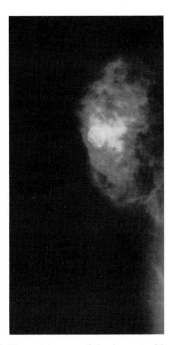

Fig. 7-11 Fibroadenoma of the breast with a well-circumscribed border in a 49-year-old woman.
(Courtesy Riverside Methodist Hospitals, Columbus, Ohio.)

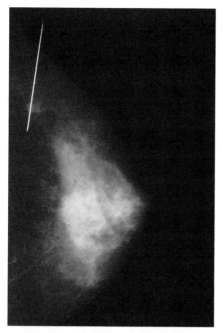

Fig. 7-12 Needle localization of fibroadenoma of the breast pinpoints the location of the mass for surgical biopsy. (Courtesy Riverside Methodist Hospitals, Columbus, Ohio.)

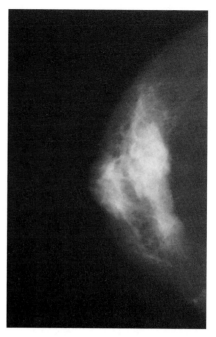

Fig. 7-13 Mammogram of a 35-year-old woman demonstrates a fibrocystic breast pattern. (Courtesy Riverside Methodist Hospitals, Columbus, Ohio.)

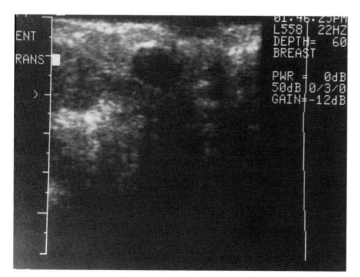

Fig. 7-14 Sonogram demonstrating a large cystic lesion within the breast of a 35-year-old woman with a fibrocystic breast pattern. Notice the well-circumscribed borders of the cyst. (Courtesy Riverside Methodist Hospitals, Columbus, Ohio.)

of the fluid. If the aspiration is unsuccessful, surgical biopsy is often performed. Although controversy exists about the correlation of fibrocystic breasts and an increased incidence of breast cancer, it is well known that a fibrocystic condition may mask a coexistent cancer. Treatment of the condition is largely symptomatic, including a monthly breast self-examination, and proper support.

CARCINOMA OF THE BREAST

Breast carcinoma is a very common malignancy among women in the United States and the second leading cause for female cancer deaths, behind only lung cancer. Current literature suggests that one of every nine women in the United States will develop breast cancer during her lifetime, with an increased incidence between the ages of 30 and 50. The incidence continues to rise throughout the postmenopausal years because of changes in estrogen levels, with the mean age for breast cancer at age 60. Approximately 50% of all lesions occur in the upper, outer quadrant of the breast.

Although the exact etiology of breast cancer is unknown, it is believed to be a multifactorial disorder. Heredity, endocrine influence, dietary habits, oncogenic factors (such as viruses), and environmental factors (such as chemical carcinogens) appear to play a role in the development of this disease. In terms of endocrine influence, current research suggests the amount of biologically available estrogen and progesterone is a key factor in the development of breast cancer. A strong family history of certain cancers also places a woman at increased risk in developing breast cancer.

Scirrhous, infiltrating, papillary, and medullary breast cancers generally begin as slow-growing, relatively painless masses, but as they grow, they may infiltrate the suspensory ligaments, causing them to shorten and retract the overlying skin. Physical signs of breast cancer include nipple retraction and distorted breast contour. The neoplasm may infiltrate and block lymphatic vessels, the major route of metastases, especially to the axilla. This infiltration causes edema in the overlying skin and enlargement of the axillary or supraclavicular lymph nodes. The skin edema may cause the normal cutaneous hair follicles to appear as multiple small depressions on the skin surface, known as a *peau d'orange* appearance. As the tumor progresses, it may attach to surrounding fascia and ulcerate the surrounding skin.

Mammography plays a very important role in the diagnosis and management of breast cancer. The tumors commonly appear radiographically as dense, irregular, stellate masses that infiltrate surrounding tissue (Fig. 7-15). Many of these neoplasms contain numerous calcifications that are radiographically visible (Fig. 7-16). Needle local-

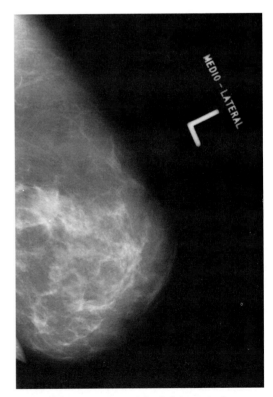

Fig. 7–15 Mammogram of the left breast of a 63-year-old woman demonstrating a stellate mass commonly associated with carcinoma of the breast. Notice the irregular borders of the mass. (Courtesy Riverside Methodist Hospitals, Columbus, Ohio.)

ization of mammographically detected, non-palpable cancerous breast lesions is reliable in directing the surgeon to the lesion in question and allows excision of the suspect tissue. The tissue specimen is radiographed and forwarded to a pathologist for histologic evaluation. Statistics demonstrate that this method of localization causes minimal morbidity, and the development and refinement of mammographic localization has greatly increased the percentage of positive findings upon surgical biopsy. This invasive technique allows more accurate diagnosis and treatment of early stage carcinoma of the breast. If the tumor can be removed before the lesion is palpable, the survival rate is greatly increased.

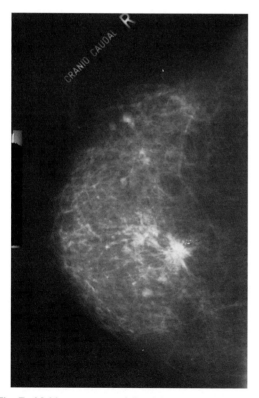

Fig. 7–16 Mammogram of the right breast in an elderly woman demonstrating a stellate mass containing microcalcifications commonly associated with carcinoma of the breast. (Courtesy Riverside Methodist Hospitals, Columbus, Ohio.)

Treatment of breast carcinoma depends on the extent of the disease. Once the carcinoma is confirmed by surgical biopsy, an axillary lymph node resection is performed to assist in the staging of the disease. Much controversy exists in terms of determining the best approach to management and treatment of breast cancers. In the past 40 years, the 5-year survival rate for breast cancer has remained virtually unchanged. Currently, two surgical options are recommended for stage I and stage II breast cancers: (1) modified radical mastectomy or (2) breast-conserving surgery followed by radiation therapy. Both methods require axillary lymph node resection; randomized clinical trials have not demonstrated a significant difference in the survival rate between these two surgical options.

Though indications for chemotherapy are continuously under review, most experts agree that patients should be referred to a medical oncologist after surgery. Treatment with an established combination of chemotherapeutic drugs is considered standard care for premenopausal females with lymph node involvement. Breast carcinomas are also classified by a hormone receptor test. Many tumors require hormones for continued growth, and these carcinomas may undergo temporary regression if hormonal balances are altered.

Disorders During Pregnancy

Diagnostic medical sonography is often used in the diagnosis of multiple and ectopic pregnancies. Ultrasonic examination is also indicated if the pregnant uterus is too small or too large for the calculated delivery date.

AMNIOTIC FLUID

Amniotic fluid is produced by various physiologic functions within the mother and the fetus. The amount of amniotic fluid present varies with the stage of pregnancy. **Oligohydramnios** occurs when too little amniotic fluid is present, and **polyhydramnios** occurs with an excess of amniotic fluid. The normal fetus swallows several hundred milliliters of fluid per day. This fluid is absorbed by the fetal intestines, with a portion excreted via the fetal urinary system and a portion transferred across the placenta into the mother's circulatory system. The major source of amniotic fluid arises from the fetus urinating fluid once the kidneys are developed. Therefore, oligohydramnios often results from poor fetal kidney function or blockage of the ureters. If a fetus is unable to swallow, polyhydramnios may occur. Two causes of this disorder are anencephaly and a high gastrointestinal obstruction.

ECTOPIC PREGNANCY

Ectopic pregnancy refers to the development of an embryo outside the uterine cavity. It occurs in approximately 1% of all pregnancies. The most common site for an ectopic pregnancy is the uterine tube (Fig. 7-17), but it may also occur in the ovary, cervix, or abdominal cavity. In the case of a tubal pregnancy, the uterine tube distends to accommodate the growing embryo, causing the blood vessels to rupture. This may produce serious internal hemorrhage and can be life threatening. If a tubal pregnancy goes untreated, the embryo will develop and survive for only 2 to 6 weeks.

Common signs and symptoms associated with ectopic pregnancy are the same as early pregnancy, but distention of the tube causes abdominal pain and tenderness. If internal hemorrhage occurs, loss of blood can cause fainting and shock. Ectopic pregnancies are more common in women who have had pelvic inflammatory disease or have a partial obstruction of the uterine tube. The etiology of tubal pregnancies is obstruction of the normal passageway for the ovum. Although ultrasound is useful in assessing ectopic pregnancies, diagnosis is confirmed via laparoscopy. The treatment is surgical removal of the embryo and the affected uterine tube.

PLACENTA DISORDERS

The placenta is a temporary organ associated with pregnancy. Its purpose is to exchange nutrients and oxygen from mother to fetus, and waste products from fetus to mother for excretion. **Placenta previa** is a condition in which the placenta develops in the lower half of the uterus and encroaches on and partially or completely covers the internal cervical os. In cases of placenta previa (Fig. 7-18), the mother experiences bleeding during the later stages of pregnancy because of the partial separation of the placenta from the uterine wall. Hemorrhage can occur, and this condition can be life-threatening to both the mother and fetus. Ultrasound is a good method of determining placenta location in cases of suspected previa and useful in the management of the pregnancy. Normal delivery cannot occur in patients with placenta previa so a cesarean section is normally performed.

Occasionally, a normally implanted placenta may prematurely separate from the uterus. This condition is termed **placental abruption** and may be life-threatening to the fetus. **Placental accreta** is an abnormal adhesion of the placenta to the uterine wall. In rare cases, failure of the placenta to separate following birth results in

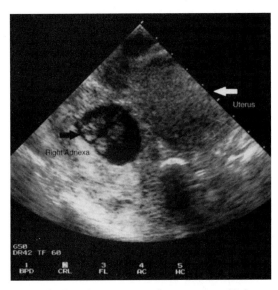

Fig. 7–17 Ectopic pregnancy shown on a sagittal ultrasound image reveals twin fetuses in the uterine tube. (Courtesy Riverside Methodist Hospitals, Columbus, Ohio.)

heavy bleeding and the need for an immediate hysterectomy.

HYDATIFORM MOLE

Hydatiform mole represents an abnormal conception in which there is usually no fetus. It occurs in about 1 in 2000 pregnancies in North America, although the incidence is much greater in certain other parts of the world for unknown reasons. With this condition, the uterus is filled with cystically dilated chorionic villi that resemble a bunch of grapes (Fig. 7-19). These villi absorb fluid and become swollen, demonstrating a characteristic pattern on ultrasound as well as

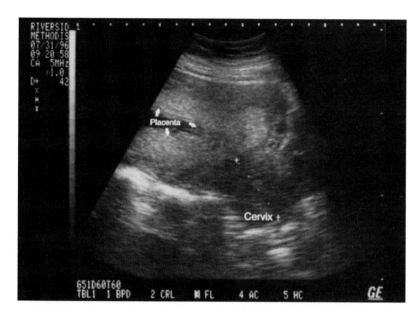

Fig. 7-18 Placenta previa seen on this sagittal ultrasound view reveals the placenta covering the internal os of the cervix. (Courtesy Riverside Methodist Hospitals, Columbus, Ohio.)

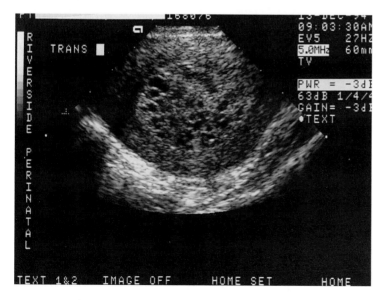

Fig. 7-19 Hydatiform mole revealed as a grapelike cluster in the uterus on this transverse ultrasound image. (Courtesy Riverside Methodist Hospitals, Columbus, Ohio.)

absence of heart sounds. Usually, these abort spontaneously in the second trimester. If they do not, suction curettage is done and most patients require no further treatment.

THE MALE REPRODUCTIVE SYSTEM

Anatomy and Physiology Review

The male reproductive system is composed of glands, ducts, and supporting structures. The glands of the male reproductive system include a pair of testes, a pair of seminal vesicles, a pair of bulbourethral glands, and one prostate gland. The testes are enclosed by a white, fibrous covering within the scrotum. They are responsible for the production of sperm and hormone secretion, mainly testosterone. The prostate gland lies just inferior to the bladder, and the urethra actually passes through this gland (Figs. 7-20 and 7-21). The prostate gland is responsible for secreting the majority of the seminal fluid and is normally about the size of a walnut.

The ducts that connect the glands include a pair of epididymides, a pair of vasa deferentia, a pair of ejaculatory ducts, and one urethra. The testes are divided into lobules that contain seminiferous tubules, which converge into larger ducts and emerge at the head of the epididymis. The epididymides lie superior and lateral to the testes and serve as a passageway for sperm. They are also responsible for secreting a portion of the seminal fluid. The vasa deferentia extend from the epididymides and pass through the inguinal canal into the pelvic cavity. They pass superior to the bladder and continue down the posterior surface of the bladder to join the ducts emerging from the seminal vesicles. This junction forms the ejaculatory ducts. These ducts eventually empty into the urethra, which is responsible for delivering the seminal fluid to the exterior of the body.

Imaging Considerations

Radiographic investigation of the male reproductive system is limited mainly to urethrograms, intravenous urography, and CT. However, ultrasound is commonly used to evaluate testicular

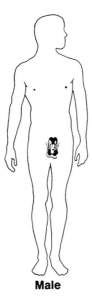

Male

Fig. 7-20 The male reproductive system. (From Bontrager KL: *Textbook of radiographic positioning and related anatomy,* ed 3, St Louis, 1993, Mosby.)

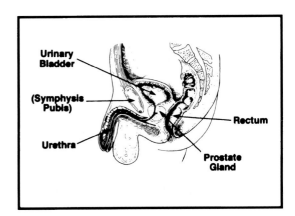

Fig. 7-21 The male urinary bladder, anterior cutaway. (From Bontrager KL: *Textbook of radiographic positioning and related anatomy,* ed 3, St Louis, 1993, Mosby.)

masses or an enlarged scrotum and to help differentiate between, on one hand, epididymitis and orchiditis and, on the other, testicular torsion. Nuclear medicine is also useful in distinguishing between epididymitis and testicular torsion. Prostatic ultrasound via a rectal probe is used to evaluate nodules and guide the physician during biopsies of the prostate.

Neoplastic Diseases

CONGENITAL ANOMALIES

As the end of gestation occurs, the male testes normally descend through the inguinal canal into the scrotum. Cryptorchidism is a condition of undescended testes. The rate of malignancy is much greater in males with this condition, so the treatment involves either bringing the testicle down and fixing it surgically or removing it. Ultrasound is often used to locate the testicle.

PROSTATIC HYPERPLASIA

Prostatic hyperplasia is a common benign enlargement, palpable through the rectum, of the prostate gland caused by the development of discrete nodules within the organ. The etiology of prostatic hyperplasia is unknown, but it is thought to be caused by hormonal changes associated with aging in that it generally affects men after age 50. The benign nodules most frequently occur in the median lobe and central portions of the lateral lobes of the prostate gland. Because of to this location, the nodules often compress the portion of the urethra passing through the prostate gland, thus interfering with urination.

Symptoms associated with this disorder include difficulty in starting, stopping, and maintaining a flow of urine and inability to completely empty the bladder. Residual urine retained in the bladder tends to become infected, threatening the kidneys with infection. In some cases, urinary tract obstructions may result from an overgrowth of the prostate gland. The most common treatment of prostatic hyperplasia is partial excision of the prostate gland, although nonsur-

gical treatment is available for some cases. A transurethral resection of the prostate (**TURP**) is performed by passing an endoscope through the urethra to core out the gland. Prostatic enlargement may be demonstrated on an intravenous urographic examination as a filling defect at the base of the bladder. Hyperplastic changes are also readily visible on CT of the pelvic area (Fig. 7-22). There is no conclusive evidence to suggest that development of prostatic hyperplasia increases an individual's chance of developing prostatic carcinoma.

Many men over the age of 50 develop small, multiple calcifications within the prostate. These are termed **prostatic calculi** and may be radiographically visible on plain abdominal or pelvic images. The development of these calculi is of no clinical significance.

CARCINOMA OF THE PROSTATE

Adenocarcinoma of the prostate is a common cancer in males. It most frequently affects elderly men, with the incidence increasing with age. The etiology of prostate cancer is unknown, but it generally affects the outer group of prostate glands and occurs more frequently in the posterior lobe of the prostate. This disease is most frequently diagnosed by physical examination and an elevation of acid phosphatase levels

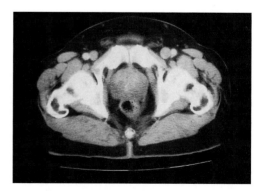

Fig. 7-22 Pelvic CT of a 68-year-old man demonstrating prostatic hyperplasia. Notice the indentation into the urinary bladder. (Courtesy Riverside Methodist Hospitals, Columbus, Ohio.)

in the blood. Common signs and symptoms associated with prostate cancer include urinary tract obstructions, a hard, enlarged prostate upon rectal palpation, and low back pain, often caused by metastatic spread to the pelvis and lumbar spine.

Some types of prostate cancer are fairly dormant, but others are very aggressive and yield a higher mortality rate. If it is diagnosed in an early stage, the initial treatment is surgical removal of the tumor. Additionally, this neoplasm is very testosterone dependent, so the testes are often removed along with the prostate. In some instances, female hormones may be administered to control the growth of the tumor by interfering with the testosterone. A new treatment modality involves planting radioactive seeds in the prostate, guided by ultrasound, to destroy the tumor.

Prostate cancer is staged A to D and graded I to III, depending on the extent of the disease. It tends to infiltrate surrounding structures early and extensively, particularly the skeletal system. Skeletal metastases occur in approximately 75% of all cases and manifest on plain radiographs as sclerotic lesions within the bone (Fig. 7-23). Bone pain in an elderly main is particularly suspect for prostate cancer. As the third leading

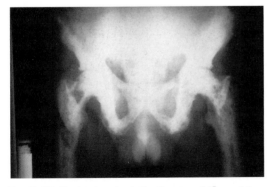

Fig. 7-23 Skeletal metastatic disease of the pelvis and spine secondary to prostate cancer. (Courtesy Riverside Methodist Hospitals, Columbus, Ohio.)

cause of cancer deaths in males, it has a 5-year survival rate of approximately 33%.

TESTICULAR MASSES

Testicular torsion occurs if a testicle twists upon itself, inducing severe pain and swelling. Failure to correct surgically in an immediate fashion can result in severe compromise of testicular vascularity. The condition is often evaluated with a nuclear medicine scan, which shows decreased uptake in the affected side (Fig. 7-24). Inflammation of the epididymis, or epididymitis, can similarly lead to scrotal swelling. The increased blood flow resulting from it can be detected by ultrasound or a nuclear medicine scan, which demonstrates increased uptake (Fig. 7-25).

Benign masses of the testes may be associated with **epididymoorchitis.** Other common benign masses include **hydroceles,** a collection of fluid in the testis or along the spermatic cord (Fig. 7-26), and **spermatoceles,** a cystic dilation of the epididymis (Fig. 7-27). Ultrasound may be used to differentiate between benign hydroceles or spermatoceles and solid, malignant neoplasms.

Malignant testicular tumors comprise approximately 1% of all male cancers. It is the most common malignancy among 15- to 34-year-olds and has a peak incidence around age 30 and a second smaller peak around age 75. The etiology of malignant tumors of the testes is unknown, but research has shown a strong hereditary association. The most common signs include enlargement or palpable hardness of the testis. As with other cancers, testicular tumors are staged I to III, depending on the size and extent of the disease. All types of malignant testicular neoplasms are treated with surgical resection. Chemotherapy, radiation therapy, or both may also be used in conjunction with surgery, depending on the type and staging of the disease. There are four types of malignant germ cell tumors: **seminomas, embryonal carcinomas, teratomas,** and **choriocarcinomas.**

Seminomas arise from the seminiferous tubules and account for approximately 40% of

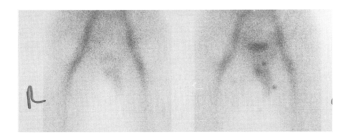

Fig. 7-24 Torsion as seen on a nuclear medicine testicular scan, which reveals a relative absence of blood flow to the right testicle. (Courtesy Riverside Methodist Hospitals, Columbus, Ohio.)

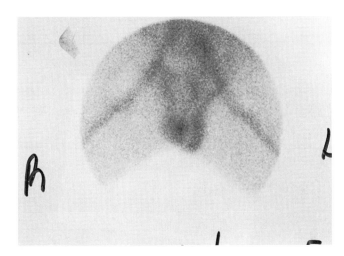

Fig. 7-25 Epididymitis as revealed on a testicular scan, which shows increased uptake in the left testicle. (Courtesy Riverside Methodist Hospitals, Columbus, Ohio.)

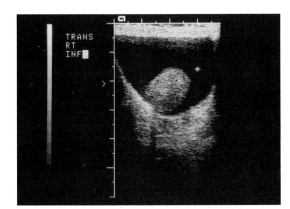

Fig. 7-26 A hydrocele is visualized as the dark collection of fluid surrounding the testicle, as seen on ultrasound of this 52-year-old man. (Courtesy Riverside Methodist Hospitals, Columbus, Ohio.)

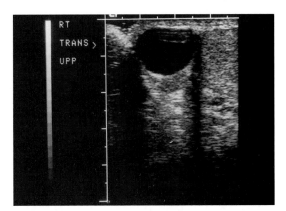

Fig. 7-27 A spematocele, evidenced by a large fluid collection on the epididymis, as seen on a testicular ultrasound scan of this 33-year-old man.

malignant testicular tumors (Fig. 7-28). Seminomas grow rapidly but tend to remain localized for a fairly long time before metastasizing. These neoplasms have an excellent prognosis because of their extreme radiosensitivity. If treated with radiation therapy, seminomas carry a 10-year survival rate of approximately 90%.

Teratomas arise from primitive germ cells and account for approximately 25% of the malignant testicular masses (Fig. 7-29). These neoplasms are composed of various cell types such as connective tissue, muscle, and thyroid glandular tissue. Teratomas are associated with a poorer prognosis than seminomas and carry a 10-year

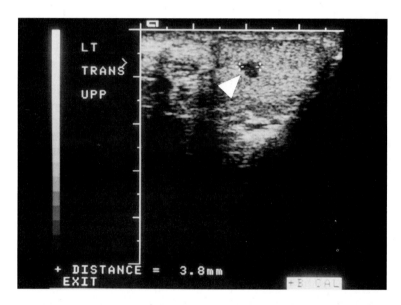

Fig. 7-28 The hypoechoic mass seen in the superior aspect of the testicle on this testicular ultrasound of a 31-year-old man is strongly suggestive of a seminoma. (Courtesy Riverside Methodist Hospitals, Columbus, Ohio.)

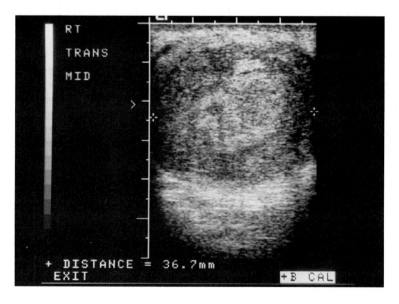

Fig. 7-29 A large, echogenic heterogeneous mass in the right testicle is highly suspicious for a teratoma in the testicular ultrasound scan of this 27-year-old man. (Courtesy Riverside Methodist Hospitals, Columbus, Ohio.)

survival rate of approximately 50% to 75%. Like seminomas, teratomas are highly malignant, spreading to the renal hilum via lymphatics and hematogenous spread.

Embryonal carcinomas make up approximately 20% of malignant testicular tumors. They are smaller than seminomas; however, they are very invasive and metastasize fairly quickly. Embryonal carcinomas carry a 10-year survival rate of approximately 35%.

Choriocarcinomas compose the smallest portion of malignant testicular tumors, accounting for only 1% of malignant neoplasms of the testes. However, choriocarcinomas are very small and aggressive neoplasms. They are often nonpalpable and metastasize very early. Choriocarcinomas carry the worst prognosis, with a 10-year survival rate of approximately 10%.

QUESTIONS

1. Imaging studies performed on a nongravid female include:
   a. hysterosalpingography
   b. IUD localization examinations
   c. pelvic sonography
   d. all of the above

2. Regular, yearly mammographic screening should occur in women _____ years of age or older.
   a. 20   c. 40
   b. 30   d. 50

3. The congenital disorder resulting in a complete duplication of the uterus, cervix, and vagina is:
   a. bicornuate uterus
   b. retroflexed uterus
   c. unicornuate uterus
   d. uterus didelphys

4. The formation of which of the following cystic ovarian masses may occur as a part of the normal menstrual cycle?
   1. luteum cysts
   2. cystadenomas
   3. cysts
      a. 1 and 2   c. 2 and 3
      b. 1 and 3   d. 1, 2 and 3

5. All of the following may result in sterility *except:*
   a. cystic teratoma   c. polycystic ovaries
   b. endometriosis   d. PID

6. A malignant neoplasm of the ovary is a:
   a. cystoadenocarcinoma
   b. cystadenoma
   c. leiomyoma
   d. fibroadenoma

7. Diagnosis of which type of neoplastic disease is often made via a Pap smear and confirmed by surgical biopsy?
   a. adenocarcinoma of the endometrium
   b. cervical carcinoma
   c. leiomyoma of the uterus

8. The majority of breast masses occur in which anatomical region of the breast?
   a. lower, inner quadrant
   b. lower, outer quadrant
   c. upper, inner quadrant
   d. upper, outer quadrant

9. Physical signs of breast cancer include:
   a. nipple discharge
   b. peau d'orange appearance
   c. massive weight loss
   d. all of the above

10. The presence of excessive amniotic fluid is termed:
    a. abruptio placentae
    b. oligohydramnios
    c. placenta previa
    d. polyhydramnios

11. The most common site for an ectopic pregnancy is in the:
    a. abdominal cavity
    b. cervix
    c. ovary
    d. uterine tube

12. Prostatic hyperplasia most frequently occurs in men:
    a. under the age of 30
    b. between the ages of 30 and 50
    c. over the age of 50
    d. prostatic hyperplasia is a female condition

13. The most common sites for skeletal metastases of adenocarcinoma of the prostate are the:
    1. lumbar spine
    2. pelvis
    3. ribs
       a. 1 and 2
       b. 1 and 3
       c. 2 and 3
       d. 1, 2 and 3

14. Benign tumors of the testes include:
    1. hydroceles
    2. seminomas
    3. spermatoceles
       a. 1 and 2
       b. 1 and 3
       c. 2 and 3
       d. 1, 2 and 3

15. Which type of malignant neoplasm of the testes is associated with the best prognosis?
    a. choriocarcinoma
    b. embryonal carcinoma
    c. seminoma
    d. teratoma

16. Describe how breast parenchyma changes with age and parity and the effect these changes have on radiographic visibility of potential masses.

17. Identify two purposes for requiring a patient to have a full bladder for female sonographic examination.

18. Describe the risk of radiation exposure from routine mammography.

19. What would be the danger of leaving cryptorchidism untreated?

20. A 60-year-old man presents to his physician with complaints of frequent urination, particularly at night. An IVP is ordered. The only visible abnormality is a filling defect at the base of his bladder. What is the likely cause?

The Cardiovascular System

Anatomy and Physiology Review
  The heart
  The cardiac cycle
  Circulatory vessels
Imaging Considerations
  Controllable factors
  Uncontrollable factors
  Other imaging modalities
Congenital and Hereditary Diseases
  Patent ductus arteriosus
  Coarctation of the aorta
  Septal defects

Transposition of the great vessels
Tetralogy of Fallot
Valvular Disease
Congestive Heart Failure
  Left-sided failure
  Right-sided failure
Degenerative Diseases
  Atherosclerosis
  Coronary artery disease
  Cerebrovascular accident
Aneurysms
Venous Thrombosis

Upon completion of Chapter 8, the reader should be able to:

■ Describe the anatomic components of the cardiovascular system.

■ Explain the appearance of the various portions of the heart on conventional chest radiographs.

■ Describe each segment of the cardiac cycle.

■ Discuss the role of other imaging modalities in the diagnosis, treatment, and management of cardiovascular disorders.

■ Differentiate the major congenital anomalies of the cardiovascular system.

■ Identify the pathogenesis of the pathologies cited and typical treatments for them.

■ Describe, in general, the radiographic appearance of each of the given pathologies.

KEY TERMS

Heart
Right and left atria
Right and left ventricles
Endocardium
Myocardium
Epicardium
Systole
Diastole
Sinoatrial node
Arteries
Adventitia
Media
Intima
Lumen
Veins
Capillaries
Cardiomegaly
Cardiac series
Stress echocardiography
Transesophageal
  echocardiography (TEE)
Thrombolysis
Urokinase

Embolization
Transjugular intrahepatic
  portosystemic stent
  (TIPSS)
Stent
Percutaneous transluminal
  angioplasty (PTA)
Permanent catheterization
Greenfield filter
Ultrafast CT
Foramen ovale
Ductus arteriosus
Murmur
Patent ductus arteriosus
Coarctation of the aorta
Rib notching
Atrial septal defect
Ventricular septal defect
Transposition of the great
  vessels
Tetralogy of Fallot
Rheumatic fever
Valvular stenosis

Congestive heart failure
Atherosclerosis
Atheroma formations
Ischemia
Coronary artery disease
Infarct
Cerebrovascular accident
  (CVA)
Ischemic stroke
Hemorrhagic stroke
Thrombus
Embolus
Lacunar infarction
Atherothrombic brain
  infarction
Transient ischemic attack
Aneurysm
Saccular aneurysm
Fusiform
Dissecting aneurysm
Venous thrombosis
Phlebitis
Thrombophlebitis

ANATOMY AND PHYSIOLOGY REVIEW

The cardiovascular system consists of the heart, arteries, capillaries, and veins and may be further divided into two subsystems of circulation. The pulmonary circulation transports blood between the heart and lungs for exchange of blood gases, whereas the systemic circulation transports blood between the heart and the rest of the body.

The Heart

The **heart** acts as a pump to propel the blood throughout the body via the circulatory vessels. It lies in the anterior chest within the mediastinum and is generally readily visible on a chest radiograph. The interior of the heart is divided into two upper chambers, termed the **right and left atria,** and two lower chambers termed the **right and left ventricles** (Fig. 8-1). Note that

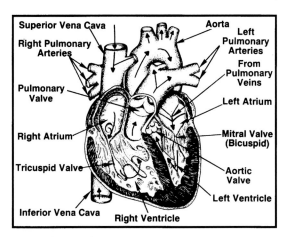

Fig. 8-1 Blood flow through the heart. (From Bontrager KL: *Textbook of radiographic positioning and related anatomy*, ed 3, St Louis, 1993, Mosby.)

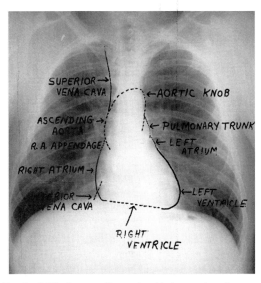

Fig. 8-2 PA chest radiograph with heart chambers and great vessels outlined. (Courtesy the American College of Radiology, Reston, Virginia.)

the heart lies in an oblique plane within the mediastinum; a conventional posteroanterior (PA) chest radiograph does not clearly demonstrate all chambers of the heart.

A frontal projection of the chest shows a cardiac silhouette, with two thirds of the heart lying to the left of midline; the right side is composed of mainly the right atrium and the left side is composed mainly of the left ventricle. The right ventricle lies midline within the cardiac shadow and is located anterior to the right atrium and left ventricle. The left atrium is located midline and is the most posterior aspect of the heart (Fig. 8-2). Therefore, it is necessary to obtain a lateral projection of the chest to best demonstrate the right ventricle and left atrium. On a lateral projection of the chest, the right ventricle constitutes the anterior portion of the cardiac silhouette, and the left atrium and left ventricle constitute the posterior portion of the cardiac shadow (Fig. 8-3).

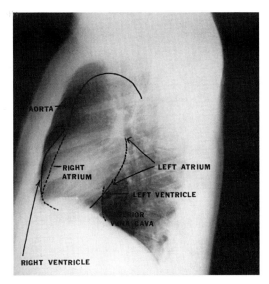

Fig. 8-3 Lateral chest radiograph with heart chambers and great vessels outlined. (Courtesy the American College of Radiology, Reston, Virginia.)

The heart contains three tissue layers. The innermost layer, termed the **endocardium,** is smooth. The valves located within and between the various chambers are also composed of endocardium. Although the valve tissue is relatively thin, in a normal heart it is able to prevent the backflow and passage of blood when the valve is closed. The middle layer is muscular and is termed the **myocardium.** This is the thickest layer of heart tissue, and the muscle receives blood supply from the right and left coronary arteries that arise directly from the aorta, just superior to the aortic valve. Maximum blood flow through the coronary arteries occurs during diastole, while the heart is relaxed. The outermost layer is a protective covering termed the **epicardium.** The entire heart is enclosed within a pericardial sac, which contains a small amount of fluid to lubricate the heart as it contracts and relaxes, thus reducing friction between the heart and other mediastinal structures.

In the normal heart, the right atrium receives deoxygenated blood from the body via the superior and inferior venae cavae. The deoxygenated blood passes through the right atrioventricular or tricuspid valve into the right ventricle. The right ventricle contracts during systole, thus propelling the blood to the lungs through the pulmonary valve and pulmonary trunk, which bifurcates into the right and left main pulmonary arteries, respectively. Approximately 60% of the deoxygenated blood enters the right lung, and approximately 40% enters the left lung.

The exchange of gases occurs at the capillary-alveolar level within the lungs, and the now-oxygenated blood is returned to the left atrium via the four pulmonary veins. The oxygenated blood flows from the left atrium to the left ventricle via the left mitral valve. The left ventricle is responsible for pumping the oxygenated blood throughout the systemic circulatory system; therefore, the left ventricle has a thicker layer of myocardium and contracts with greater force than does the right ventricle. The oxygenated blood flows through the aortic valve into the aorta when the left ventricle contracts.

The Cardiac Cycle

The contraction of the myocardium is termed **systole** and the subsequent relaxation is termed **diastole.** The pacemaker of the heart is the **sinoatrial** (SA) **node,** which is located in the upper portion of the right atrium near the superior vena cava. An electrical current is transmitted through the myocardium, resulting in a heartbeat.

Electrocardiography graphically displays this electrical activity. The elements of an electrocardiogram include the P wave, PR interval, QRS complex, T wave, and QT duration (Fig. 8-4). The P wave is the graphic display of the spread of the electrical impulse from the atria. The PR interval shows the amount of time required for the electrical impulse to travel from the SA node to the ventricular muscle fibers. The spread of the electrical impulse through the ventricles is displayed by the QRS complex, and the period in which the ventricles recover from the spent electrical impulse is graphically displayed by the T wave. The QT duration represents the total time from ventricular depolarization (QRS) to ventricular repolarization (T).

Circulatory Vessels

Arteries are blood vessels that carry blood away from the heart and are generally named for their location or the organ they supply (e.g., splenic artery). They are composed of three layers. The outermost layer is termed the **adventitia,** the middle layer is the **media,** and the innermost layer is the **intima.** The internal, tubular structure of the vessel is termed the **lumen. Veins** are blood vessels that carry blood to the heart. They are composed of the same three layers; however, venous walls are thinner than arterial walls, and veins contain valves at set intervals to help with blood return to the heart. **Capillaries** are microscopic vessels that connect the arteries and veins (Fig. 8-5). They are responsible for the exchange of substances necessary for nutrient and waste transport.

IMAGING CONSIDERATIONS

A number of imaging modalities play an important role in evaluation of the cardiovascular system. Radiography continues to play a very important role in the diagnosis and management of cardiovascular disease. Chest radiographs obtained through traditional film screen imaging or through computed radiography provide information concerning heart shape and size.

However, the technologist must be aware that many factors may affect the cardiac image. Some factors can be controlled by the technologist, whereas others cannot.

Controllable Factors

Factors that the technologist can control include patient posture, degree of inspiration,

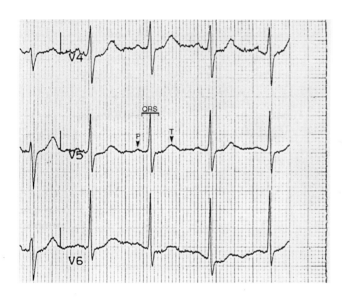

Fig. 8–4 Electrocardiograph demonstrating the P wave, QRS wave, and T wave. (Courtesy Riverside Methodist Hospitals, Columbus, Ohio.)

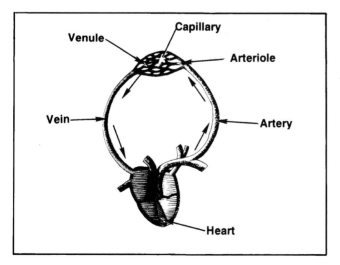

Fig. 8–5 General systemic circulation. (From Bontrager KL: *Textbook of radiographic positioning and related anatomy,* ed 3, St Louis, 1993, Mosby.)

correct positioning, geometric factors, and exposure technique selection. Whenever possible, chest radiographs should be taken with the patient in an erect position. If a patient is semirecumbent or recumbent, the heart appears to be enlarged because the abdominal organs push the diaphragm and heart up into the thoracic cavity. It is important to identify cases in which the patient is not erect to aid the physician in diagnosis and interpretation.

Chest radiographs obtained without a good inspiration also distort heart shape and size (Figs. 8-6 and 8-7). Remember that at least 10 posterior ribs should be visible within the lung fields on a good inspiratory chest radiograph. The sternoclavicular joints should be an equal distance from the spine and the scapulae should be rolled out of the lung fields on a well-positioned PA chest radiograph. To position a patient for a lateral chest, the arms and shoulders should be placed above the patient's head to ensure that they are above the apices.

Geometric factors affecting heart shape and size include source-to-image receptor distance (SID) and object-to-image receptor distance (OID). Conventional chest radiographs are generally obtained using a 72-inch SID to decrease magnification of the heart to an approximate

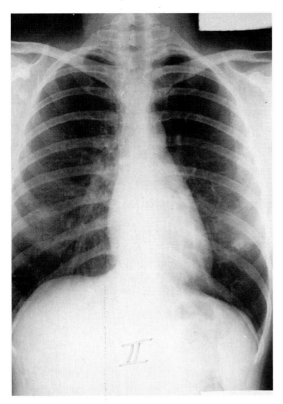

Fig. 8-6 PA chest radiograph with good inspiration. (Courtesy the American College of Radiology, Reston, Virginia.)

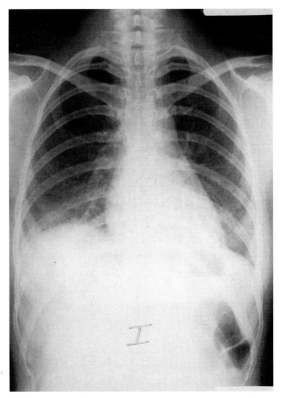

Fig. 8-7 PA chest radiograph with expiration on the same patient as in Fig. 8-6; notice the enlargement of the cardiac shadow on this radiograph. (Courtesy the American College of Radiology, Reston, Virginia.)

factor of 10%. Again, it is important to document variations in SID to aid in the proper diagnosis of heart disorders. Because the heart is fairly anterior in the mediastinum, it is preferable to obtain PA chest images whenever possible. This places the heart closest to the image receptor, allowing for the smallest OID. Positioning the patient for a PA projection also helps decrease magnification of the cardiac silhouette. A third geometric factor that is frequently overlooked is the anode-heel effect. Technologists can use this phenomenon to their advantage by placing the anode over the apical region and the cathode toward the base of the lungs, thus distributing the radiographic density more evenly throughout the chest radiograph.

Adequate penetration of the mediastinal structure is also critical in chest radiography and requires the use of a relatively high kilovoltage. A minimum of 100 kilovolts peak (kVp) should be used. Compensating filters, such as trough filters, may also be used to ensure adequate penetration of the mediastinum while maintaining optimum visualization of the vascular markings within the lung fields. Vascular markings within the chest help the physician assess ventricular function. The pulmonary vessels also provide information about pulmonary artery pressure. Dilatation of these vessels often indicates problems with the right ventricle. Exposure times of a second or less should be used whenever possible to decrease involuntary cardiac motion. It has been documented that heart motion may increase the size of the cardiac shadow. The heart may look larger if the radiograph is exposed during diastole.

In most institutions, chest radiography is the most commonly performed procedure, and technologists all too often underestimate the importance of these basic radiographic principles. Well-positioned diagnostic chest radiographs are crucial in the diagnosis and treatment of cardiovascular disorders. In a normal adult, the transverse diameter of the cardiac shadow should be less than half the transverse diameter of the thorax on a PA erect chest radiograph. An enlarged heart is termed **cardiomegaly** (Fig. 8-8), which

is indicative of many cardiovascular disorders and is a nonspecific finding.

Uncontrollable Factors

Factors affecting cardiac shape and size that are not under the technologist's control include patient body habitus, bony thorax abnormalities, and pathologic conditions, such as a pneumothorax or pulmonary emphysema. Bony abnormalities of special concern include scoliosis and pectus excavatum. Individuals with pectus excavatum present with a funnel-shaped depression of the sternum. The abnormal placement of the xiphoid causes displacement of the heart to the left and distortion of the cardiac shadow.

Other Imaging Modalities

Although largely relegated to historical interest, a **cardiac series** is an examination in which the esophagus was filled with barium sulfate to

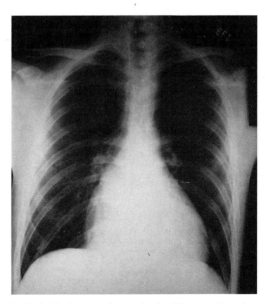

Fig. 8-8 PA chest radiograph of a 53-year-old male with aortic insufficiency resulting in cardiomegaly. (Courtesy the American College of Radiology, Reston, Virginia.)

better demonstrate the borders of the heart (Figs. 8-9 and 8-10). For this study, a 45-degree right anterior oblique position projects the heart shadow into the left lung field free from the other mediastinal structures. However, it is necessary to use approximately a 60-degree left anterior oblique position to project the heart into the right lung field so that it is not superimposed on other mediastinal structures.

Fluoroscopy may be used to visualize cardiac calcifications and chamber motion. In general, however, cardiac fluoroscopy is of limited value in the diagnosis of heart disease.

Echocardiography is a noninvasive allied procedure that can provide detailed information about heart anatomy and function and vessel patency (Fig. 8-11). Echocardiography uses ultra-

sound to provide a good examination of the left atrium, left ventricle, and aortic root and allows evaluation of left ventricular function. Cardiac sonography is also used to measure the thickness of the ventricular walls and provides an accurate assessment of cardiac motion and valve function using Doppler sonography. In addition, it is an excellent modality for visualizing the ascending and abdominal aorta in cases of suspected aneurysm. **Stress echocardiography** combines an exercise test with an echocardiogram to check the heart's contraction ability and its pumping efficiency. If exercise is not possible, a drug, dobutamine, can be used to increase the cardiac output to assess how well the heart pumps during infusion. Similarly, another drug, dipyridamole (Persantine), can be used in con-

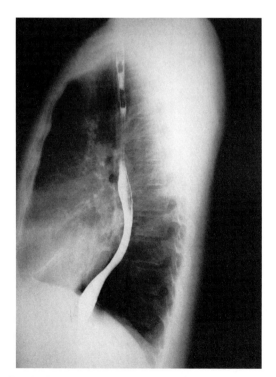

Fig. 8-9 Lateral projection of the chest with barium sulfate outlining the left atrium of the heart. (Courtesy Riverside Methodist Hospitals, Columbus, Ohio.)

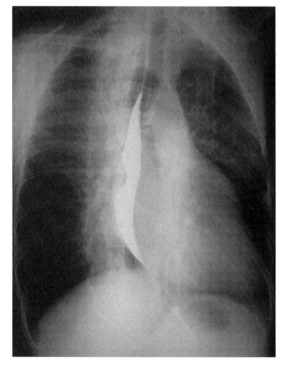

Fig. 8-10 Right anterior oblique position of the chest with barium sulfate outlining the left atrium of the heart. (Courtesy Riverside Methodist Hospitals, Columbus, Ohio.)

junction with a nuclear isotope to produce a stress test without exercise. By maximizing blood flow in the heart, this test allows any disparity in blood flow due to blockage to be readily detected with the nuclear medicine imaging. **Transesophageal echocardiography (TEE)** is a newer type of echocardiography procedure in which the patient swallows a mobile, flexible probe. The heart's structure can then be readily visualized without inteference from structures such as the skin, rib cage, and chest muscles.

Like echocardiography, Doppler sonography is adjunct, noninvasive procedure used to study peripheral vasculature. Doppler sonography has been a mainstay of vascular imaging since the 1970s and is used to determine the velocity, as well as the presence or absence, of blood flow in both arteries and veins. Using ultrasound, the Doppler effect is the principle that sound coming toward you has a higher pitch than sound going away. The return of pulsed ultrasound allows calculation of the shift in the direction of blood flow and creates a spectral display from which velocity is calculated (Fig. 8-12). With Doppler sonography, the flow of blood is not affected until any obstruction present is at least 60% complete. The percentage of stenosis present dictates the treatment of vascular disease, and usually this consists of surgery (e.g., endarterectomy). Such vascular imaging is said to be *duplex* in that the Doppler sonography helps reveal physiologic characteristics, and the imaging component defines anatomy, for example, plaque morphology. The most common conditions imaged by Doppler sonography are carotid

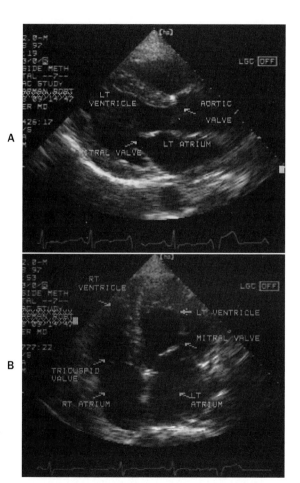

Fig. 8–11 A, Echocardiography visualization of heart anatomy of a 47-year-old male, as seen in a parasternal, sagittal view; **B,** A coronal view of the same heart via echocardiography. (**A** and **B** Courtesy Riverside Methodist Hospitals, Columbus, Ohio.)

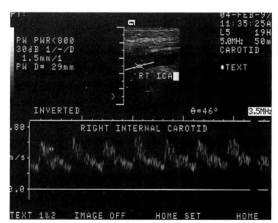

Fig. 8–12 Illustration of the Doppler effect with normal arterial flow in the internal carotid artery depicted above a graph of the arterial flow. (Courtesy Riverside Methodist Hospitals, Columbus, Ohio.)

stenosis (significantly reducing carotid angiography) (Figs. 8-13 and 8-14), lower extremity arterial stenosis, and deep venous thrombosis (Figs. 8-15 and 8-16), largely supplanting traditional venography.

Nuclear medicine procedures used in the assessment of cardiovascular disease include myocardial perfusion scans, gated cardiac blood pool scans, and radionuclide angiocardiography. A myocardial perfusion scan is the most widely

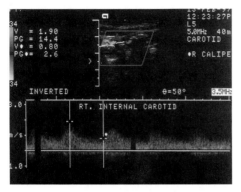

Fig. 8-13 A Doppler sonogram of an abnormal internal carotid artery spectrum due to heterogeneous calcified plaque. Note the difference of appearance of the graphical representation as compared to Fig. 8-12. (Courtesy Riverside Methodist Hospitals, Columbus, Ohio.)

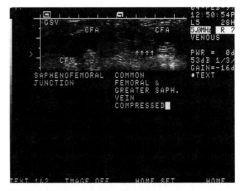

Fig. 8-15 Doppler sonographic portrayal of normal flow on the left of the image through the greater saphenous vein (GSV), common femoral vein (CFV), and common femoral artery (CFA). Compression on the right side of the image depicts normal closure of the common femoral vein and greater saphenous vein, as expected. (Courtesy Riverside Methodist Hospitals, Columbus, Ohio.)

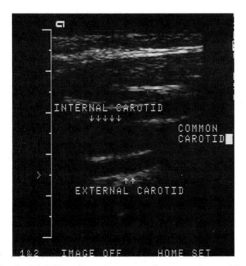

Fig. 8-14 A Doppler sonogram of a normal carotid bifurcation from the common carotid into the internal and external carotid arteries. (Courtesy Riverside Methodist Hospitals, Columbus, Ohio.)

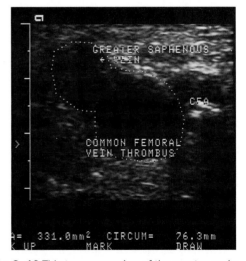

Fig. 8-16 This transverse view of the greater saphenous vein and common femoral vein indicates their failure to close upon compression, as due to the large venous thrombus contained within. (Courtesy Riverside Methodist Hospitals, Columbus, Ohio.)

used procedure in nuclear cardiology. It is especially useful in detecting regions of myocardial ischemia and scarring (Figs. 8-17 and 8-18). In this study, a special agent is used to dilate the coronary arteries, and then a radionuclide is injected. It concentrates in the areas of the heart that have the best blood flow. Those areas lacking blood flow demonstrate filling defects, visualized between images taken at rest and under stress. Myocardial perfusion scanning is particularly useful in combination with echocardiography stress evaluation. Gated cardiac blood pool scans are used to evaluate left ventricular function; radionuclide angiocardiography is mainly used in the management of congenital heart defects in pediatric patients. In addition, positron emission tomography (PET), where available, plays a role in demonstrating myocardial viability and metabolic imaging.

Angiography is still the most commonly performed procedure for cardiovascular disease. It may be performed for diagnostic purposes or for therapeutic reasons. Some traditional diagnostic angiography is being challenged by less invasive magnetic resonance imaging (MRI) and computed tomography (CT) angiography. Therapeutic angiography is, however, steadily increasing through expanded use of interventional

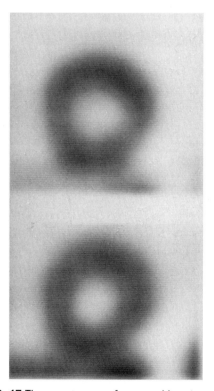

Fig. 8–17 The appearance of a normal heart on a nuclear medicine perfusion scan of a 58-year-old female, with the isotope distribution equal throughout the myocardium on both an unstressed (bottom) and stressed (top) image. (Courtesy Grant Medical Center, Columbus, Ohio.)

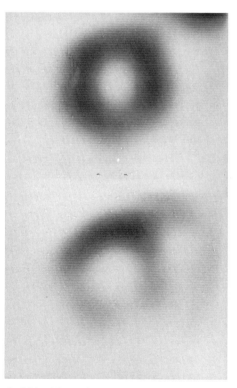

Fig. 8–18 In this nuclear medicine perfusion scan of this 69-year-old male, note the ischemia of the septum, anterior and apical portions of the left ventricle, as demonstrated by the lack of isotope uptake in the myocardium during stress (top). Compare this appearance to the normal uptake in the nonstressed image (bottom). (Courtesy Grant Medical Center, Columbus, Ohio.)

procedures. One such of these is **thrombolysis**, a procedure in which **urokinase**, a high-intensity anticoagulant, is dripped over a period of hours directly onto a clot to dissolve it (Fig. 8-19). With **embolization**, devices such as coils are used to clot off vessels (Fig. 8-20). Common examples of the use of embolization include clotting of vessels feeding brain tumors, arteriovenous malformations, or other abnormalities of the brain to prevent excessive bleeding dur-

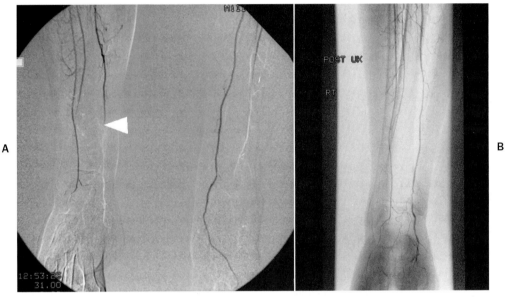

Fig. 8-19 A, An apparent embolus in the right popliteal artery prevents blood flow to the foot in this 91-year-old female; **B,** In this thrombolysis procedure, urokinase is sprayed onto the embolus and then allowed to drip over a 30-minute period. Patency is restored. (**A** and **B** Courtesy Riverside Methodist Hospitals, Columbus, Ohio.)

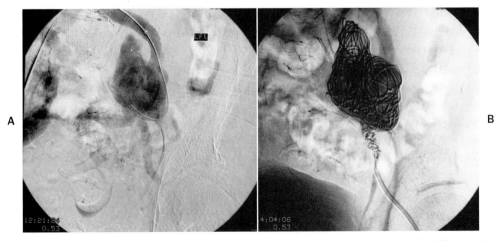

Fig. 8-20 A, A large aneurysm is seen angiographically in the left common iliac artery of this 74-year-old male; **B,** Embolization of this large aneurysm was accomplished by progressive insertion of a variety of coils and guide wire fragments. (**A** and **B** Courtesy Riverside Methodist Hospitals, Columbus, Ohio.)

ing open cranial surgery. In a **transjugular intrahepatic portosystemic stent (TIPSS)** procedure, a catheter is used to connect the jugular vein to the portal vein to reduce the flow of blood through a diseased liver (Fig. 8-21). Arterial **stents** are devices placed in arteries (Fig. 8-22), typically the iliac, aorta, renal, and coronary, to open occluded vessels. Insertion of a stent is often in preceded by **percutaneous transluminal angioplasty (PTA)** with a

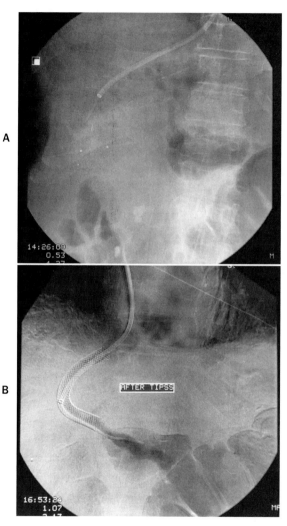

Fig. 8-21 **A,** A specialized catheter is used to create an opening through a cirrhotic liver of a 69-year-old male for the beginning of a TIPSS procedure; **B,** Following dilation of the pathway using standard angioplasty technique, a shunt is installed to connect the right hepatic vein to the right portal vein, restoring blood flow. (**A** and **B** Courtesy Riverside Methodist Hospitals, Columbus, Ohio.)

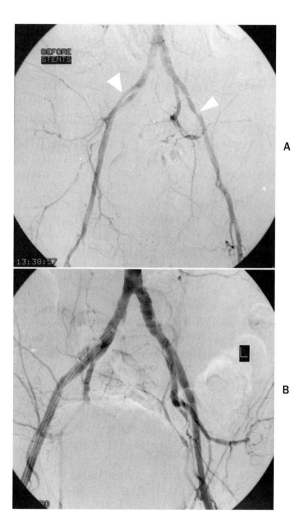

Fig. 8-22 **A,** A bilateral lower extremity arteriogram reveals stenosis of both external iliac arteries.
B, Following balloon angioplasty, stent placement in each external iliac artery results in restored flow of blood. (**A** and **B** Courtesy Riverside Methodist Hospitals, Columbus, Ohio.)

balloon catheter to open up the vessel's occlusion prior to stent placement (Fig. 8-23). In **permanent catheterization,** a catheter is placed in the subclavian or jugular vein and tunneled under the skin to allow for improved dialysis access. **Greenfield filters** are baskets placed in the inferior vena cava to catch clots before they enter the heart (Fig. 8-24). Besides typical contrast media, some of these procedures utilize carbon dioxide as the contrast agent for patients

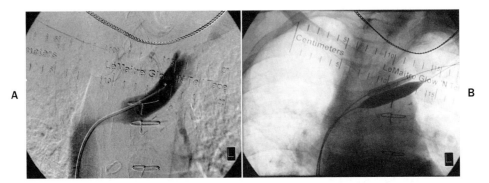

Fig. 8-23 A, Catheterization and angiography of the left brachiocephalic vein of this 56-year-old male reveal significant narrowing. **B,** Balloon angioplasty and a stent are used to open up the stenotic left brachiocephalic vein. Excellent blood flow was restored in subsequent images. (**A** and **B** Courtesy Riverside Methodist Hospitals, Columbus, Ohio.)

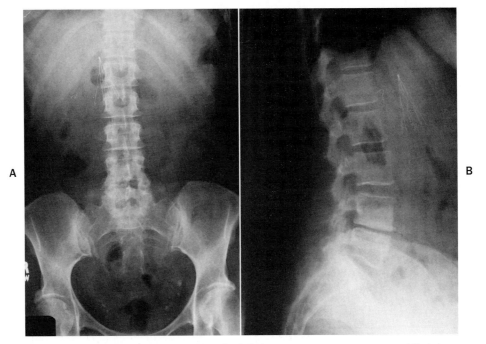

Fig. 8-24 A, Greenfield filter placement in the inferior vena cava, as seen on an AP abdomen radiograph. **B,** Greenfield filter placement in the inferior vena cava, as seen on a lateral abdomen radiograph. (**A** and **B** Courtesy Riverside Methodist Hospitals, Columbus, Ohio.)

who do not tolerate normal agents (Fig. 8-25). The role of interventional angiography will continue to grow and reduce costs and complications from certain surgical procedures it replaces.

Ultrafast CT, also known as *electron beam CT* is a newer technique to examine the heart, particularly as related to coronary artery calcifications. Uses expected in the next 2 to 3 years include noninvasive contrast-enhanced angiography, assessment of cardiac interventions, full evaluation of the left ventricle, and assessment of pulmonary emboli, pericardial disease, and congenital heart disease. The ultrafast CT unit uses a scanning focused x-ray beam to provide complete cardiac imaging in 50 ms—fast enough to "freeze" heart motion without the need for ECG gating. An electron gun produces an electron stream that is magnetically focused onto four tungsten targets. Each target emits two fan beams of x-rays, which are directed through the patient and registered on detectors arranged in a semicircle above the patient. The net result is that extremely thin slices are readily demonstrated, either as a cine loop or single images. These show calcifications, if present, which may represent a predictor of atherosclerosis and current heart disease. Despite its availability for a number of years, ultrafast CT has yet to make a major impact in diagnosis of cardiac disease.

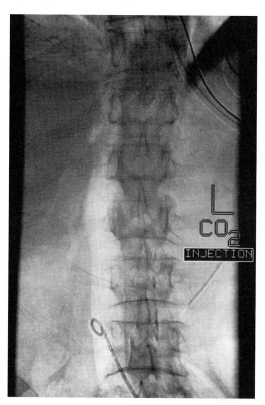

Fig. 8-25 Use of carbon dioxide (CO_2) as a contrast medium is demonstrated in this inferior vena cavagram (appearing white along the right of the spine) on a frail 75-year-old male. (Courtesy Riverside Methodist Hospitals, Columbus, Ohio.)

CONGENITAL AND HEREDITARY DISEASES

Because fetal circulation and blood-gas exchange occur within the placenta, certain characteristics are present in the fetal circulatory system that should normally disappear at birth. These characteristics include an opening in the septum between the atria, termed the **foramen ovale,** which allows the blood to bypass the pulmonary circulatory system, and a small vessel termed the **ductus arteriosus,** which connects the pulmonary artery and the descending aorta. If these anatomic structures persist, a variety of congenital anomalies can develop in the newborn. The incidence of congenital cardiovascular anomalies is approximately 8 per 1000 live births.

Etiology of congenital heart disease includes heritable disorders, chromosomal aberrations (such as Down syndrome), and environmental factors (such as drugs, infection, radiation, and maternal disease). In addition, individuals presenting with congenital anomalies of the heart are at an increased risk of developing endocardial infections. Approximately one third of all infants born with congenital anomalies of the heart die within the first month of life. Therefore, immediate diagnosis and treatment are vital. Radiography and diagnostic medical sonography play a critical role in the diagnosis and treatment of congenital anomalies, along with the diagnosis of heart murmurs by physical examination and abnormal heart rates demonstrated by electrocardiography. A **murmur** is an abnormal heart sound resulting from disturbed or turbulent flow, often through malformed valves.

Patent Ductus Arteriosus

The **ductus arteriosus** is a temporary vessel that serves during in utero life. It shunts blood from the pulmonary artery into the systemic circulation because the pulmonary circulation is unneeded during this time. If it does not close at birth, **patent ductus arteriosus** results (Fig. 8-26). Chest radiographs of the infant demonstrate cardiomegaly and increased pulmonary vascular congestion. This condition is more common in premature infants, especially in those who have respiratory distress syndrome.

Because the left ventricle contracts with more force than the right ventricle, the arterial blood within the aorta is shunted into the pulmonary trunk via the open ductus arteriosus instead of out into the systemic circulation. This increases the volume of blood propelled into the lungs, thus increasing pulmonary vascular congestion and the volume of blood returning to the left atrium. Infants with this condition generally display cyanotic features resulting from the shunting. Echocardiography is the imaging method of choice for evaluating the severity of this anomaly.

Coarctation of the Aorta

Although the ductus arteriosus may close normally at birth, a narrowing of the aorta may occur at the junction site. This anomaly is termed **coarctation of the aorta.** It occurs anatomically inferior to the vessels responsible for circulation to the head, neck, and upper extremities, so circulation to these anatomic regions is not affected. However, blood flow to the abdomen and lower extremities is compromised, and the femoral pulse is very weak in most individuals possessing this anomaly. Radiographically, two

bulges of the aorta are demonstrated in the aortic arch region, one superior to and one inferior to the stenosis. **Rib notching,** another radiographic indication of coarctation of the aorta (Fig. 8-27), refers to well-defined bony erosions along the lower rib margins as a result of the enlargement of anastomotic vessels. Coarctation of the aorta may be successfully treated surgically by removing the narrowed region of the aorta and reattaching the normal aorta superior and inferior to the coarctation.

Septal Defects

A defect in either the ventricular or atrial septum allows the blood to be shunted between the two chambers (Fig. 8-28), mixing pulmonary and systemic blood. The blood is generally shunted from the left to the right chamber because of increased pressure in the left side of the heart. This shunting of the blood results in an enlargement of the right side of the heart and increased pulmonary vascularitis as the lungs overload with blood.

Atrial septal defects are the most common congenital heart defect. If the foramen ovale does not close at birth, an opening remains between the right and left atria. In most cases, this does not require surgical intervention. **Ventricular septal defects** involve a defect between the two ventricles and are more serious because the pressure difference is greater between the ventricles than between the atria. Surgical intervention depends on the size of the defect and the risk of developing bacterial endocarditis at the site of the defect.

Transposition of Great Vessels

Transposition of the great vessels is an anomaly in which the aorta arises from the right ventricle instead of the left ventricle and the pulmonary trunk arises from the left ventricle instead of the right ventricle (Fig. 8-29). This serious congenital defect does not allow the pulmonary and systemic subsystems to communicate. Deoxygenated blood returns to the right atrium, travels through the right ventricle, and is

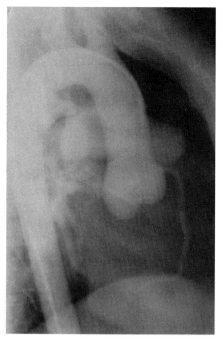

Fig. 8-26 Aortogram demonstrating patent ductus arteriosus. Notice filling of the pulmonary vessels as well as the aorta. (Courtesy Riverside Methodist Hospitals, Columbus, Ohio.)

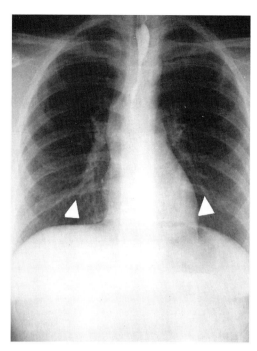

Fig. 8-27 Rib notching as seen with coarctation of the aorta. Other radiographic indicators include the considerable prominence of the aorta, and the indentation of the barium column just below the aortic knob. (Courtesy the American College of Radiology, Reston, Virginia.)

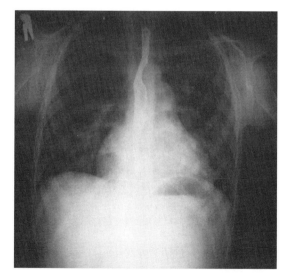

Fig. 8-28 Chest radiograph depicting ventricular septal defect. Notice the enlargement of the right heart border. (Courtesy Children's Hospital, Columbus, Ohio.)

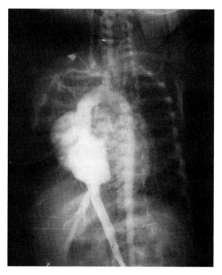

Fig. 8-29 Angiogram demonstrating transposition of great vessels. Notice the "closed" system of the right side of the heart. The blood is returned via the vena cavae, and redistributed via the aorta, thus bypassing the lungs. (Courtesy Children's Hospital, Columbus, Ohio.)

pumped through the aorta back into the systemic subsystem without becoming oxygenated. The oxygenated blood returns to the left atrium, travels through the right ventricle, and is pumped through the pulmonary trunk back to the lungs for gas exchange to occur. Obviously, this anomaly is incompatible with life. Because immediate recognition and treatment of this defect is imperative, emergency cardiac catheterization and balloon septostomy must be performed to enlarge the opening between the atria to increase mixing of venous and arterial blood and to decompress the left atrium. Surgical correction of this anomaly is indicated after the age of 6 months.

Tetralogy of Fallot

Tetralogy of Fallot is a combination of four defects: pulmonary stenosis, ventricular septal defect, overriding aorta, and hypertrophy of the right ventricle. The narrowing of the pulmonary valve prevents passage of a sufficient volume of blood from the right ventricle to the lungs and results in the most common cause of cyanosis in infants with cardiovascular anomalies. Normally, the aorta should arise from the left ventricle, but, in patients with tetralogy of Fallot, the aorta arises from a ventricular septal defect. In other words, it overrides the right ventricle, which, in turn, results in hypertrophy of the right ventricle. Enlargement of the right ventricle is demonstrated radiographically as a boot-shaped cardiac shadow caused by displacement of the heart apex (Fig. 8-30). Corrective surgery is usually performed after the age of 1 year.

VALVULAR DISEASE

Abnormalities of the heart's valves often cause cardiac symptoms such as dyspnea, fatigue, or chest pain, and signs such as murmurs. Additionally, valvar lesions often result in abnormal pulses detectable through palpation. Clinicians are often able to diagnose most valve abnormalities by assimilating historical and physical findings. Nonivasive techniques add to the precision

of diagnosis, and invasive studies are reserved for surgical candidates.

The most common cause of chronic valve disease of the heart is **rheumatic fever.** This condition most frequently affects the bicuspid (mitral) and aortic valves and is more common in females than in males. Because of advances in pharmaceuticals, technology, and medical care, the incidence of rheumatic heart disease is on the decline. Rheumatic fever produces inflammatory changes within the connective tissues of the body, thus affecting the valves within the heart. It may result in stenosis, insufficiency, or incompetency. Individuals suffering from rheumatic heart disease present with a distinct heart murmur audible upon physical examination.

Valvular stenosis is caused by a scarring of valve cusps that eventually adhere to one another. The results of valvular stenosis become apparent in adult life because it generally takes years for the scarring to affect valve function. Mitral valve stenosis inhibits blood flow from the left atrium into the left ventricle. It slows the blood flow through the lungs and the right side of the heart, resulting in an enlargement of the right side of the heart and the left atrium. Insufficiency and incompetency occur when the valves do not close properly and allow blood to

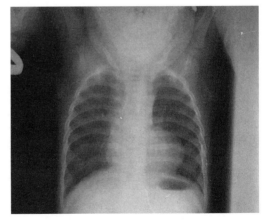

Fig. 8-30 Chest radiograph on an infant with tetralogy of Fallot. Notice the "boot-shaped" cardiac shadow. (Courtesy Children's Hospital, Columbus, Ohio.)

reflux during systole. This complication often follows endocarditis and most commonly affects the mitral or aortic valve.

Radiographically, manifestations of mitral stenosis may be subtle. More progressed cases may show the heart silhouette as enlarged, and the diseased valves may contain small calcifications. In severe cases, the diseased valves are replaced with prosthetic devices that are clearly visible on conventional chest radiographs (Fig. 8-31).

CONGESTIVE HEART FAILURE

Congestive heart failure occurs when the heart is unable to propel blood at a sufficient rate and volume. This results in congestion of the subcirculatory systems and does not allow a sufficient supply of blood to reach the tissues of the body. Congestive heart failure is most commonly caused by hypertension but may result from other disease processes that overburden the heart, such as valvular disease. Congestive heart failure may affect either side of the heart, but both sides are commonly affected together.

It may develop gradually or have a quick onset in combination with pulmonary edema. Regardless of the original side affected, prolonged strain on the heart eventually affects the entire organ. Signs and symptoms may vary with the extent and location of the disease. The treatment of congestive failure is usually medical but depends on the cause and severity of the disease and may include surgical intervention, especially in cases of valvular disease.

Left-Sided Failure

When the left ventricle of the heart cannot pump an amount of blood equal to the venous return in the right ventricle, the pulmonary subcirculatory system becomes overloaded. The fluid that accumulates in the capillaries of the lungs leaks into the interstitial tissues within the lungs. This results in rales and pulmonary edema, which can be a life-threatening condition. Radiographically, the heart is enlarged, and the hilar region of the lungs are congested with increased vascular markings (Fig. 8-32). Upon

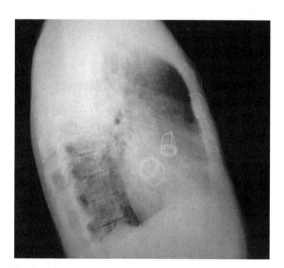

Fig. 8-31 Lateral chest radiograph demonstrating two prosthetic valve replacements clearly visible within the heart. (Courtesy the American College of Radiology, Reston, Virginia.)

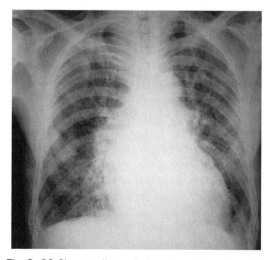

Fig. 8-32 Chest radiograph demonstrating left-sided congestive heart failure. Notice the engorgement of the pulmonary vessels and interstitial fluid accumulation within the lung tissue. (Courtesy the American College of Radiology, Reston, Virginia.)

physical examination, individuals with left-sided heart failure present with an increased heart rate because the heart tries to compensate for the deficiency. Individuals commonly complain of difficulty in breathing or shortness of breath upon exertion and respiratory distress severe enough to awaken them during the night. As the disease progresses, sleeping in a recumbent position becomes impossible. The most common cause of left-side failure is hypertension, but other causes include aortic and mitral valvular disease and coronary artery disease.

Right-Sided Failure

Right ventricular failure is not as common as left-sided failure and occurs when the right ventricle cannot pump as much blood as it receives from the right atrium. This causes the venous blood flow to slow down, producing engorgement of the superior and inferior venae cavae and edema of the lower extremities. A common complaint from individuals with right-sided failure is swelling of their ankles. Radiographically, the right atrium and right ventricle appear enlarged. Common causes of true, right-sided failure are pulmonary valve stenosis, emphysema, and pulmonary hypertension secondary to pulmonary emboli.

DEGENERATIVE DISEASES

Atherosclerosis

Atherosclerosis is a degenerative condition affecting the major arteries of the body, often termed *hardening of the arteries*. It is the most prevalent disease in humans, occurring in epidemic proportions in the United States. The etiology of atherosclerosis is unknown, and researchers are not sure whether it is genetic in origin or an acquired, environmental disease. It affects sexes equally; however, it tends to affect males at an earlier age than females. Atherosclerosis may occur in any artery (Fig. 8-33), but it has a predilection for the aorta, coronary arteries, and cerebral arteries (Fig. 8-34). Risk factors

associated with this disorder include increased age, increased serum lipoproteins and cholesterol, hypertension, increased blood sugar levels, cigarette smoking, and a sedentary lifestyle. In addition, some other disease processes, such as diabetes mellitus, predispose individuals to atherosclerotic disease.

The cause of the development of **atheroma formations** (fibro-fatty plaques) within the vessel is currently being deleted.. The most common theory suggests that the disease process first affects the intima or inner layer of the artery, which narrows the lumen, and secondarily affects the media or middle layer, causing a weakening in the vessel wall. As the disease progresses, the atheroma may calcify, hemorrhage, ulcerate, or

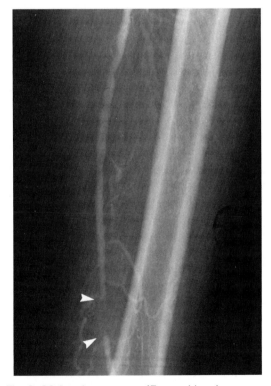

Fig. 8–33 Arteriogram on a 47-year-old male demonstrates how atherosclerosis occludes the femoral artery. (Courtesy Riverside Methodist Hospitals, Columbus, Ohio.)

include a superimposed thrombosis. These arterial changes often occur silently, and symptoms may not be present until atheroma formation occludes more than two thirds of the vessel. In some cases, this slow narrowing allows enough time for the formation of collateral vessels to maintain blood supply distal to the stenotic site. If normal blood supply is decreased or stopped completely, **ischemia** occurs. Unfortunately, the most common signs and symptoms associated with atherosclerotic disease result from ischemia of a vital organ, such as the heart or brain, or a weakening of a vital artery resulting in an aneurysm. Atherosclerotic disease is the most common cause of coronary heart disease and cerebrovascular accidents.

Cardiovascular angiography is often used in the diagnosis and treatment of atherosclerosis through the use of percutaneous transluminal angioplasty. Doppler sonography also plays a major role in diagnosis of atherosclerosis (Fig. 8-35). MRI and echocardiography are both noninvasive modalities that may also visualize blood flow without the use of contrast agents.

Coronary Artery Disease

Coronary artery disease (CAD) results from the deposition of atheromas in the arteries supplying blood to the heart muscle. As the plaques accumulate in the coronary arteries, blood supply to the heart muscle is decreased, resulting in ischemia, a local and temporary impairment of circulation due to obstruction of circulation, and myocardial damage as an **infarct**, an area of ischemic necrosis. Major complications of coronary artery disease include angina pectoris (chest pain), myocardial infarction, and subsequent

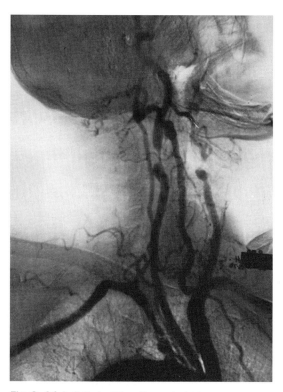

Fig. 8–34 A digital subtraction arteriogram demonstrating atherosclerotic disease of carotid artery. Notice that the carotid artery is almost completely occluded. (Courtesy the American College of Radiology, Reston, Virginia.)

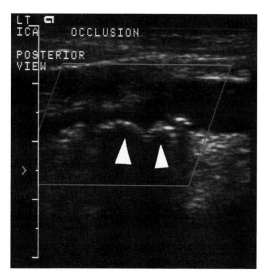

Fig. 8–35 Atherosclerosis as seen in Doppler sonography of the internal carotid artery in a 75-year old male. Arrows point to the"hilly" plaque deposit on the lower surface of the artery; the lack of echo signal underneath them indicates calcium contained within the plaque. (Courtesy Riverside Methodist Hospitals, Columbus, Ohio.)

myocardial necrosis, if the patient survives the heart attack. Acute myocardial infarction causes approximately 35% of the deaths in men in the United States between the ages of 35 and 50 years. It is the single most frequent cause of death in the United States. Most cases, upon autopsy, demonstrate significant widespread atherosclerotic disease of the coronary arteries.

Clinical signs and symptoms of myocardial infarction include a sudden onset of severe crushing chest pain that may radiate down the left arm or up into the neck. It may be accompanied by profuse sweating, shortness of breath, nausea, or vomiting. In milder cases, it may be passed off as indigestion. Immediate medical attention is critical to the survival of individuals experiencing a myocardial infarction. Approximately 20% to 25% of these patients die before reaching the hospital. Early medical intervention significantly increases survival. Survival rates are approximately 85% for those first attack victims receiving medical attention within the first 30 minutes after the attack. The prognosis of coronary artery disease is variable, depending largely on the location of the occlusion, the extent of damage to the heart muscle, and the amount of collateral circulation available. Cardiac angiography plays a major role in the diagnosis of stenotic or occluded heart vessels (Figs. 8-36 and 8-37). In some cases, percutaneous transluminal angioplasty may be performed to open these vessels.

Medical treatments of coronary artery disease may include antianginal drugs to improve circulation and decrease the amount of oxygen consumed by the myocardium. Other cases may be treated surgically with coronary artery bypass grafts, which involve bypassing the obstruction with a segment of the saphenous vein. A portion of the saphenous vein is removed from the patient's leg, and one end is attached to the aorta above the level of the coronary arteries. The lower end of the graft is attached to the coronary artery, beyond the site of the occlusion.

Nuclear medicine studies such as myocardial perfusion scans and gated examinations are im-portant noninvasive methods of determining the presence and extent of coronary artery disease; these studies also assist in the clinical management of postmyocardial patients. In addition, echocardiography may be used to provide needed clinical information in the diagnosis, treatment, and management of coronary artery disease.

Cerebrovascular Accident

Atherosclerotic disease affecting the blood supply to the brain results in a **cerebrovascular accident (CVA)**, commonly referred to as a *stroke*. There are essentially two ways a stroke occurs. In an **ischemic stroke,** a blood clot blocks a blood vessel in the brain. Ischemic strokes account for 83% of all strokes. In a **hemorrhagic stroke,** a blood vessel in the brain breaks or ruptures.

Under normal circumstances, blood clotting slows and eventually stops bleeding and is beneficial. In a stroke, however, blood clots are dangerous because they can block blood flow and cause ischemia. An ischemic stroke can occur in two ways: infarction caused by thrombosis of a cerebral artery or embolism to the brain from a thrombus elsewhere in the body. A **thrombus** is a blood clot that obstructs a blood vessel, and an **embolus** is a mass of undissolved matter (solid, liquid, or gas) present in a blood vessel brought there by blood current. Vessel occlusion by an embolus usually results in development of an infarct.

The most frequent type of CVA results from thrombosis, accounting for about 52% of all strokes. These may be easily diagnosed with angiography. Two types of thrombosis can cause stroke: large vessel thrombosis and small vessel disease, also known as **lacunar infarction.** Large vessel thrombosis most often occurs in the large arteries as a result of long-term atherosclerosis followed by rapid blood clot formation. Typical sites are the bifurcation of the common carotid artery, within the carotid sinus, or the termination of the internal carotid artery, giving rise to the cerebral arteries (Fig. 8-38). An infarct caused by thrombosis of a cerebral artery is

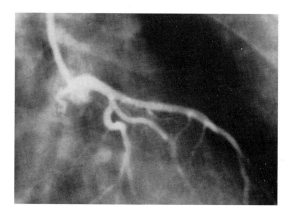

Fig. 8–36 Coronary angiography demonstrates a normal left anterior descending artery as shown in this RAO projection. (Courtesy Riverside Methodist Hospitals, Columbus, Ohio.)

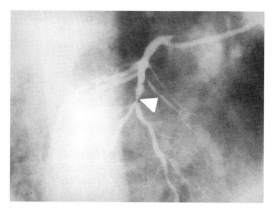

Fig. 8–37 A major stenosis is seen in this coronary arteriogram in an LAO projection, just as the left coronary artery bifurcates into the left anterior desending artery to the right and a major diagonal branch to the left. (Courtesy Riverside Methodist Hospitals, Columbus, Ohio.)

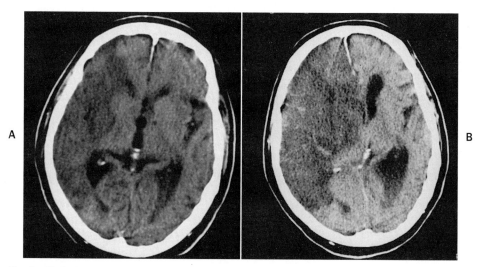

A   B

Fig. 8–38 A, An unenhanced C.T. of the brain of a 83-year-old female reveals a large infarct along the distribution of the middle cerebral artery on the right side; **B,** A similar unenhanced CT taken 4 days later reveals worsening of the edema with early shift of the right lateral and third ventricles to the left. (**A** and **B** Courtesy Riverside Methodist Hospitals, Columbus, Ohio)

termed an **atherothrombic brain infarction** (ABI). Symptoms associated with ABI develop slowly over a period of hours or days and include confusion, hemiplegia, and aphasia. This type of CVA may be preceded by a temporary episode of neurologic dysfunction termed a **transient ischemic attack** (TIA), which includes hemiparesis, hemiparesthesia, or monocular blindness. These symptoms should clear within 24 hours. Patients with a thrombotic stroke are also likely to have coronary artery disease, and heart attack is a frequent cause of death for those who have a thrombotic stroke.

Small vessel disease (i.e., lacunar infarction) occurs when blood flow is blocked to a very small arterial vessel. *Lacune* is French for "hole" and describes the small cavity that remains after products of a deep infarct have been removed by other cells. Although little is known about small vessel disease, it is closely linked to hypertension. About 20% of all strokes are caused by small vessel disease.

Infarction may also be caused by an embolism to the brain from a thrombus elsewhere in the body, most commonly from the left side of the heart. Those CVAs resulting from cerebral embolism have a sudden onset of symptoms without warning. The prognosis is much better for CVAs caused by infarct than for those from hemorrhage. The 30-day survival rate associated with infarct is approximately 73%. Angiography, Doppler sonography, CT, and MRI (Fig. 8-39) all play vital roles in the diagnosis and management of CVAs.

In a hemorrhagic stroke, brain hemorrhage results from a weakening in the diseased vessel wall. Typically, the ruptured vessel has been weakened by arteriosclerosis from hypertension. The onset of this type of CVA is sudden and often lethal because it expands rapidly. Brain hemorrhages account for approximately 10% to 15% of all cerebrovascular accidents and are of two types: subarachnoid and intracerebral. Most bleeds occur in the cerebrum and bleed into the

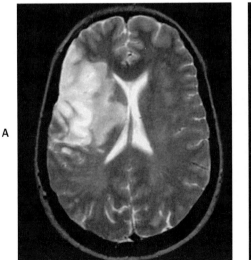
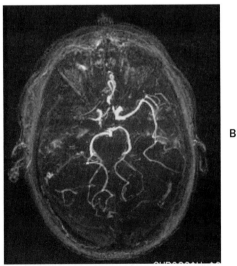

A

B

Fig. 8-39 **A,** An MRI of the head of a 54 year-old female who experienced sudden left facial paralysis and slumped forward while shopping reveals a large infarct along the distribution of the middle cerebral artery. **B,** An MR angiogram of the same patient demonstrates occlusion of the middle cerebral artery, thought likely to be secondary to an embolus from carotid artery disease. (**A** and **B** Courtesy Riverside Methodist Hospitals, Columbus, Ohio.)

lateral ventricle. Most commonly, they are preceded by an intense headache that is often accompanied by vomiting. Loss of consciousness follows within minutes and leads to total contralateral hemiplegia or death. The prognosis of this type of CVA is very poor; it has a 30-day survival rate of approximately 17%.

ANEURYSMS

A localized "ballooning" or outpouching of a vessel wall is called an **aneurysm.** It results when the vessel wall has been weakened by atherosclerotic disease, trauma, infection, or congenital defects. Aneurysms are usually classified as saccular, fusiform, or dissecting. A **saccular aneurysm** is a localized bulge involving one side of the arterial wall (Fig. 8-40). Usually, it is lo-

cated in a cerebral artery. If this bulging includes the entire circumference of the vessel wall, it is termed **fusiform.** This type is often found in the distal abdominal aorta. A **dissecting aneurysm** results when the intima tears and allows blood to flow within the vessel wall, thus forming an intramural hematoma (Fig. 8-41). Symptoms of a dissecting aneurysm often mock those of a

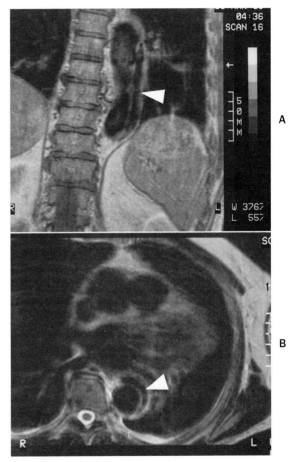

Fig. 8-41 A, A dissecting aneurysm in a 79-year-old male seen in a coronal MRI view, with clear depiction of the extraluminal flow. **B,** A dissecting aneurysm in a 79-year old male, seen as extraluminal flow in this transverse MRI view, which represents a view looking down into the aorta. (**A** and **B** Courtesy Riverside Methodist Hospitals, Columbus, Ohio.)

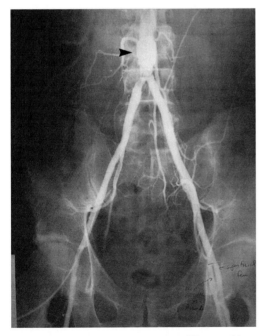

Fig. 8-40 Abdominal aortogram on a 53-year-old male demonstrating a saccular abdominal aneurysm and bilateral areas of stenosis at the bifurcation of the aorta into the common iliac arteries. (Courtesy Riverside Methodist Hospitals, Columbus, Ohio.)

heart attack. Angiography is often used in the diagnosis of aneurysms. Diagnostic medical sonography and CT are often of value, especially in the case of a dissecting aneurysm.

VENOUS THROMBOSIS

The formation of blood clots within a vein is called **venous thrombosis.** These clots commonly form in the veins of the lower extremities (Fig. 8-42) and result from a slowing of the blood return to the heart. The contraction of the leg muscles assists with venous blood return; therefore, postoperative or bedfast patients are especially prone to this disorder. **Phlebitis,** an inflammation of the vein, is often associated with venous thrombosis. The medical term used to specify the combination of these disorders is **thrombophlebitis.**

Venography is often performed to determine the location and the extent of this disease. One major complication associated with deep vein thrombosis is a pulmonary embolism. Filters may be placed in the patient's inferior vena cava to prevent these clots from reaching the kidneys and chest. These filters may be inserted under fluoroscopic control and are clearly visible on plain radiographs of the abdomen (Fig. 8-43).

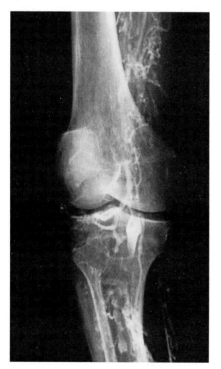

Fig. 8-42 Venogram of the left lower extremity demonstrating deep vein thrombosis. (Courtesy Riverside Methodist Hospitals, Columbus, Ohio.)

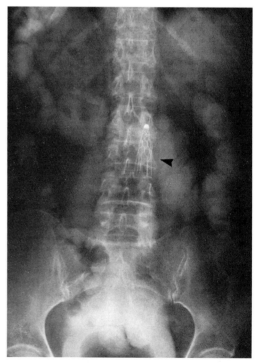

Fig. 8-43 Abdominal radiograph on an elderly female demonstrating the proper placement of a vena cava filter. (Courtesy Riverside Methodist Hospitals, Columbus, Ohio.)

QUESTIONS

1. The heart chamber located most anteriorly and comprising the anterior border of the cardiac shadow on a lateral chest radiograph is the:
   a. left atrium
   b. left ventricle
   c. right atrium
   d. right ventricle

2. The bicuspid valve is also known as the:
   a. left atrioventricular valve
   b. right atrioventricular valve
   c. aortic valve
   d. pulmonary valve

3. Contraction of the myocardium is termed:
   a. diastole
   b. systole
   c. peristole
   d. myostol

4. How many posterior ribs should be visible on a good inspiration PA chest radiograph?
   a. 12
   b. 10
   c. 8
   d. 6

5. In a fetus, the ductus arteriosus connects which two structures?
   a. aorta and SVC
   b. aorta and pulmonary trunk
   c. right and left atria
   d. right and left ventricles

6. Tetralogy of Fallot includes which of the following defects?
   a. pulmonary stenosis
   b. ventricular septal defect
   c. hypertrophy of right ventricle
   d. a and c
   e. a, b and c

7. Which valves are most commonly affected by rheumatic heart disease?
   a. mitral
   b. pulmonary
   c. tricuspid
   d. all of the above

8. A condition in which the left ventricle cannot pump an amount of blood equal to the venous return of the right ventricle is:
   a. coronary artery disease
   b. left-sided congestive heart failure
   c. right-sided congestive heart failure
   d. patent ductus arteriosus

9. Risk factors associated with atherosclerosis include:
   1. low blood sugar levels
   2. hypertension
   3. cigarette smoking
      a. 1 and 2
      b. 1 and 3
      c. 2 and 3
      d. 1, 2 and 3

10. A decrease in tissue blood supply is termed:
    a. atheroma
    b. infarction
    c. ischemia
    d. necrosis

11. The single most frequent cause of male deaths in the United States is:
    a. congestive heart failure
    b. coronary artery disease
    c. transposition of great vessels
    d. valvular disease

12. Clinical signs of a myocardial infarction include:
    1. shortness of breath
    2. crushing chest pain
    3. neck pain
       a. 1 and 2
       b. 1 and 3
       c. 2 and 3
       d. 1, 2 and 3

13. Which type of vessels are used as the graft material for coronary artery bypass grafts?
    a. arteries
    b. capillaries
    c. veins

14. The term *atherothrombic brain infarction* denotes:
    a. brain hemorrhage due to atherosclerosis
    b. infarction caused by thrombosis of a cerebral artery
    c. an embolism to the brain from a left heart thrombus
    d. none of the above

15. Imaging procedures that may be used to demonstrate an abdominal aneurysm include:
    a. angiography
    b. CT
    c. diagnostic sonography
    d. a and b
    e. a, b and c

16. Which type of aneurysm results when the intima tears and allows blood to flow within the vessel wall?

17. An elderly patient presents with shortness of breath upon exertion and overall respiratory distress. A chest radiograph reveals an enlarged heart and a congested hilar region, with some pulmonary edema. What is a likely cause?

18. Identify at least two common sites for atherosclerosis to occur.

19. What is the cause of ischemia in coronary artery disease?

20. What is the most common cause for CVA and the most common site for it to occur?

The Hemopoietic System

Anatomy and Physiology Review
Imaging Considerations
Acquired Immune Deficiency Syndrome

Neoplastic Disease
  Multiple myeloma
  Leukemia
  Hodgkin's disease

Upon completion of Chapter 9, the reader should be able to:

- Identify the major constituents of blood and describe the function of each constituent.

- Specify the various blood types.

- Explain the role of the lymphatic system in terms of immunity.

- Describe the pathogenesis, prognosis, and signs and symptoms of the disease processes discussed in this chapter.

KEY TERMS

Erythrocytes
Anemia
Hematocrit
Hemocytoblasts
Reticuloendothelial
   system
Agglutination
Rh factor
Rh-positive

Rh-negative
Leukocytes
Thrombocytes
Lymph
Lymph nodes
Lymphocytes
Lymphadenogram
Acquired immune deficiency
   syndrome

Human immunodeficiency
   virus
Pneumocystis carinii
   pneumonia
Kaposi's sarcoma
Multiple myeloma
Leukemia
Hodgkin's disease
Reed-Sternberg cells

ANATOMY AND PHYSIOLOGY REVIEW

The hemopoietic system consists of blood, lymphatic tissue, bone marrow, and the spleen. The circulating blood contains both plasma and blood cells, with the plasma comprising approximately 55% of the total blood volume. The plasma is about 90% water and 10% solutes such as proteins, glucose, amino acids, and lipids. Three basic types of blood cells—erythrocytes, leukocytes, and thrombocytes (Table 9-1)—make up the remaining 45% of the total blood volume.

The **erythrocytes** or red blood cells are very small in relation to the other blood cells. They do not possess a nucleus and are shaped like biconcave disks. Erythrocytes are responsible for transporting oxygen and carbon dioxide to and from the various organs of the body. This is accomplished via the hemoglobin in the erythrocytes, which allows oxygen or carbon dioxide molecules to attach to the cell for transport. Individuals with a hemoglobin level of less than 12 g per 100 ml of blood have **anemia** and are considered "anemic" because they have less than normal oxygen or carbon dioxide transportation occurring. The total percent of red blood cells in blood volume is determined by a laboratory test termed **hematocrit.**

Erythrocytes are formed by specialized cells called **hemocytoblasts** that are located in the myeloid tissue found within red bone marrow.

Table 9-1   Blood Cell Types

Type	Formed by	Function	Life Span
Erythrocyte	Myeloid tissue within red bone marrow	Transporting O_2 and CO_2	120 days
Leukocyte	Granular: red bone marrow Nongranular: lymphatic tissue	Body defense, immunity	Granular: 2 weeks Nongranular: years
Thrombocyte	Myeloid tissue within red bone marrow	Blood clotting	10 days

These cells live approximately 120 days and are phagocytosed by the **reticuloendothelial system,** which consists of specialized cells in the liver, spleen, and bone marrow. During the phagocytosis, the iron within the hemoglobin is released and bilirubin is formed. The iron is used again in the development of new erythrocytes, and the bilirubin is excreted in the bile.

Erythrocytes may contain various antigens that determine blood type. This is especially critical for blood transfusions because blood type incompatibility can have fatal results. Erythrocytes may contain no antigens, either the A or B antigen, or both the A and B antigens. The resulting blood types are O (no antigen), A, B, and AB. If incompatible blood types are mixed (e.g., a type O patient receives type AB blood), the erythrocytes from the donor clump together in the serum of the recipient. Because the type O recipient does not possess the A or B antigen, antibodies are formed to fight against the foreign red blood cells. This is termed **agglutination.** Eventually, the recipient destroys the donor erythrocytes with the rejection, possibly resulting in immediate shock. In some cases, the reaction may be delayed, resulting in fever, pain, and ultimate renal failure as the kidneys try to excrete the by-products produced from the destruction of the erythrocytes. Crossmatching of blood types to eliminate the chance of a recipient's receiving incompatible blood is essential.

Type O blood is considered the universal donor because it does not contain any antigens and can be given to anyone, regardless of blood type. Type AB is considered the universal recipient because it possesses both antigens and can receive any type of blood (Table 9-2). In addition, the Rh blood factor should also be considered. The **Rh factor** is termed such because it was first discovered in the blood of the rhesus monkey. Approximately 85% of the human population contains this factor and are classified as **Rh-positive.** Individuals not possessing the Rh factor are **Rh-negative.** The Rh factor becomes a problem if an Rh-positive father transmits the Rh factor to a fetus carried by an Rh-negative mother. The first pregnancy generally progresses normally, but in subsequent pregnancies the mother's anti-Rh antibodies, made during the first pregnancy, attack the Rh-positive fetal blood. This scenario can be avoided by Rh immunization of the mother before pregnancy.

Leukocytes or white blood cells may be classified as granular or nongranular. Granular leukocytes contain cytoplasmic granules and irregular nuclei. They are formed within the red bone marrow and include basophils, neutrophils, and eosinophils. The names of these cells correspond to the manner in which they respond to certain dyes for microscopic inspection. Nongranular leukocytes do not contain cytoplasmic granules, and they possess regular nuclei. They are mainly formed in the lymphatic tissue of the spleen and include lymphocytes and monocytes. Leukocytes play an important role in the body's defense system. They are able to move out of capillaries into tissue to "attack" and phagocytose foreign substances. The life span of leukocytes varies, depending on the type of cell. Granular leukocytes live for only about 2 weeks, whereas lymphocytes may live for years. Normal blood contains between 5000 and 9000 leukocytes per cubic milliliter. Changes in the number of leukocytes often indicate the presence of disease.

The third major type of blood cells is the **thrombocytes** or platelets. These cells are

Table 9-2 Cross-Matching of Blood Types

Recipient Blood Type	Acceptable Donor Type			
	A	**B**	**AB**	**O†**
A	yes	no	no	yes
B	no	yes	no	yes
AB*	yes	yes	yes	yes
O†	no	no	no	yes

*AB-Universal Recipient
†O-Universal Donor

necessary for blood to clot properly and respond within seconds to initiate the coagulation process. The thrombocytes are also formed in the myeloid tissue within the red bone marrow and have a life span of approximately 10 days.

The lymphatic system is a subsystem of the circulatory system. Its major function is in assuring immunity through production of lymphocytes and antibodies, but it is also responsible for absorbing fat from the intestinal tract and for manufacturing blood under certain circumstances. The lymphatic system is comprised by both lymphatic vessels and nodes. Lymphatic vessels contain a milky liquid substance termed **lymph.** The **lymph nodes** are small ovoid bodies attached in a chainlike pattern along the vessels. They filter out particles and foreign materials from the blood. Major areas of lymph node chains include the neck, mediastinum, axillary, retroperitoneal, pelvic, and inguinal regions. These lymph nodes often become enlarged when the body is invaded by an infectious agent and in cases of neoplastic disease.

The spleen, which is also part of the lymphatic system, is an oval organ in the left upper quadrant. Its chief function is production of lymphocytes and plasma cells. Additionally, it stores red blood cells and functions in phagocytosis. It is occasionally ruptured in abdominal trauma and can be removed without detrimental effects.

Mature **lymphocytes** are the most important cell in the development of immunity. T lymphocytes are derived from lymphatic tissue of the thymus gland, and B lymphocytes are derived from the bone marrow. These two types of lymphocytes work together with macrophages to ingest foreign substances and process the specific foreign antigens. Via a complex process, an antibody is formed capable of attacking the foreign antigen. An antibody is an immunoglobulin produced by plasma cells and can be categorized into one of five classifications: IgG, IgM, IgA, IgD, and IgE. This is the systemic response that can have a negative effect on tissue grafts and organ transplants. The human body sees the transplant as foreign; therefore, the lymphocytes and macrophages try to destroy the foreign antigens, resulting in rejection of the graft or organ.

Although the risk of whole-body radiation exposure is of little concern in diagnostic radiology, it is important for the radiographer to remember that exposure to x-rays or gamma rays can have a harmful effect on the blood marrow and lymphoid tissue. It takes a whole-body dose of approximately 50 to 75 rads to cause a detectable change in the blood cells. The most radiosensitive blood cells are the lymphocytes, followed by the leukocytes and thrombocytes.

IMAGING CONSIDERATIONS

Radiography plays a limited role in the diagnosis and treatment of hemopoietic disorders. Skeletal radiography may be used in cases of multiple myeloma and for some types of leukemia. Chest radiographs are helpful in identifying lymphatic changes within the mediastinum and various opportunistic infections associated with acquired immune deficiency syndrome (AIDS). Abdominal computed tomography (CT) is also of great value in the assessment of lymph node enlargement (Fig. 9-1) and may be followed by lymphography to further determine the location and extent of neoplastic diseases of the lymphatic system.

During lymphography, an oily medium is injected through cut-down of the foot into a lymph vessel readily visualized through earlier injection of an indicator dye. Initial radiographs or lymphangiogram films are taken immediately following the injection of contrast material to visualize the lymphatic vessels (Fig. 9-2, *A*). The patient then returns in approximately 24 hours for additional radiographs, termed **lymphadenograms,** which visualize the lymph nodes (Fig. 9-2, *B*). Contrast usually leaves the lymph vessels within a matter of hours, but nodes can retain contrast media for a month or longer, particularly when diseased. Patients with significantly compromised pulmonary function are contraindicated for lymphography as the lungs receive the overflow of oily contrast media through the thoracic duct.

Magnetic resonance imaging (MRI) is proving to be quite useful in imaging bone marrow and the diseases that affect the marrow. Although MRI produces a signal void in areas of compact bone, changes in the marrow pattern are quite visible and useful in the diagnosis of many disorders (Fig. 9-3).

Many bloodborne pathogens may be transmitted to the health care worker. Therefore, it is of utmost importance that radiographers always practice universal precautions in terms of blood and other body fluids. Precautions must be taken when the radiographer may come into contact with blood or other body fluids, and

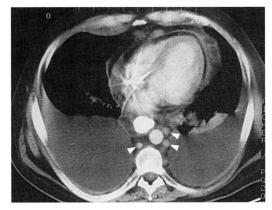

Fig. 9-1 CT of the lower chest and upper abdomen demonstrating enlargement of lymph nodes on a 27-year-old man with lymphoma. (Courtesy Ohio State University Hospitals, Columbus, Ohio.)

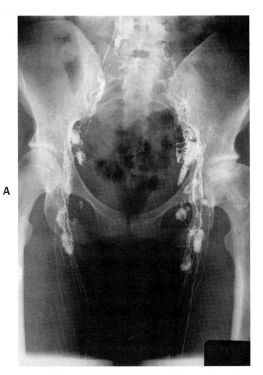

A

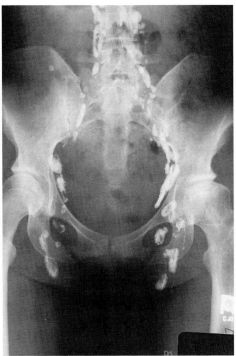

B

Fig. 9-2 A, Lymphogram film of a 24 year-old man suspected of having Hodgkin's disease, taken after contrast injections, shows collection in the lower extremity lymph vessels.
B, Lymphogram film of the same patient taken 24 hours later reveals collection of the contrast medium in the pelvic and abdominal lymph nodes, with no obvious deformity of the nodes. (**A** and **B** Courtesy Riverside Methodist Hospitals, Columbus, Ohio.)

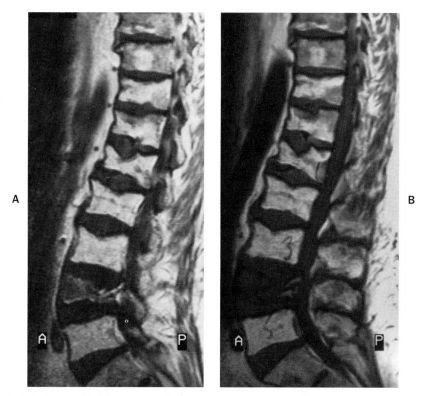

Fig. 9-3 A, A T$_2$ weighted sagittal MRI view without gadolinium demonstrates an obvious L4 lesion. **B,** A T$_2$ weighted sagittal MRI view with gadolinium demonstrates L4 destruction, consistent with multiple myeloma in this 55-year-old man. (**A** and **B** Courtesy Riverside Methodist Hospitals, Columbus, Ohio.)

gloves should be worn whenever the possibility of contamination exists. Additional protective apparel may be necessary if large amounts of body fluids may be encountered. Needles should not be recapped; they should be placed in puncture-proof containers for hazardous waste disposal. Handwashing cannot be over-emphasized because it plays an important role in good infection control practices. It is the single most significant factor in infection control.

ACQUIRED IMMUNE DEFICIENCY SYNDROME

Acquired immune deficiency syndrome (AIDS) was first recognized in 1981. It is caused by the

human immunodeficiency virus (HIV) and acts to paralyze the normal immune mechanisms within the human body. This virus inhibits the body's response to the presence of a variety of diseases; thus, one major sign of AIDS is the presence of unusual opportunistic infections such as *Pneumocystis carinii, Toxoplasma gondii,* cryptococci, *Mycobacterium avium,* herpes, and Kaposi's sarcoma. Other signs and symptoms include generalized lymphadenopathy, malaise, fever, and weight loss. It may also affect the central nervous system resulting in apathy, memory loss, inability to concentrate, and dementia.

With no known cure and approximately a 90% mortality rate, AIDS remains a major health crisis. The virus may lie dormant in an in-

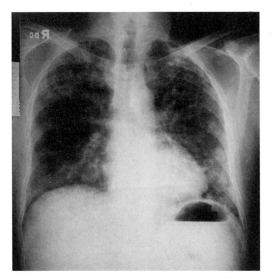

Fig. 9-4 Chest radiograph of a 53-year-old man diagnosed with AIDS. The radiograph demonstrates *Pneumocystis carinii* pneumonia with diffuse bilateral airspace parenchymal infiltrative densities. (Courtesy American College of Radiology, Reston, Virginia.)

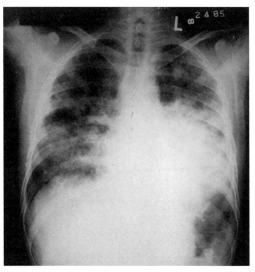

Fig. 9-5 Chest radiograph of a 27-year-old man with Kaposi's sarcoma of the skin and pulmonary involvement showing nodular diffuse patchy parenchymal infiltration with nodular densities in the upper lobes. (Courtesy American College of Radiology, Reston, Virginia.)

dividual for years; however, this does not happen in most patients. Emerging treatments are extending the lives of individuals, hence the 90% mortality rate. Although it can affect anyone, regardless of age or sexual orientation, HIV most frequently affects homosexual and bisexual males and intravenous drug users. The virus is transmitted through sexual contact and exposure to infected blood and body fluids.

One of the most common life-threatening infections associated with AIDS is *pneumocystis carinii* pneumonia, often in combination with a cytomegalovirus. It occurs in over half of all AIDS patients. Chest radiographs (Fig. 9-4) reveal bilateral perihilar reticular-interstitial infiltrates that rapidly progress within 3 to 5 days to diffuse consolidation.

Kaposi's sarcoma is the most common malignancy in AIDS patients. It is present in approximately 25% to 30% and may affect the connective tissue in various sites within the body. It most often affects the skin, lymph nodes, and gastrointestinal system. About 20% of patients with Kaposi's sarcoma also demonstrate pulmonary involvement. Radiographically, the patients present with hilar adenopathy, nodular pulmonary infiltrates, and pleural effusion (Fig. 9-5). Endobronchial Kaposi's sarcoma is frequent and may result in atelectasis or postobstruction pneumonia.

NEOPLASTIC DISEASE

Multiple Myeloma

Multiple myeloma is a neoplastic disease of the plasma cells that results in cell proliferation. It is usually confined to the bone marrow and forms discrete tumors that weaken the affected bone. Multiple myeloma most frequently affects the pelvis, spine, ribs, and skull. The abnormal plasma cells produce large amounts of protein, specifically the immunoglobulins, which create a variety of problems in addition to skeletal involvement. This protein is excreted via the urine and disrupts normal renal function. The protein can be detected in both blood and urine.

Typically seen in persons over the age of 50, the signs and symptoms of multiple myeloma include progressive bone pain, anemia, fatigue, bleeding disorders, renal insufficiency or failure, hypercalcemia, and recurrent bacterial infections, especially pneumococcal pneumonia. Radiography plays a vital role in the diagnosis and treatment of multiple myeloma because skeletal radiographs demonstrate diffuse osteoporosis with discrete osteolytic regions (Fig. 9-6). Chemotherapy and palliative radiation therapy may be prescribed, but the prognosis is poor because

as the disease progresses it leads to multiple bone lesions, renal failure, and infections. The median survival of patients with multiple myeloma is approximately 2 to 3 years.

Leukemia

Leukemia is a term associated with neoplastic disease of leukocytes that results in an overproduction of white blood cells. This increase in leukocytes interferes with normal blood cell production and may lead to anemia, bleeding, and infection. Leukemias can infiltrate lymphatic tissue and organs such as the liver and spleen. The cause of leukemia is unknown, but exposure to irradiation and certain chemicals (especially benzene) seem to predispose individuals to developing this disorder.

Leukemias are classified according to cell type and cell maturity. Granulocytic or myelocytic leukemias develop from primitive or stem cells. Monocytic leukemias develop from precursor cells (the cells from which leukocytes are derived) and are the least common type of leukemia. Lymphocytic leukemias arise from lymphoid cells. Additionally, leukemias are classified as either acute or chronic. Acute leukemias have an abrupt onset and may present as a hemorrhagic episode. They generally are associated with primitive or poorly differentiated cells. Chronic leukemias progress at a relatively slow pace with nonspecific signs such as fatigue and weakness. They are associated with mature or well-differentiated cells. These terms are used in combination to describe the specific type of leukemia. Acute lymphocytic leukemia (ALL) predominantly affects children. Chronic lymphocytic leukemia (CLL) predominantly affects individuals over age 50. Chronic myelocytic leukemia (CML), also called *chronic granulocytic leukemia* (CGL), most often affects adults between the ages of 20 and 50. Acute myelocytic leukemia (AML) and acute monoblastic leukemia (AMOL) can affect anyone at any age. Leukemias, in general, account for

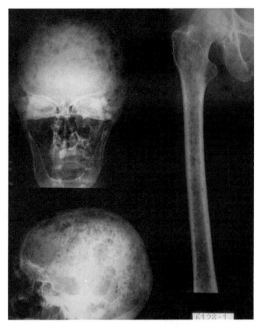

Fig. 9-6 Radiographs of a 65-year-old man with multiple myeloma demonstrating the presence of innumerable, discrete, lytic, well-circumscribed skeletal defects. (Courtesy American College of Radiology, Reston, Virginia.)

approximately 33% of all cancer deaths in children under the age of 15 years.

In many cases, proper therapy can stop the pathologic process. Regardless of the type of leukemia, all forms require the destruction of cells by either radiation or antileukemic drug therapy that renders the patient severely immunosuppressed. In some cases, bone marrow transplants may be attempted. Most patients with acute leukemias die within 6 months without treatment. More than 90% of acute lymphocytic leukemias carry a 5-year remission rate of 50% or better following treatment. Acute myelocytic and acute monoblastic leukemias result in 70% to 85% remission following treatment. In all cases, survival depends on complete remission. Chronic granulocytic leukemia, however, is progressive, with an average survival of about 3 to 4 years after the onset of the disease and a 5-year survival rate of approximately 20%.

Radiography plays a limited role in the diagnosis and treatment of most leukemias. Diagnostic medical ultrasound and CT are of value in assessing lymphatic disease. Additionally, lymphography (Fig. 9-7) may be helpful in staging the disease.

Hodgkin's Disease

Hodgkin's disease is another neoplastic disease affecting the lymphoid tissue and is a type of lymphoma. In general, lymphomas are divided into Hodgkin's and non-Hodgkin's lymphoma (NHL), which can have a different nodal distribution as seen on CT. Hodgkin's disease is generally retroperitoneal with less mesenteric involvement, and NHL involves the mesentery.

Hodgkin's disease has an unknown etiology, commonly affects individuals between the ages of 20 and 40, and tends to affect men slightly more often than women. Common signs and symptoms associated with Hodgkin's disease are general malaise, fever, anorexia, and enlarged lymph nodes. Mediastinal lymph nodes are often visible on a chest radiograph and definitive diagnosis is made via biopsy of the lymphatic tissue. **Reed-Sternberg cells** differentiate Hodgkin's lymphomas from other types of lymphatic disease. As with other neoplastic disorders, Hodgkin's disease is staged according to the extent of the disease. Stage I denotes one anatomic node location, and stage IV denotes extranodal spread to the bone marrow, the lungs, or the liver. There are four histoplastic types of Hodgkin's lymphomas, with the prognosis varying with the type.

Hodgkin's disease is most commonly treated with a combination of radiation and chemotherapy. Stage I Hodgkin's lymphoma is associated with a 5-year survival rate of 90%. Stage IV Hodgkin's disease only has approximately a 20%, 5-year survival rate. The overall prognosis is associated with a 5-year survival rate of approximately 42%. Again, ultrasound, CT, lymphography, and nuclear medicine studies are of value in staging and following the course of the disease.

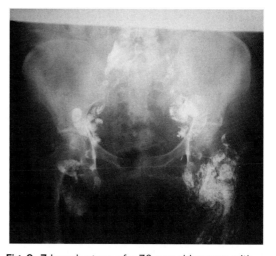

Fig. 9-7 Lymphogram of a 70-year-old woman with lymphosarcoma. Notice the enlarged lymph nodes with partial obstruction of the left channels at the hip area and extravasation of contrast material. (Courtesy Ohio State University Hospitals, Columbus, Ohio.)

QUESTIONS

1. The majority of blood volume is comprised of:
   a. erythrocytes   c. plasma
   b. leukocytes   d. thrombocyte

2. Bilirubin is formed during the destruction of:
   a. erythrocytes   c. plastocytes
   b. leukocytes   d. thrombocytes

3. Which type of blood is considered to be a universal donor?
   a. A   c. AB
   b. B   d. O

4. Which cells are most important in the development of immunity?
   a. erythrocytes   c. platelets
   b. lymphocytes   d. thrombocytes

5. Which type of pneumonia is commonly associated with AIDS?
   a. pneumococcal
   b. *Pneumocystis carinii*
   c. streptococcal
   d. all of the above

6. Kaposi's sarcoma is frequently associated with AIDS, and it may affect the:
   a. gastrointestinal system
   b. lymph nodes
   c. skin
   d. all of the above

7. A neoplastic disease of the plasma is:
   a. Hodgkin's disease
   b. leukemia
   c. lymphoma
   d. multiple myeloma

8. Which type of leukemia predominately affects children?
   a. acute lymphocytic
   b. chronic lymphocytic
   c. chronic myelocytic
   d. acute myelocytic

9. Reed-Sternberg cells are associated with what type of neoplastic disease?
   a. leukemia
   b. Hodgkin's disease
   c. multiple myeloma
   d. Hodgkin's

10. Hodgkin's disease affects what type of blood cells?
    a. erythrocytes   c. plastocytes
    b. lymphocytes   d. thrombocytes

11. A patient has a lymphangiogram, and films are taken from the feet through the abdomen. Should the diagnostician be alarmed if the abdominal lymph nodes are not readily visible in the first set of films? Why or why not?

12. Identify two means of transmission for the AIDS virus.

13. What is the difference in cellular origin between multiple myeloma and leukemia?

14. What is the risk of using radiation or antileukemic drug therapy in treating leukemias?

15. Identify at least three signs and symptoms of Hodgkin's disease.

The Central Nervous System

Anatomy and Physiology Review
Imaging Considerations
Congenital and Hereditary Diseases
    Meningomyelocele
    Hydrocephalus
Inflammatory Diseases
    Meningitis
    Encephalitis
Degenerative Diseases
    Degenerative disk disease and herniated nucleus
       pulposus
    Cervical spondylosis
    Multiple sclerosis
Neoplastic Diseases
    Gliomas
    Medulloblastoma
    Meningioma
    Pituitary adenoma
    Craniopharyngioma
    Tumors of central nerve sheath cells
    Metastases from other sites
    Spinal tumors

Upon completion of Chapter 10, the reader should be able to:

- Describe the anatomic components of the central nervous system (CNS) and their general function.

- Discuss the role of the various imaging modalities in evaluation of the CNS, particularly magnetic resonance imaging (MRI) and computed tomography (CT).

- Discuss common congenital anomalies of the CNS.

- Characterize a given condition as inflammatory, degenerative, or neoplastic.

- Identify the pathogenesis of the pathologies cited and typical treatments for them.

- Describe, in general, the radiographic appearance of each of the given pathologies, as possible, or alternative means of imaging.

KEY TERMS

Blood-brain barrier	Herniated nucleus pulposus	Meningioma
Annulus fibrosis	Cervical spondylosis	Pituitary adenoma
Nucleus pulposus	Multiple sclerosis	Sylvian triangle
Meningocele	Glioma	Craniopharyngioma
Myelocele	Astrocytoma	Acoustic neurilemoma
Meningomyelocele	Glioblastoma multiforme	Acoustic neuroma
Hydrocephalus	Oligodendroglioma	Schwannoma
Meningitis	Ependymoma	Meningiomas
Encephalitis	Medulloblastoma	Neurofibromas

ANATOMY AND PHYSIOLOGY REVIEW

The central nervous system (CNS) comprises the brain and the spinal cord. It is composed of neurons (nerve cells) and neuroglia (the interstitial tissue). The CNS extends peripherally through nerves that carry motor messages through efferent nerves to the muscles and sensory messages from the skin and elsewhere back to the spinal cord and brain through afferent nerves. This chapter concentrates on conditions involving the brain and spinal cord.

The brain consists of the cerebrum (right and left hemispheres), cerebellum, diencephalon (including the hypothalamus), and the brainstem. The brainstem, composed of the midbrain, pons, and the medulla oblongata, serves to connect the cerebrum with the spinal cord. The innumerable motor and sensory nerves pass through the brain stem into the spinal cord. The spinal cord originates as an extension of the medulla oblongata at the foramen magnum in the base of the skull. It extends to approximately the level of the second or third lumbar vertebra to terminate with a cone-shaped area called the *conus medullaris* (Fig. 10-1). Spinal nerves beyond this point are referred to as the *cauda equina*.

Both the brain and the spinal cord are invested by the meninges, which consist of three distinct layers (Fig. 10-2). The dura mater is the outermost and is tough and fibrous. It has three major extensions: the falx cerebri, which divides the cerebral hemispheres; the falx cerebelli, which similarly divides the cerebellar hemispheres; and the tentorium cerebelli, which separates the occipital lobe of the cerebrum from

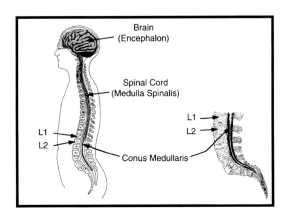

Fig. 10-1 Central nervous system. (From Bontrager KL: *Radiographic positioning and related anatomy*, ed 3, St Louis, 1993, Mosby.)

the cerebellum. The arachnoid is the middle layer of the meninges and has the appearance of cobwebs. The pia mater is innermost and adheres directly to the cortex of the brain and the spinal cord. The subarachnoid space, at its deepest at the base of the brain, is located between the arachnoid and the pia mater. It is filled with cerebrospinal fluid (CSF) to continuously bathe the brain and spinal cord with nutrients and to cushion them against shocks and blows. The CSF is secreted by the choroid plexus, a network of capillaries located in the brain's ventricles.

The ventricles are four interconnected cavities within the brain. As noted, they house the choroid plexus that secretes CSF. The right and left lateral ventricles are located in their respective cerebral hemispheres (Fig. 10-3, *A* and *B*). They may be further divided into anterior, posterior, and inferior horns, as well as a body and a trigone. The CSF flows from the lateral ventricles into the third ventricle via interventricular foramina (of Monro). The third and fourth ventricles are midline structures connected to each other by the cerebral aqueduct (Fig. 10-3, *C*). From there, it flows through a median and two lateral foramina (Magendie and Luschka, respectively) into the

subarachnoid space surrounding the brain and the spinal cord.

Most of the brain's blood is supplied anteriorly via the bilateral internal carotid arteries and posteriorly via the bilateral vertebral arteries. After entering the cranial vault through the foramen magnum, the vertebral arteries converge to form the basilar artery. The basilar artery and portions of the internal carotid arteries form

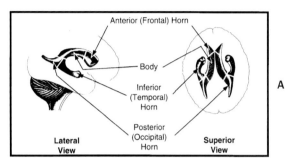

A

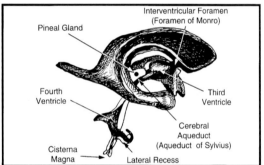

B

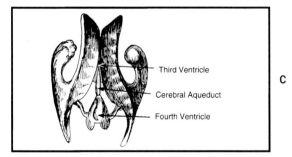

C

Fig. **10-3 A,** Lateral and superior views of the lateral ventricles; **B,** a lateral view of the ventricular system; **C,** a superior view of the ventricular system. (A, B, and C From Bontrager KL: *Radiographic positioning and related anatomy,* ed 3, St Louis, 1993, Mosby.)

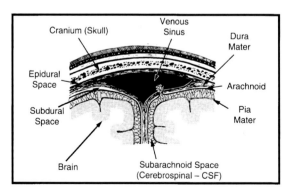

Fig. **10-2** Coronal perspective of meninges and meningeal spaces. (From Bontrager KL: *Radiographic positioning and related anatomy,* ed 3, St Louis, 1993, Mosby.)

the circle of Willis (Fig. 10-4) to distribute oxygenated, arterial blood through various branches to all parts of the brain. Venous blood is returned to large venous sinuses in the dura mater, which ultimately drain into the internal jugular veins (Fig. 10-5).

The capillaries that connect the arteries and veins function somewhat differently in the brain than in other organs. Here, they prevent the passage of unwanted substances into the brain through a special function called the **blood-brain barrier.** This is accomplished in a number

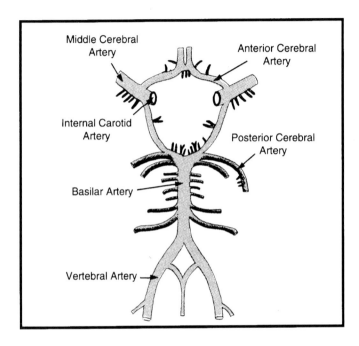

Fig. 10-4 The circle of Willis. (From Bontrager KL: *Radiographic positioning and related anatomy,* ed 3, St Louis, 1993, Mosby.)

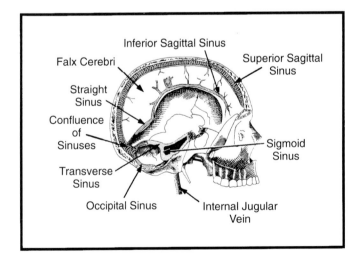

Fig. 10-5 Dura mater sinuses and venous drainage of the brain. (From Bontrager KL: *Radiographic positioning and related anatomy,* ed 3, St Louis, 1993, Mosby.)

of ways but especially as a result of these capillary cells having a very tight junction that prevents macromolecules and fluids from leaking out into the brain parenchyma. This protects the brain by keeping toxins out, yet it allows removal of the waste products of brain metabolism. These specialized capillaries are found everywhere in the brain except the pineal and pituitary glands and the choroid plexus. The significance of the blood-brain barrier in terms of imaging is that contrast media enhancement in the brain occurs where the barrier breaks down from inflammation, ischemia, or neoplastic growth (with its new vascularity). Also, glucose readily passes over this barrier and is the primary agent used so far in positron emission tomography (PET) scanning.

Although the intervertebral disks are not part of the CNS, they may impact on it when they herniate and impinge on adjacent spinal nerves. Disks cushion movement of the vertebral column. They comprise a tough outer covering, known as the **annulus fibrosus,** and a pulpy center, called the **nucleus pulposus** (Fig. 10-6).

IMAGING CONSIDERATIONS

Conventional radiographic demonstration of the various cranial structures can provide information important in evaluation of the CNS. Its role, however, has largely been reduced to evaluation of cranial trauma because of the rapid as-

cent of MRI and continued refinements in CT. Other studies important in evaluation of the CNS include angiography, sonography, nuclear medicine, and PET scanning.

In addition to visualization of fractures caused by trauma, plain skull films may also reveal normal variants. Blood vessels such as the middle meningeal artery commonly cause radiolucent impressions on the inner table of the cranial vault (Fig. 10-7). Their linear progression and bilateral appearance help distinguish them from fractures. Visualization of an enlarged or deformed pituitary fossa can

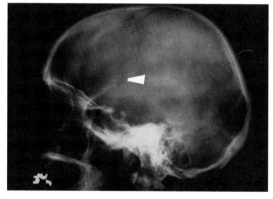

Fig. 10-7 Normal appearance of the middle meningeal artery as indicated on this lateral skull radiograph. (Courtesy the American College of Radiology, Reston, Virginia.)

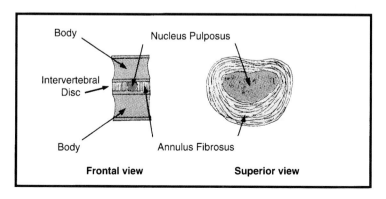

Fig. 10-6 An intervertebral disk. (From Bontrager KL: *Radiographic positioning and related anatomy,* ed 3, St Louis, 1993, Mosby.)

provide information concerning the presence of a pituitary tumor or increased intracranial pressure (Fig. 10-8). A calcified pineal gland situated in the midline can be seen on about 60% of all plain skull films (Fig. 10-9). Its displacement can indicate the presence of a pathologic lesion if it is greater than 2 to 3 mm. The choroid plexus (Fig. 10-10), falx cerebri (Fig. 10-11), and falx cerebelli may also be calcified.

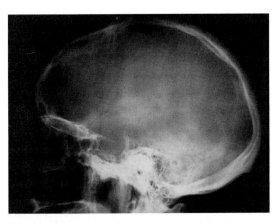

Fig. 10-8 An enlarged sella turcica on this lateral skull radiograph evidences a pituitary macroadenoma. (Courtesy the American College of Radiology, Reston, Virginia.)

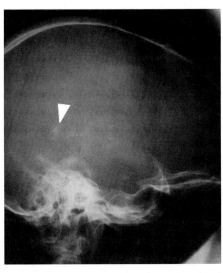

Fig. 10-10 Normal calcification of the choroid plexus in the posterior horn of the lateral ventricle as seen in this lateral skull radiograph of a 60-year-old woman. (Courtesy the American College of Radiology, Reston, Virginia.)

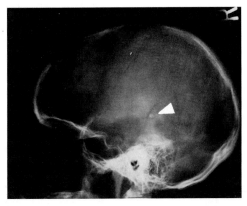

Fig. 10-9 Normal calcification of the pineal gland as seen on this lateral skull radiograph of a 44-year-old man. (Courtesy the American College of Radiology, Reston, Virginia.)

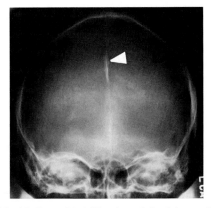

Fig. 10-11 Normal calcification of the falx cerebri as seen in this PA skull projection of a 59-year-old man. (Courtesy the American College of Radiology, Reston, Virginia.)

The role of plain films in the evaluation of the spine was described in Chapter 2. A number of conditions that impact on the spinal cord can readily be demonstrated. The fluoroscopic procedure of myelography has been a staple of radiology for years, allowing visualization of conditions (such as herniated disks) that impinge on the spinal cord. Its role, however, is greatly diminishing because of the significant specificity of MRI.

For a wide variety of conditions related to the CNS, MRI has emerged as the modality of choice (Fig. 10-12). Its sensitivity is excellent in evaluation of all types of spinal disease, including tumors and disk disease. The ability of MRI to evaluate brain tumors and conditions such as

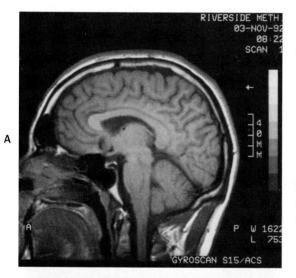

A

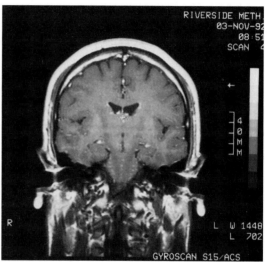

C

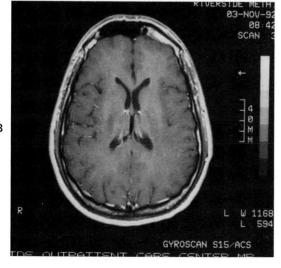

B

Fig. 10-12 A, Normal MRI of a young female with a history of seizures as seen in a sagittal, T_1 weighted view without gadolinium contrast; **B,** a normal T_1 weighted axial view with gadolinium contrast of the same patient; **C,** a normal T_1 weighted coronal view with gadolinium contrast of the same patient.
(**A, B,** and **C** Courtesy Riverside Methodist Hospitals, Columbus, Ohio.)

stroke, cranial tumors, and infection surpasses that of CT. Evaluation of demyelinating disease such as multiple sclerosis is substantively enhanced by MRI. Despite rapid evolution in technology, it currently has only a small role in the evaluation of trauma, mainly limited to evaluation of spinal cord compression and in some instances, vertebral fractures.

Computed tomography continues to play a significant role in the evaluation of the CNS. It is rapid, noninvasive, safe, and quite accurate. It is particularly useful in evaluating cerebral bleeding after trauma because it readily reveals the extent of any hematoma present. Other related roles include any kind of routine anatomic evaluation, such as assessment of shunt functioning or the sinuses (as discussed in Chapter 3). Postmyelographic CT of the spine is also fairly prevalent but is decreasing with the more widespread use of MRI. As bony detail is not seen as well on MRI, CT is also used to evaluate vertebral fractures.

Other modalities used to evaluate the CNS include angiography, ultrasound, nuclear medicine, and PET scanning. As elsewhere in the body, angiography is used to study the vasculature. A variety of conditions involving cerebral circulation can have wide effects on the brain, as discussed in Chapter 9. Ultrasound is useful in evaluating the brain of neonates before closure of the fontanelles because the fibrous tissue covering the fontanelles provides a ready window into the brain. It is also useful intraoperatively in evaluation of tumors and guidance for shunt placement (Fig. 10-13). New efforts are being made to apply ultrasound to assessment of blood flow through the intracranial parts of the carotid arteries. In nuclear medicine, technetium-labeled flow agents are being used in combination with single positron emission computed tomography

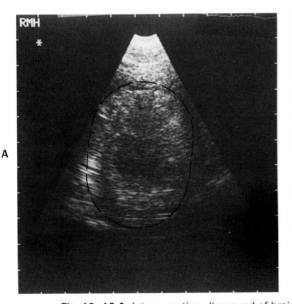

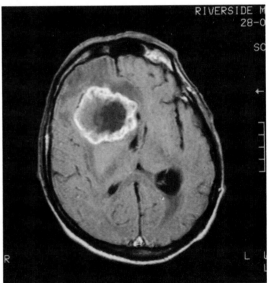

Fig. 10-13 A, Intraoperative ultrasound of brain tumor (glioblastoma) in a 61-year-old man showing the tumor size and location in a transverse plane for the operating surgeon; **B,** a T$_1$ weighted axial MRI view with contrast demonstrates the same lesion. (**A** and **B** Courtesy Riverside Methodist Hospitals, Columbus, Ohio.)

(SPECT) to assess tumors, areas of stroke and ischemia, and Alzheimer's disease (Fig. 10-14). The brain scan, once a staple of nuclear medicine, has yielded completely to CT. To complement the more traditional anatomic evaluation of other modalities, PET scanning allows imaging of the body's normal chemical processes and provides physiologic evaluation (Fig. 10-15). Significant cost-benefit issues arise in its use and may ultimately limit its usefulness.

CONGENITAL AND HEREDITARY DISEASES

Meningomyelocele

As mentioned in Chapter 2, spina bifida is a condition in which the bony neural arch that encloses and protects the spinal cord is not completely closed. It most commonly occurs in the lumbar region, and the spinal cord and its meninges may or may not herniate through the resultant opening. Complications depend on the

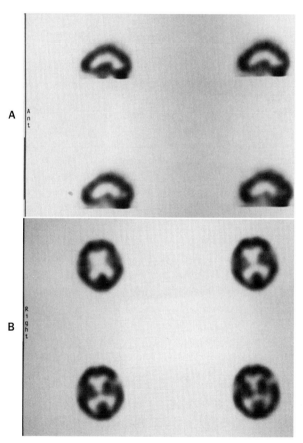

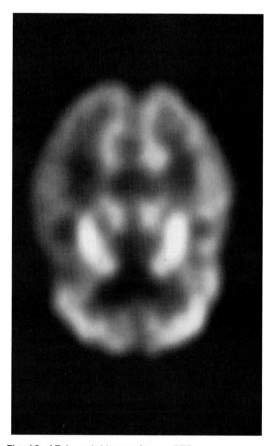

Fig. 10-14 **A,** Transaxial views of the head of a 77-year-old woman seen on a SPECT scan reveal no pathology; **B,** Lateral views of the head from the same SPECT scan. (**A** and **B** Courtesy Riverside Methodist Hospitals, Columbus, Ohio.)

Fig. 10-15 An axial image from a PET scan demonstrating an infarct in the posterior left parietotemporal region, with shunting of blood to hypermetabolic basal ganglia. (Courtesy the Christ Hospital, Cincinnati, Ohio.)

extent of protrusion and range from treatable to life-threatening. Any opening of the sac to the exterior of the body risks meningeal infection, so surgical closure is critical. If only the meninges protrude, the condition is termed a **meningocele** (Fig. 10-16). These are treated surgically without difficulty, and usually with an excellent prognosis. A **myelocele** is a protrusion of the spinal cord, which may be treatable surgically. A **meningomyelocele** is the most serious of possible conditions and consists of a protrusion of both the meninges and the spinal cord into the skin of the back (Fig. 10-17 and 10-18). These patients often present with severe neurologic deficit, the extent of which depends on the level of herniation. Associated neurologic difficulties include paraplegia and diminished control of the lower limbs, bladder, and bowel. Hydrocephalus occurs in most of these patients.

Hydrocephalus

Normally, CSF flows around the spinal cord and over the convexity of the brain before resorption into the venous sinuses. This normal circulation can be interrupted by causes such as an obstruction to flow and impaired absorption; increased CSF production can also disturb the normal circulation. As a result, the ventricles distend proximal to the site of obstruction, resulting in compression atrophy of the brain tissue around the dilated ventricles. In such cases, the sulci are obliterated and the gyri are flattened. **Hydrocephalus** refers to an excessive accumulation of CSF within the ventricles and can be either congenital or acquired.

In noncommunicating hydrocephalus, an obstruction can result congenitally or from tumor growth, trauma, or inflammation. It interferes with or blocks the normal CSF circulation from the ventricles to the subarachnoid space. Poor resorption of CSF by the arachnoid villi results in communicating hydrocephalus. It can arise from a number of factors, including increased intracranial pressure caused by tumor compression, raised intrathoracic pressure impairing venous drainage, inflammation from meningitis, or after a subarachnoid hemorrhage. Hydrocephalus can also occur from overproduction of CSF, although this is the least common cause.

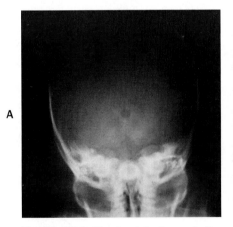

A

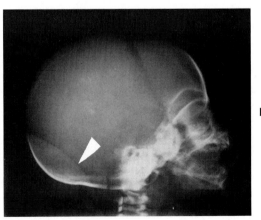

B

Fig. 10-16 **A,** Circular defect seen in the middle of the occipital bone of this newborn is the site of a meningocele. **B,** A lateral skull radiograph demonstrates the soft tissue density associated with the meningocele superimposed over the occipital bone. (**A** and **B** Courtesy the American College of Radiology, Reston, Virginia.)

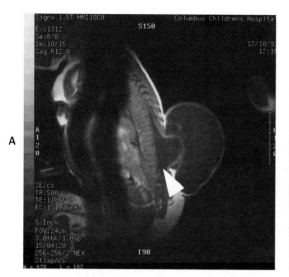

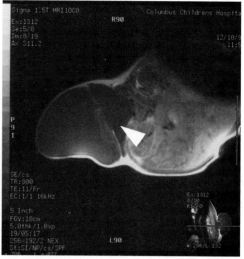

Fig. 10-17 A, A T$_1$ weighted sagittal MRI view without gadolinium in this newborn readily demonstrates a meningomyelocele, with the *arrow* indicating the herniated spinal cord.
B, A T$_1$ weighted axial MRI view without gadolinium of the same patient similarly demonstrates the meningomyelocele, with the *arrow* indicating the herniated spinal cord. (**A** and **B** Courtesy Children's Hospital, Columbus, Ohio.)

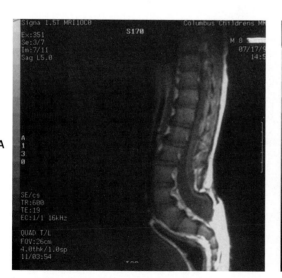

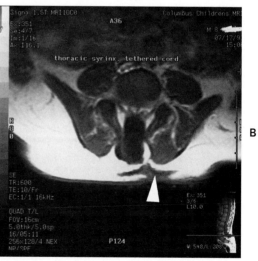

Fig. 10-18 A, A T$_1$ weighted sagittal MRI view without gadolinium in this infant demonstrates a surgically repaired meningomyelocele. **B,** A T$_1$ weighted axial MRI view without gadolinium similarly demonstrates the surgically repaired meningomyelocele, with the *arrow* pointing to the surgical site. (**A** and **B** Courtesy Children's Hospital, Columbus, Ohio.)

Computed tomography provides excellent visualization of this disorder (Fig. 10-19). In neonates, sonography is used to demonstrate the ventricular system through the infant's fontanelles, which permit passage of the beam until their eventual closure. Treatment may consist of surgery. In some cases, a shunt (an artificial passageway) is surgically inserted to divert excess fluids. Placed between the ventricles and either the internal jugular vein, the heart, or the peritoneum, it drains excess CSF. The shunt contains a one-way valve to prevent the backflow of blood into the ventricles. Radiographs are taken to demonstrate shunt placement after insertion, and CT is used to follow up on a periodic basis to evaluate ventricular size, which indirectly assesses shunt function.

INFLAMMATORY DISEASES

Meningitis

An inflammation of the meningeal coverings of the brain and spinal cord is termed **meningitis.** It can be caused by bacteria, viruses, or other organisms that reach the meninges from elsewhere in the body via blood or lymph, as a result of trauma and penetrating wounds, or from adjacent structures (e.g., the mastoids) that become infected. Bacterial infection is the most common cause of meningitis (Fig. 10-20). Pathogens responsible for bacterial meningitis include meningococci, streptococci, and pneumococci. These are pus-forming (pyogenic) types of bacteria, and they may be carried to the meninges via the middle ear or frontal sinus. In addition, a few cases result from infection by the tubercle bacillus, which is not pus-forming. This type of bacterial meningitis is more difficult to diagnose because it does not have the same acute symptoms as the other types of bacterial meningitis. Tuberculous meningitis is usually metastatic from the lung in association with miliary tuberculosis.

In cases of meningitis, CSF is under increased pressure and can contribute to hydrocephalus. The primary means of diagnosing meningitis is

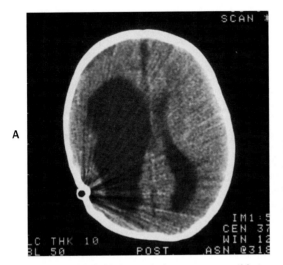
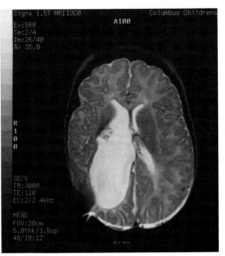

Fig. 10-19 A, Hydrocephalus as seen on this transverse CT view of a 6-month-old girl with only mild dilatation of the left ventricle. Streaking artifacts originate from the shunt being checked for placement. **B,** A T$_2$ weighted axial MRI view without gadolinium demonstrates the hydrocephalus in the same patient. (**A** and **B** Courtesy Children's Hospital, Columbus, Ohio.)

the increased intracranial pressure detectable via the results of a spinal tap. Upon laboratory examination, the CSF contains both the bacteria responsible for the infection and a large amount of polymorphonuclear leukocytes (pus cells). Signs and symptoms of meningitis include a sudden onset of severe headache, neck stiffness, and fever. Antibiotics in particular have been

greatly successful against many forms of meningitis. However, meningitis may be fatal, especially in the neonate or the elderly.

Encephalitis

An infection of the brain tissue is termed **encephalitis.** In contrast to meningitis, which is

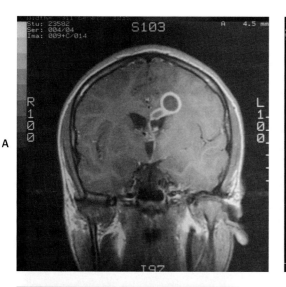

A

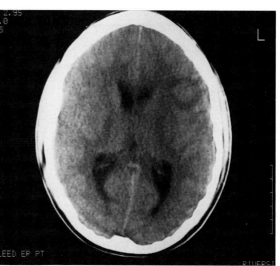

C

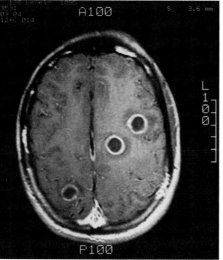

B

Fig. 10–20 **A,** A T$_1$ weighted coronal MRI view with gadolinium demonstrates a ring lesion that communicates with the left lateral ventricle in this 17-year-old boy, creating meningitis as a result of transplantation into the brain of a bacterial (staph) infection; **B,** A T$_1$ weighted axial MRI view with gadolinium of the same patient demonstrates the presence of multiple infectious lesions. **C,** An axial CT view of the same patient demonstrates the presence of an infectious lesion as well as slightly widened ventricles, as characteristic with meningitis. (**A, B,** and **C** Courtesy Riverside Methodist Hospitals, Columbus, Ohio.)

most frequently a bacterial infection, encephalitis is usually viral in nature (Fig. 10-21) and may also occur subsequent to conditions such as chickenpox, smallpox, influenza, or measles. The symptoms and signs most commonly associated with encephalitis are headache and coma. This condition is more serious than meningitis because individuals who acquire encephalitis more frequently develop permanent neurologic disabilities. The viral infection results in cerebral edema with numerous hemorrhagic spots scattered throughout the cerebral hemispheres, the brainstem, and cerebellum. In some instances, it may even be fatal because there is no specific treatment for viral encephalitis.

DEGENERATIVE DISEASES

Degenerative Disk Disease and Herniated Nucleus Pulposus

A **herniated nucleus pulposus,** or herniated disk, may result from either degenerative disease or trauma. A weakened or torn annulus fibrosus is subject to rupture, which allows the nucleus pulposus to ooze out and compress spinal nerve roots. The disk may prolapse in any direction and in some instances may not produce pain. However, pressure may be placed on the spinal cord as the nucleus pulposus spreads beyond its normal confines posteriorly (Fig. 10-22), resulting in pain along the course of adjacent nerve

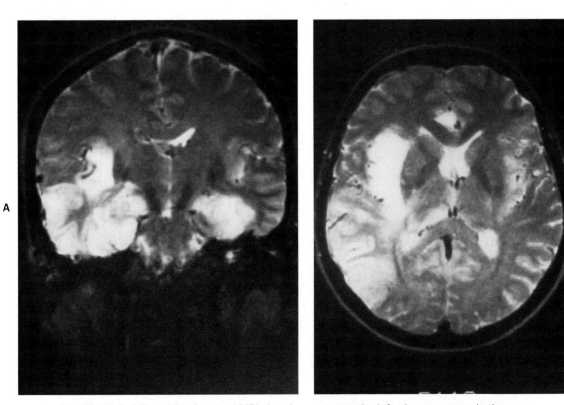

A   B

Fig. 10-21 A, A T$_2$ weighted coronal MRI view demonstrates the infectious response in the brain of this boy with herpes encephalitis; **B,** A T$_2$ weighted axial MRI view demonstrates the extent of the infectious process in the same patient with herpes encephalitis. (**A** and **B** Courtesy Riverside Methodist Hospitals, Columbus, Ohio.)

roots and a weakening of the muscles supplied by these nerves. The most common locations for disk herniation are in the lower cervical and lower lumbar regions.

Symptoms may include a sudden and severe onset of pain in the distribution of the compressed nerve root in combination with weakened muscles, although at times symptoms may be more insidious. Compression of the nerve root may be demonstrated through myelography, CT, and MRI. The imaging modality of choice has become MRI (Fig. 10-23), largely supplanting the roles of myelography and CT in diagnosis of disk disease. However, with normal aging, the nucleus pulposus tends to dehydrate, and change the water content, which alters the relaxation times on an MR study. Bed rest, traction, physical therapy, and analgesics can be used as treatment. If these fail to relieve pain, surgical laminectomy with spinal fusion may be performed. Chemonucleolysis is a procedure formerly used to dissolve part of the diseased

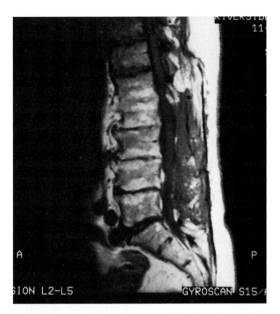

Fig. 10-22 T_1 weighted sagittal MRI view of the spine in this 75-year-old man readily demonstrates severe degenerative disk disease as well as fusion of L1 and L2. (Courtesy Riverside Methodist Hospitals, Columbus, Ohio.)

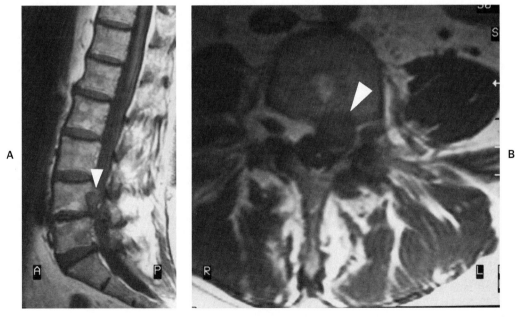

Fig. 10-23 A, Herniated nucleus pulposus at L4-L5 interspace seen on a T_1 weighted sagittal MRI view of the lumbar spine; **B,** the axial view of the same herniated nucleus pulposus demonstrates disk herniation to the left of midline on this T_1 weighted MRI image. (**A** and **B** Courtesy Riverside Methodist Hospitals, Columbus, Ohio.)

disk. Although still used in some places, it has largely fallen out of favor because of complications. Aspiration of the disk is a relatively new technique that holds promise for relief of this condition.

Cervical Spondylosis

Osteoarthritic conditions may also affect the vertebral column, leading to nerve disorders caused by chronic nerve root compression. These osteoarthritic changes of the neck are referred to as **cervical spondylosis** and are readily visible radiographically. Osteophytes (spurs) form in the articular facets of the cervical vertebrae and compress the nerves located in the interver-tebral foramina. They may also compress the spinal cord (Fig. 10-24). Magnetic resonance imaging excels at visualization of spinal cord compression as a result of cervical spondylosis. As with degenerative disk disease, treatment is conservative at first but may include laminectomy and decompression procedures.

Multiple Sclerosis

Multiple sclerosis (MS) is a chronic, progressive disease of the nervous system most commonly affecting individuals between the ages of 20 and 40. The origin of this disease is unknown, but MS involves degeneration of the myelin sheath covering the nervous tissue of

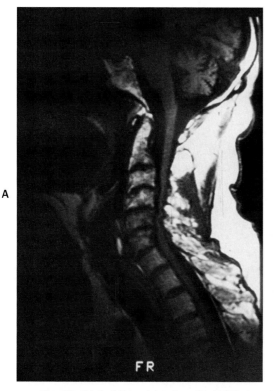
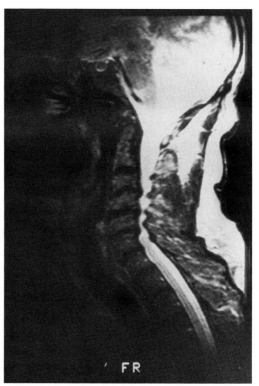

Fig. 10-24 A, A T_1 weighted sagittal MRI view demonstrates compression of the spinal cord in this elderly man with cervical spondylosis. CSF is dark adjacent to the gray spinal cord.
B, A T_2 weighted sagittal MRI image indicates the constriction of CSF flow *(white)* at C2 through C5. (**A** and **B** Courtesy Riverside Methodist Hospitals, Columbus, Ohio.)

the spinal cord and the white matter within the brain. This demyelination impairs nerve conduction, beginning with muscle impairment and a loss of balance and coordination. As multiple sclerosis progresses, tremors, vision impairment, and urinary bladder dysfunction develop, along with a continued weakening of the muscles. Numerous patchy areas of demyelinated nerves develop, forming scar tissue or sclerotic lesions throughout the nervous system. These scars are termed multiple sclerosis plaques and are well demonstrated upon MRI examination, making MRI the modality of choice for evaluating individuals with suspected MS. Multiple sclerosis runs a long and unpredictable course, eventually leading to permanent neurologic disabilities. There is no treatment for multiple sclerosis, but most patients benefit from physical therapy in conjunction with medication to reduce muscle spasticity.

NEOPLASTIC DISEASES

Primary tumors of the brain comprise about 10% of the deaths from cancer and may be difficult to classify as purely benign or malignant. In many cases, the location of the brain neoplasm is of equal or greater importance than its malignancy or benignancy because of the complications produced by mass effect. Edema accompanying a tumor causes an increase in intracranial pressure, which can cause headaches, vomiting, blurred vision, and seizures. Hemorrhage and brainstem herniation can occur, resulting in death as brainstem function (e.g., control of respiration) fails.

Other characteristics of primary brain tumors include a greater incidence in males and a relative infrequency of metastasis. In children, brain tumors often tend to occur in the posterior fossa, but the anterior portion of the cerebrum is a more prevalent site in adults. In addition, primary brain tumors are among the most common brain neoplasms in children, whereas metastases to the brain from other areas are more common in adults.

Two categories of brain tumors exist: glial and nonglial. Glial tumors generate from the nonnervous system (i.e., supporting tissues of the brain and spinal cord). Gliomas account for about half of all primary brain tumors. Their growth is accomplished through infiltration, making them difficult to treat surgically through resection. Nonglial tumors grow through expansion and are more treatable surgically. Meningiomas are the most frequently occurring nonglial tumor. The modalities of choice in imaging brain tumors of all types are MRI and CT. In addition to surgical intervention, radiation therapy and chemotherapy also play an important role in the treatment of brain tumors.

Gliomas

The most common type of primary brain tumor is the **glioma** (Fig. 10-25). Although derived from glial (supporting) cells, their precise classification is unsettled. Tumors may contain different types of cells in the same tumor. Gliomas

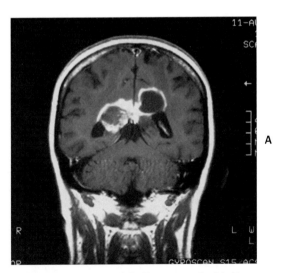

Fig. 10-25 A, A "butterfly" glioma seen in this T_1 weighted coronal MRI view with gadolinium in a 54-year-old woman; (Courtesy Riverside Methodist Hospitals, Columbus, Ohio.)

Continued

commonly occur in the cerebral hemispheres and posterior fossa, with nearly half of all gliomas classified as the malignant glioblastoma variety (Fig. 10-26). Other types of glioma include benign astrocytomas, oligodendroglio-

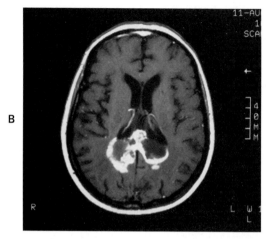

Fig. 10-25 cont'd. B, A T$_1$ weighted axial MRI view with gadolinium of the same "butterfly" glioma.
(Courtesy Riverside Methodist Hospitals, Columbus, Ohio.)

mas, and ependymomas. In terms of MRI results, gliomas are evaluated based on the associated edema (Fig. 10-27), mass effect, and the amount of contrast enhancement. There is an association between the aggressiveness of the tumor and these three factors. Malignant gliomas may be extremely vascular, demonstrating pathologic vessels upon angiographic examination. Low-grade malignant gliomas, however, are relatively avascular. The CT images generally demonstrate an ill-defined area of decreased density (attenuation) with displacement of the midline structures and ventricular compression. Without contrast enhancement, it is difficult to differentiate the surrounding edema from the actual tumor, so the use of an iodinated, IV contrast agent is necessary to enhance the lesion. Surgical biopsy generally provides the final diagnosis of the exact type of glioma. Symptoms include severe headaches, vision impairment, personality changes, and seizures.

Astrocytomas account for about a third of all gliomas (Fig. 10-28) and are composed of astrocytes, which are star-shaped neuroglial cells

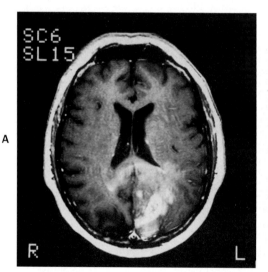

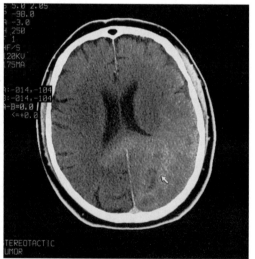

Fig. 10-26 A, A T$_1$ weighted axial MRI view with gadolinium demonstrates a glioblastoma multiforme in a 70-year-old man. **B,** CT study of the brain without contrast demonstrates an intraparenchymal hemorrhage after biopsy in the same patient with the glioblastoma multiforme. (**A** and **B** Courtesy Riverside Methodist Hospitals, Columbus, Ohio.)

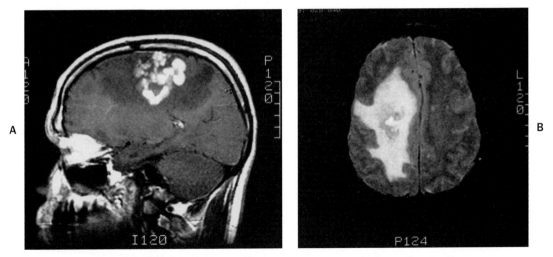

Fig. 10-27 A, A T_1 weighted sagittal MRI view with gadolinium of a large glioma with surrounding edema in a 25-year-old man; **B,** a T_2 weighted axial MRI view without gadolinium of the same glioma in the right parietal region, again with edema *(white on T_2)* surrounding the tumor. (**A** and **B** Courtesy Riverside Methodist Hospitals, Columbus, Ohio.)

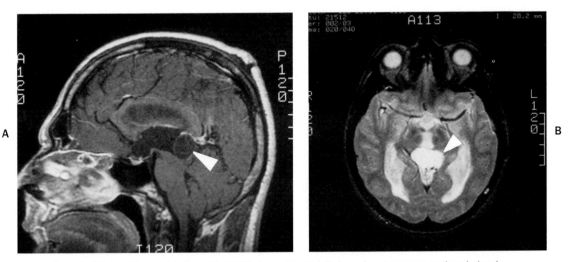

Fig. 10-28 A, A T_1 weighted sagittal MRI view with gadolinium demonstrates a pineal gland astrocytoma in this 32-year-old man; **B,** A T_2 weighted axial MRI view demonstrates the same pineal gland astrocytoma. (**A** and **B** Courtesy Riverside Methodist Hospitals, Columbus, Ohio.)

with many branching processes. Astrocytomas are white, usually slow-growing, infiltrative tumors with a low grade of malignancy. Early detection leads to a good prognosis. A **glioblastoma multiforme** (an advanced astrocytoma) is highly malignant. An **oligodendroglioma** is a slow-growing, astrocytic tumor that is usually histologically relatively benign (Fig. 10-29). It typically calcifies so that its appearance in a punctate or stippled pattern on a skull radiograph is virtually diagnostic. **Ependymoma** is a firm, whitish tumor that arises from the ependyma, the lining of the ventricles (Fig. 10-30). Typically, it derives from the roof of the fourth ventricle, but it may also appear from the central canal of the spinal cord.

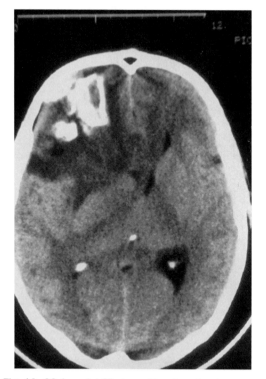

Fig. 10–29 An axial CT view without contrast demonstrates the presence of an oligodendroglioma and surrounding edema. (Courtesy Riverside Methodist Hospitals, Columbus, Ohio.)

Medulloblastoma

Like astrocytic tumors, **medulloblastomas** are soft, infiltrating tumors of neuroepithelial tissue. These rapidly growing tumors are highly malignant and most often occur in the cerebellum of children and young adults (Fig. 10-31), usually extending from the roof of the fourth ventricle. They are more common in males and rarely seen in adults. Because MRI does not image bone or demonstrate artifacts associated with the dense bone within the base of the skull, it is an excellent modality for the demonstration of a medulloblastoma on both enhanced and nonenhanced examination (see Fig. 10-31). These tumors may also be demonstrated on CT examination, with the medulloblastoma visible as a midline lesion that is denser than normal brain tissue, surrounded by edema. In addition, tumor dissemination throughout the subarachnoid space often blocks the flow of CSF, causing hydrocephalus. Shunting is used to relieve the hydrocephalus. Surgical excision of the tumor as possible, radiation therapy to the entire CNS, and chemotherapy have improved the 5-year survival rate to over 50%. Unfortunately, recurrence is common with this tumor.

Meningioma

A **meningioma** is a slow-growing, generally benign tumor that originates in the arachnoid tissue. It is the most common nonglial tumor and more frequent in women than in men. It is most often found adhering to the dura in relation to the intracranial venous sinuses. It does not invade the brain but compresses it with its growth. Resultant neurologic deficits are generally less in proportion to the tumor size than with gliomas.

In some instances, the skull may thicken over the site of the meningioma, with the increased calcification visible upon conventional skull radiographs. This area of hyperostosis may be palpable upon physical examination. Because these tumors are fed by the meningeal arteries, plain skull films may also demonstrate an enlarged

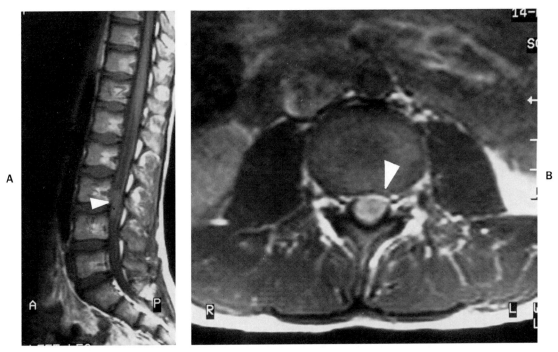

Fig. 10-30 A, A T$_1$ weighted sagittal MRI view of the lumbosacral spine demonstrates an ependymoma at L3-L4 interspace in this young male. **B,** A T$_1$ weighted axial MRI view with gadolinium demonstrates the same ependymoma. (**A** and **B** Courtesy Riverside Methodist Hospitals, Columbus, Ohio.)

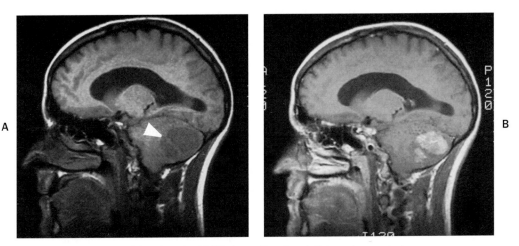

Fig. 10-31 A, A T$_1$ weighted sagittal MRI view without gadolinium demonstrates a medulloblastoma in the cerebellum of this 25-year-old man. **B,** A T$_1$ weighted sagittal MRI view with gadolinium demonstrates the medulloblastoma, illustrating more of its actual size. (**A** and **B** Courtesy Riverside Methodist Hospitals, Columbus, Ohio.)

foramen spinosum and increased meningeal vascular markings on the inner table of the skull. Computed tomographic studies demonstrate a well-defined mass of increased attenuation, with calcifications visible in approximately 20% of the lesions. The extent of the meningioma is clearly visible upon enhancement with an iodinated, IV contrast agent. Nonenhanced MRI is not as sensitive as CT at detecting meningiomas because there is not a significant contrast difference between these tumors and normal brain tissue. However, the use of an IV gadolinium contrast agent clearly demonstrates meningiomas upon MRI examination (Fig. 10-32). Surgical removal is the method of treatment for a symptomatic meningioma.

Pituitary Adenoma

A **pituitary adenoma** is a usually benign tumor of the pituitary gland. Hormones produced by the pituitary are affected, with one type of adenoma of the anterior pituitary resulting in giantism if it develops before puberty and acromegaly if it occurs in adults because of excessive production of growth hormone (GH). Prolactin-secreting adenomas cause amenorrhea-galactorrhea syndrome, in which the breasts spontaneously secrete milk and menstrual periods cease. Pituitary adenomas may grow out of the sella turcica. As they grow, they compress structures such as the optic chiasm, causing visual problems.

A common radiographic demonstration of this growth is an enlargement and erosion of the sella turcica on a lateral skull radiograph. Angiography might demonstrate a displacement of the *sylvian triangle,* but generally only after the adenoma has assumed a considerable size. The **sylvian triangle** is an anatomic landmark created by the middle cerebral artery and its branches. Computed tomography is useful to confirm the diagnosis of pituitary adenomas and to detect the extent of these lesions. Enlarge-

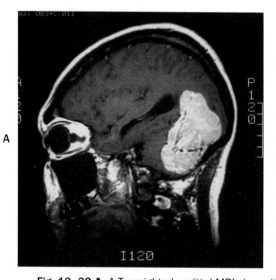 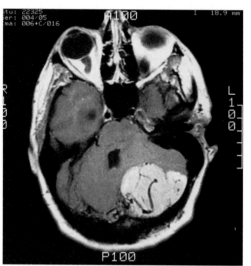

Fig. 10-32 A, A T_1 weighted sagittal MRI view with gadolinium of a large meningioma in the posterior occipital area with marked hydrocephalus in this 31-year-old woman; **B,** a T_1 weighted axial MRI view with gadolinium of the same meningioma. Displacement of the fourth ventricle is seen, as well as a distortion of the vascular structures within the meningioma. (**A** and **B** Courtesy Riverside Methodist Hospitals, Columbus, Ohio.)

ment of the sella turcica is generally demonstrated, as well as supra-sellar extension into the optic chiasm. These neoplasms are generally slightly denser than the surrounding brain tissue and show obvious enhancement upon IV injection of an iodinated contrast medium. Small microadenomas are best demonstrated on thin slice, contrast-enhanced, MRI images (Figs. 10-33 and 10-34). Generally, pituitary adenomas are treatable through surgical extraction, possibly followed by radiation therapy. Small adenomas may also be treated medically by drugs such as bromocriptine that increase prolactin inhibitory factor (PIF) and suppress the tumor growth.

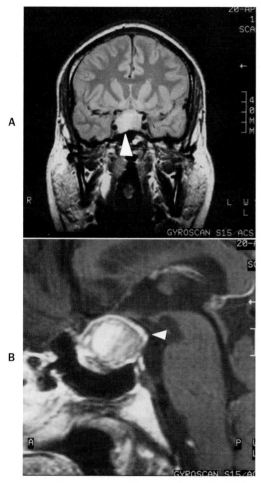

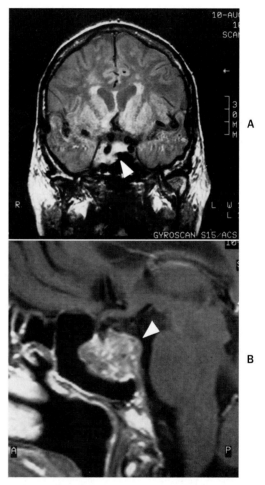

Fig. 10-33 **A,** A T_1 weighted coronal MRI view demonstrates a suprasellar macroadenoma of the pituitary in this 37-year-old man. **B,** A T_1 weighted sagittal MRI high-resolution scan with gadolinium demonstrates the same suprasellar macroadenoma of the pituitary. (**A** and **B** Courtesy Riverside Methodist Hospitals, Columbus, Ohio.)

Fig. 10-34 **A,** Large pituitary adenoma extending downward into the right cavernous sinus in a 79-year-old woman as seen on this MRI T_2 weighted coronal scan; **B,** A high-resolution T_1 weighted sagittal MRI view of the same pituitary adenoma with gadolinium. (**A** and **B** Courtesy Riverside Methodist Hospitals, Columbus, Ohio.)

Craniopharyngioma

A **craniopharyngioma** is a cystic, benign tumor growing from remnants of the development of the pituitary gland. It is thought to be developmental in origin and most commonly presents in childhood. Craniopharyngiomas usually arise above the sella and extends upward into the third ventricle (Fig. 10-35). Occasionally, they are seen within the sella, causing erosion of the sella turcica. Calcification of the wall of the cyst is common and readily identifiable on plain films of the skull. Computed tomography examinations show a midline suprasellar mass of low attenuation containing calcification. Angiography may reveal displacement of the sylvian triangle like that of a pituitary adenoma if the tumor is large. Although treated surgically, excision is often difficult because of location and proximity to structures such as the third ventricle and optic nerves. Radiation therapy is used to enhance the effects of surgery.

Tumors of Central Nerve Sheath Cells

Three tumors of the peripheral nerve sheath are the **acoustic neurilemoma, acoustic neuroma** (Fig. 10-36), and **schwannoma** (Fig. 10-37). They account for up to 10% of all intracranial tumors and are most common in middle-aged and elderly adults. The most common site is the eighth cranial (i.e., the vestibulocochlear or acoustic) nerve. At this location, the tumor compresses the adjacent brain tissue and erodes the temporal bone. Symptoms of acoustic neuromas include facial paralysis, tinnitus, and partial hearing loss on the affected side. Nerve sheath tumors can also be found on other cranial nerves, especially the trigeminal, and on spinal nerve roots and peripheral nerves. The imaging method of choice for acoustic neuromas is MRI. In extreme cases, erosion and expansion of the internal auditory canal may be visible on an AP axial projection of the skull. Surgical excision of the tumor is the method of treatment.

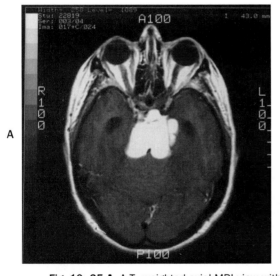
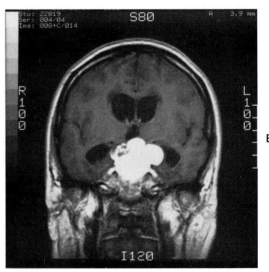

Fig. 10-35 **A,** A T$_1$ weighted axial MRI view with gadolinium demonstrates a mass, later confirmed by biopsy to be a craniopharyngioma in this 53-year-old woman. **B,** A T$_1$ weighted coronal MRI view with gadolinium demonstrates the relative size of the craniopharyngioma in the same patient. (**A** and **B** Courtesy Riverside Methodist Hospitals, Columbus, Ohio.)

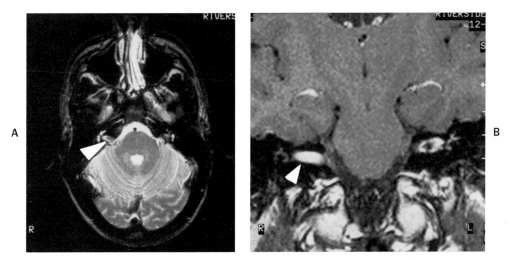

Fig. 10-36 A, A T$_2$ weighted axial MRI view of a right acoustic neuroma that is not readily visible without gadolinium in this 24-year-old man; **B,** A high-resolution, T$_1$ weighted coronal MRI view with gadolinium readily reveals the acoustic neuroma. Compare the appearance of the tumor with the appearance of the normal vasculature and anatomy on the left side. (**A** and **B** Courtesy Riverside Methodist Hospitals, Columbus, Ohio.)

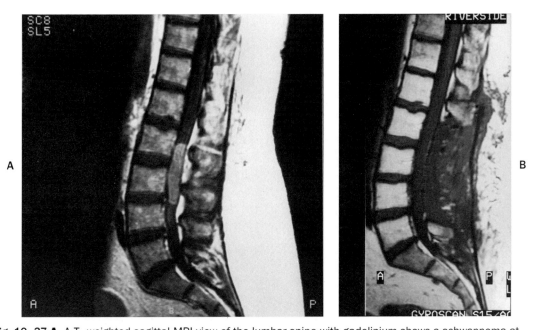

Fig. 10-37 A, A T$_1$ weighted sagittal MRI view of the lumbar spine with gadolinium shows a schwannoma at L3-L4 before surgery in this 27-year-old woman. **B,** A T$_1$ weighted sagittal MRI view of the same lumbar spine without gadolinium after surgery demonstrates apparent total excision of the tumor has been accomplished. Note also the excision of the spinous processes from the surgical site. (**A** and **B** Courtesy Riverside Methodist Hospitals, Columbus, Ohio.) *Continued*

Metastases from Other Sites

Secondary metastases from another site can involve any intracranial structure and account for about 25% of all brain tumors (Fig. 10-38). The metastatic lesions may be solitary or multiple. Brain metastasis usually arises from lung carcinoma. Other significant causes include breast cancer, colon cancer, and malignant melanoma. Signs and symptoms of brain metastasis are similar to those for other brain tumors. Patients with metastases from other sites usually present with signs of increased intracranial pressure, especially headache and ataxia; those with primary brain tumors are more likely to present with seizures. Diagnosis and follow-up are done with MRI and CT. Treatment with chemotherapy is performed, but the prognosis is generally quite poor.

Spinal Tumors

Primary tumors of the spinal cord are less common than those of the brain. They are com-

monly divided into extradural and intradural groups, with the latter further divided into extramedullary (outside the spinal cord) and intramedullary (within the spinal cord). The most common types of primary spinal neoplasms are **meningiomas** (Fig. 10-39) and **neurofibromas** (Fig. 10-40), both of which are extramedullary tumors. The most common intramedullary tumors are astrocytoma and ependymoma.

Symptoms of these tumors may be similar to those of a herniated nucleus pulposus in that spinal tumors also compress the nerve roots, leading to pain and muscular weakness. In evaluating spinal cord tumors, MRI has essentially replaced myelography. Radiation and chemotherapy are the primary means of treating spinal tumors because many are not surgically resectable.

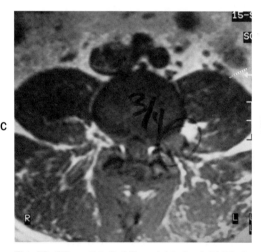

Fig. 10-37 cont'd. C, A T_1 weighted axial MRI view with gadolinium of the L3-L4 interspace demonstrates some residual tumor is present in the left neural foramina. (**C** Courtesy Riverside Methodist Hospitals, Columbus, Ohio.)

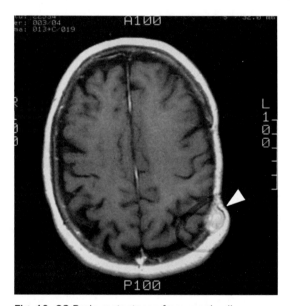

Fig. 10-38 Brain metastases from renal cell carcinoma as seen in this T_1 weighted axial MRI view with gadolinium status after craniotomy in this 59-year-old woman. (Courtesy Riverside Methodist Hospitals, Columbus, Ohio.)

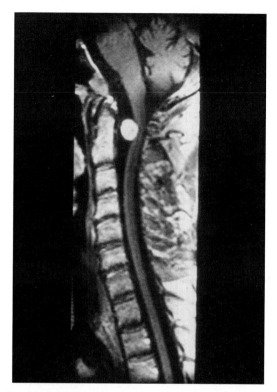

Fig. 10–39 A T$_1$ weighted sagittal MRI view of the spine with gadolinium demonstrates the presence of a meningioma in this 45-year-old woman with ataxia. (Courtesy Riverside Methodist Hospitals, Columbus, Ohio.)

A

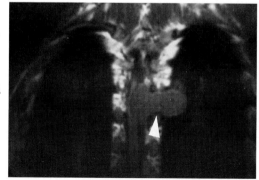

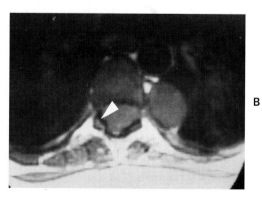

B

Fig. 10–40 A, A T$_1$ weighted coronal MRI view demonstrates the presence of a "dumbbell" neurofibroma showing clear compression of the spinal cord of this young female with back pain and leg weakness. **B,** An axial T$_1$ weighted MRI image similarly demonstrates the lesion and compression of the spinal cord *(arrow)* into a narrow space. (**A** and **B** Courtesy Riverside Methodist Hospitals, Columbus, Ohio.)

QUESTIONS

1. Under normal conditions, the central nervous system within the cranial vault is well protected from damage by all of the following *except* the:
   a. cauda equina
   b. cerebrospinal fluid
   c. diplöe
   d. dura mater

2. The correct order of meninges from outermost to innermost is:
   a. arachnoid, pia, dura
   b. dura, arachnoid, pia
   c. dura, pia, arachnoid
   d. pia, arachnoid, dura

3. The blood-brain barrier prevents passage of unwanted substances into the CNS through the cerebral:
   a. arteries   c. dura mater
   b. capillaries   d. veins

4. Erosion of the sella turcica is most commonly associated with neoplasms of the:
   a. meninges   c. pituitary
   b. pineal gland   d. pons

5. Protrusion of both the spinal cord and the meninges into the skin of the back is a:
   a. meningocele
   b. meningomyelocele
   c. myelocele
   d. spinal hydrocephalus

6. The most typical cause of meningitis is:
   a. bacterial infection
   b. trauma
   c. tumor compression
   d. viral infection

7. The imaging modality of choice for demonstration of herniated nucleus pulposus has become:
   a. CT   c. myelography
   b. MRI   d. ultrasonography

8. Which of the following neoplastic conditions are highly malignant and often occur in the cerebellum of children?
   a. astrocytoma
   b. medulloblastoma
   c. meningioma
   d. pituitary adenoma

9. A cystic, benign tumor that grows from the embryologic remnants of the pituitary gland is a(n):
   a. acoustic neurilemoma
   b. craniopharyngioma
   c. meningioma
   d. pituitary adenoma

10. The most common site for tumors of the peripheral nerve sheath (e.g., schwannoma) is on which cranial nerve?
    a. 4   c. 7
    b. 6   d. 8

11. Where is CSF manufactured and absorbed? Explain the physiologic basis for the development of hydrocephalus.

12. Why is MRI the modality of choice in demonstrating diseases in the posterior fossa?

13. List three examples of pathologies of the CNS that may be demonstrated with conventional radiographs.

14. What are the major differences between meningitis and encephalitis?

15. Explain the differences between glial and nonglial tumors and give an example of each type.

Traumatic Disease

Introduction
    Level I, II, and III trauma centers
Trauma of the Vertebral Column and Head
    Injuries to the vertebral column
    Injuries to the skull and brain
Skeletal Trauma
    Fractures
    Fractures in specific locations
    Visceral cranial fractures

Dislocations
    Battered child syndrome
    Legg-Perthes Disease
Trauma of the Chest and Thorax
    Pneumothorax
    Atelectasis
Abdominal Trauma
    Intraperitoneal air

Upon completion of Chapter 11, the reader should be able to:

■ Differentiate among level I, II, and III trauma centers and the role each plays in the emergency medical system.

■ Define common terminology associated with traumatic disease.

■ Discuss the role of various imaging modalities in the evaluation and treatment of traumatic injuries.

■ Describe, in general, the radiographic appearance of each of the given pathologies.

■ Classify skeletal fractures according to the various classifications discussed in this chapter, and describe the healing process associated with skeletal trauma.

KEY TERMS

Level I medical center
Level II medical center
Level III medical center
Compression fracture
Linear fracture
Depressed fracture
Concussion
Contusion
Coup lesion
Contrecoup lesion
Coma

Hematoma
Fracture
Open fracture
Closed fracture
Impacted fracture
Comminuted fracture
Noncomminuted fracture
Avulsion fracture
Incomplete fracture
Greenstick fracture
Torus fracture

Growth plate fracture
Stress fracture
Fatigue fracture
Occult fracture
Blow-out fracture
Dislocation
Subluxation
Pneumothorax
Atelectasis
Pneumoperitoneum

INTRODUCTION

In the United States, trauma is the most common cause of death for individuals between the ages of 1 and 45 years, prompting the Committee on Trauma of the American College of Surgeons (ACS) to develop and periodically review guidelines to ensure optimal patient care by classifying medical centers and hospitals according to their ability to treat various injuries. Trauma results primarily from motor vehicle accidents, unintentional accidents at home and in the workplace, gunshot wounds, stab wounds, physical altercations, and domestic violence and physical abuse. According to the National Center for Health Statistics, unintentional accidents are the leading cause of death in white males between the ages of 15 and 24 years, and homicide is the leading cause of death in black males within the same age range (Table 11-1).

Deaths from traumatic injuries have a trimodal distribution, with the first critical period occurring seconds after the injury. Death during this period results from lacerations of the brain and spinal cord or the heart and great vessels. The second critical period occurs during the first 4 hours following the injury, with death generally resulting from intracranial hemorrhage, lacerations of the liver and spleen, or significant blood loss from multiple injuries. The third critical period occurs days to weeks following the injury, when death results from infection and multiple organ failure.

A well-designed *emergency medical system* (EMS) provides for prehospital care, acute hospital care, and rehabilitative care. Medical facilities are classified as a level I, level II, or level III trauma center, based on the availability of specialized medical personnel and equipment. When patients are triaged at the site of an accident, their injuries are classified as life-threatening, urgent, or nonurgent. Multiple injuries most likely occur in conjunction with severe head injuries. These patients must be treated with utmost care. Before transporting trauma victims, a clear airway must be established, acute bleeding must be controlled, and the patient

Table 11–1. Numbers of Deaths and Causes for Death according to Age: United States 1994

Cause of Death	Deaths	Cause of Death	Deaths
1-4 years		**15-24 years**	
All causes	6764	All causes	34,548
Unintentional injuries	**2467**	Unintentional injuries	**13,662**
Congenital anomalies	856	Homicide and legal intervention	**8019**
Malignant neoplasms	479	Suicide	4693
Homicide and legal intervention	430	Malignant neoplasms	1809
Diseases of heart	286	Diseases of heart	968
Pneumonia and influenza	188	Human immunodeficiency virus infection	578
Human immunodeficiency virus infection	161	Congenital anomalies	450
Certain conditions originating in the perinatal period	113	Pneumonia and influenza	229
		Cerebrovascular diseases	197
Septicemia	77	Chronic obstructive pulmonary diseases	189
Anemias	65		
5-14 years		**25-44 years**	
All causes	8193	All causes	149,771
Unintentional injuries	**3388**	Unintentional injuries	**25,808**
Malignant neoplasms	1105	Human immunodeficiency virus infection	24629
Homicide and legal intervention	**587**	Malignant neoplasms	22185
Congenital anomalies	448	Diseases of heart	16121
Suicide	314	Suicide	12,181
Diseases of heart	284	Homicide and legal intervention	**11803**
Human immunodeficiency virus infection	104	Chronic liver disease and cirrhosis	4373
Pneumonia and influenza	104	Cerebrovascular diseases	3387
Chronic obstructive pulmonary diseases	100	Diabetes mellitus	2258
Benign neoplasms	97	Pneumonia and influenza	2004

From National Center for Health Statistics: Health, United States, 1994, Hyattsville, MD, 1995, Public Health Service.

must be immobilized to avoid displacing fractures of the skeletal system and the spine and to avoid further injury to the spinal cord. Immobilization is accomplished with the use of splints, backboards with head blocks, and special air splint suits.

This system ensures that the trauma victim is taken to the closest appropriate medical facility to receive the proper medical care for the injuries, but not necessarily to the closest hospital. Once the patient arrives at the proper medical facility, careful assessment is necessary. This assessment includes evaluation of the patient's state of consciousness, vital signs (blood pressure, pulse, temperature, and respirations), pupil size and reaction to light, and motor activity of the extremities. A cross-table lateral cervical spine radiograph is necessary to assess damage to the cervical spine before the patient is moved. Additionally, radiographs of the chest, abdomen, and skeletal system must be obtained to evaluate the extent of injuries. Although statistics show that only 5% of all trauma victims have life-threatening injuries, these types of injuries are responsible for 50% of all in-hospital trauma deaths.

Level I, II, and III Trauma Centers

The primary hospital in the trauma system is a **level I medical center.** These medical centers can provide total care for all injuries. Level I centers require 24-hour per day in-house coverage by a radiologic technologist to perform emergency and surgical radiographic and fluoroscopic procedures and computed tomographic examinations. Technologists must be available on call to perform angiographic, sonographic, and nuclear medicine studies as required. Level I trauma centers are generally located in large metropolitan areas and serve as both primary care and tertiary care institutions.

Level II medical centers are the most common trauma facilities serving as community trauma centers. These institutions can handle the majority of trauma cases and transport patients to level I facilities only when necessary. Level II facilities have a radiologic technologist in-house 24 hours per day to perform emergency and surgical radiographic and fluoroscopic procedures, with technologists on call to perform CT, angiographic, sonographic, and nuclear medicine examinations as needed. These medical centers are generally community hospitals located in smaller cities and towns and provide a valuable service. **Level III medical centers** are usually located in remote rural areas and serve communities that do not have a level II center. Radiologic technologists are generally in-house for most of the day but may be available on call during late evening and night time hours.

TRAUMA OF THE VERTEBRAL COLUMN AND HEAD

Injuries to the Vertebral Column

The causes of vertebral column injuries include direct trauma and hyperextension-flexion injuries (whiplash). Radiographic indications of spinal column injuries include the interruption of smooth, continuous lines formed by the vertebrae stacking on each other (Fig. 11-1). Also, the vertebral bodies may lose some height, or the interspace may narrow. Muscle spasm as a result of trauma may cause a reversal or straightening of the normal spinal curvatures.

Perhaps the most common condition of the vertebral column is generalized back pain, typically in the lumbar area. Such back pain may not always result from bony involvement. Disk disease can cause muscle spasm with pain referral throughout the back. Finally, back pain may be secondary to referred pain from the hip.

Compression fractures are the most frequent type of injury involving a vertebral body.

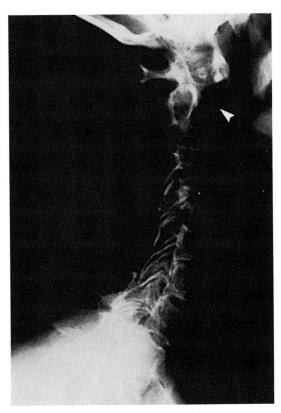

Fig. 11-1 A lateral cervical spine radiograph of an individual involved in a motor vehicle accident, demonstrating subluxation of the first and second cervical vertebrae as evidenced by the uneven alignment of the vertebral bodies. (Courtesy the American College of Radiology, Reston, Virginia.)

Usually the damage is limited to the upper portion of the vertebral body, particularly to the anterior margin. Such fractures generally occur in the thoracic and lumbar vertebrae (Fig. 11-2) with the most common site being T11-T12 in the thoracic spine and T12-L1 in the lumbar spine.

Cervical spine injuries may involve the odontoid process, usually at the junction of the odontoid and the body of the second cervical vertebra. A *hangman's fracture* (Fig. 11-3) is a fracture of the arch of the second cervical vertebra and is usually accompanied by anterior subluxation of the second cervical vertebra on the third cervical vertebra. A hangman's fracture, sometimes referred to as *traumatic spondylosis,* results from acute hyperextension of the head.

Radiography of the trauma patient with vertebral trauma is critical. Fractures and dislocations of the spine are classified as stable or unstable. The spine may be visualized as two columns, with the anterior column composed of the vertebral bodies and intervertebral disks and the posterior column composed of the posterior elements (e.g., spinous processes, lamina). If either the anterior column or the posterior column of the spine is fractured or dislocated, the injury is classified as stable. However, if both columns are involved in the injury, it is classified as unstable. In all cases, the patient should be immobilized until cross-table lateral radiographs have been obtained and cleared by a physician. To rule out possible fractures and dislocations, the lateral cervical spine radiograph must include all seven vertebrae in their entirety, including spinous processes and intervertebral disk spaces. At times, this may require assistance in depressing the patient's shoulders or the use

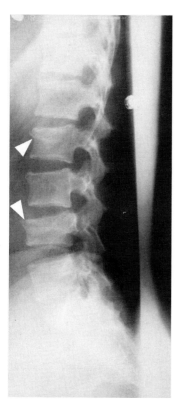

Fig. 11-2 A lateral lumbar radiograph demonstrating compression fractures of the second and fourth lumbar vertebral bodies with no apparent fracture of the posterior elements of the spine. (Courtesy the American College of Radiology, Reston, Virginia.)

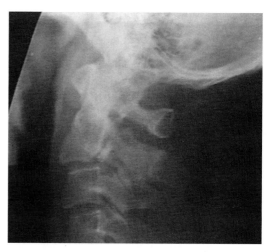

Fig. 11-3 A lateral cervical spine radiograph demonstrating a typical hangman's fracture with disruption of the spinal laminar line at C2 with the spinous process of C2 displaced posteriorly. (Courtesy the American College of Radiology, Reston, Virginia.)

of the twining (swimmer's method) projection to clearly demonstrate the entire seventh cervical vertebra. A twining projection may also be necessary to demonstrate the upper thoracic vertebra in a lateral projection. Additional trauma projections of the cervical spine such as the pillar projection or trauma oblique projections may be requested to better demonstrate the complex anatomy of the spine.

Spinal injury often results in a loss of neurologic function. It may be temporary or permanent depending on the cause of the dysfunction. Compression of the spinal cord due to contusion or hemorrhage leads to rapid swelling of the spinal cord. This causes a rise in the intradural pressure and causes temporary neurologic dysfunction. This temporary loss of neurologic function usually resolves in several days. However, lacerations of the spinal cord or transection of the cord results in permanent damage because the severed nerves do not regenerate. Laceration of the spinal cord above the fifth cervical vertebra is almost always fatal, and lacerations below this region result in permanent paralysis. Patients with lacerations or transection of the cord develop immediate flaccid paralysis with loss of all sensation and reflex activity, which gradually changes to spastic paraplegia within days.

Fractures or dislocations of the vertebrae may impinge on the spinal cord and cause significant damage. The responsibility of the technologist in terms of proper patient handling and obtaining of diagnostic-quality images cannot be overemphasized. Often, tomography of the vertebral column may be used to better demonstrate vertebral anatomy. Computed tomography (CT) also plays a vital role in the diagnosis and treatment of vertebral fractures, dislocations, and associated problems. There is still a role for conventional tomography in spinal fractures, especially with horizontal fractures. In certain situations, magnetic resonance imaging (MRI) may be used to evaluate the extent of ligamentous and soft tissue injury or injury to the spinal cord.

Stable injuries to the spine are treated with complete bed rest until the swelling and pain subside. Unstable injuries are immobilized with traction until the bone and soft tissue structures have healed. Cervical radiographs are often performed to demonstrate proper alignment while the patient is in traction. Surgery may also be necessary for internal fixation of the fractures or to remove displaced fragments and decompress the spinal cord. Computed tomography of the spine may be used preoperatively to serve as a road map to the surgeon because this imaging modality clearly demonstrates the size, number, and location of various fracture fragments. It may also be used postoperatively to demonstrate the outcome of the surgery.

Injuries to the Skull and Brain

The anatomy surrounding the delicate brain generally protects it well under normal conditions. The diploic arrangement of the calvaria, the mechanical buffering action of cerebrospinal fluid (CSF), and the tough dura mater all work to prevent brain injury. Despite this protection, sufficient force to the skull can cause injury to the brain. Head trauma is the major neurologic cause of mortality and morbidity in individuals under 50 years of age.

Head trauma can result in skull fractures, brain injury, or a combination of the two. The role of plain film radiography in evaluation of head trauma is rather limited, as CT allows rapid assessment of the nature of any brain injury. Assessment of the state of the brain following head injury is more crucial than that of the skull. Routine skull radiography on trauma victims may be delayed to allow treatment of the complications of brain injury readily diagnosed by CT. Skull fractures visualized by either modality are often seen with accompanying hematomas. If patients sustain an open skull fracture, they are at risk for development of meningitis or brain abscesses. Regardless of the imaging modality used, the technologist must constantly observe a patient with a head injury while performing an examination. Any change noted in the patient's condition should be reported immediately.

CEREBRAL CRANIAL FRACTURES

Cerebral cranial fractures usually refer to those in the calvaria of the skull. Vascular markings in the skull, either venous or arterial, are routinely demonstrated as linear translucencies and can occasionally be mistaken for cerebral cranial fractures (Fig. 11-4). In most cases, a fracture appears more translucent than a vascular marking because a fracture traverses the full thickness of the skull. Although the edges of the fractures may branch abruptly, they can be seen to fit together, whereas venous channels have irregular edges that cannot be fitted together. The sutures between the individual cranial bones remain visible radiographically, even after they become fused. To an untrained eye, these sutures may also resemble a fracture.

In most cases, the location of the skull fracture is more important than the extent of the fracture. If the fracture crosses an artery, an arterial bleed may occur, resulting in an epidural hematoma. A fracture that enters the mastoid air cells or a sinus communicates with a potentially infected space, which would allow the contamination to spread throughout the cranium, possibly resulting in encephalitis or meningitis.

Fractures visible after skull trauma are generally classified as either linear, depressed, or basilar skull fractures. **Linear fractures** appear as straight, sharply defined, nonbranching lines and are intensely radiolucent (Fig. 11-5). Up to 80% of all skull fractures are linear fractures. A **depressed fracture** appears as a curvilinear density because the fracture edges are overlapped (Fig. 11-6). These fractures are caused by high-velocity impact from small objects. Injury to the cerebral cortex may result, causing bleeding into the subarachnoid space. A depressed fracture is best demonstrated when the x-ray beam is directed tangential to the fracture.

Basilar skull fractures are very difficult to demonstrate radiographically. Air-fluid levels in the sphenoid sinus or clouding of the mastoid

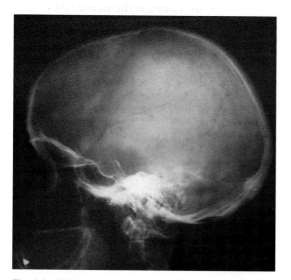

Fig. 11-4 A lateral skull radiograph demonstrating normal vascular markings within the cerebral cranium. (Courtesy the American College of Radiology, Reston, Virginia.)

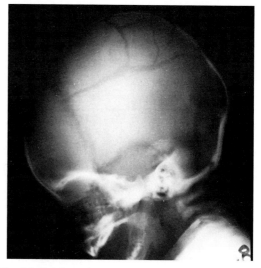

Fig. 11-5 A lateral skull radiograph of a 3-month-old infant with a history of striking his head on a bath tub. The radiograph reveals linear skull fracture of the parietal bone. (Courtesy Riverside Methodist Hospitals, Columbus, Ohio.)

air cells is often the only radiographic finding suggesting a fracture. Therefore, it is important to include a cross-table lateral skull radiograph with the trauma skull radiographic series.

BRAIN TRAUMA

In addition to brain injury from a penetration wound (as could happen with a fracture), it can also occur from an acceleration and rapid deceleration of the head, which is termed a *closed head injury.* With head trauma, the brain is traumatically shaken within the cranium and subjected to forces of compression, acceleration, and deceleration. Brain tissues are injured from compression, tension, and shearing, with the last perhaps most important (Fig. 11-7). The superficial cerebrum in the frontal, temporal, and occipital regions is most often affected.

Following a blow to the head, an individual may experience a temporary loss of consciousness and reflexes. This widespread paralysis of brain function is known as a **concussion** and is characterized by headache, vertigo, and vomiting. Higher mental functions may be impaired for several hours, with the patient remembering little of the events surrounding the concussion. There is a strong tendency toward spontaneous and complete recovery because of the lack of structural damage to the brain. Recovery generally occurs in less than 24 hours. Treatment is conservative once assessment (usually by CT) has ruled out any hemorrhage or fracture. Bed rest and possible admission to the hospital are the usual means of dealing with concussion.

A brain **contusion** can also result from a direct blow to the head. This bruising of brain parenchyma is more serious than a concussion. A contusion formed on the side of the head where the trauma occurs is called a **coup lesion,** and one formed on the opposite side of the skull in reference to the site of trauma is a **contrecoup lesion.** Contusions are characterized by neuron damage, edema, and punctate (pinpoint punctures or depressions) hemorrhaging. On CT, contusions appear as small, ill-defined foci of increased density (Fig. 11-8). Subdural or epidural hematomas can occur in conjunction with a contusion and result in increased intracranial pressure that can be life-threatening. Signs seen in the patient with a contusion include drowsiness, confusion, and agitation. Hemiparesis and unequal pupil size may also be seen. Computed tomography plays a major role

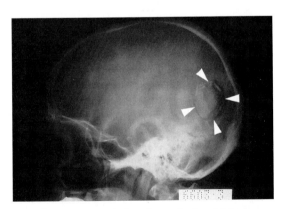

Fig. 11-6 A lateral skull radiograph of a child who was struck in the head with a baseball bat. The radiograph demonstrates a depressed fracture of the frontal bone. (Courtesy Riverside Methodist Hospitals, Columbus, Ohio.)

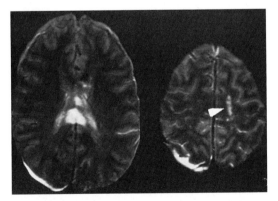

Fig. 11-7 A T$_2$ weighted MRI image demonstrates a shearing injury of the corpus callosum *(arrow)* and a small subdural hematoma on the lateral margins of the brain in this young male who fell and failed to regain consciousness. (Courtesy Riverside Methodist Hospitals, Columbus, Ohio.)

in the diagnosis of hematomas resulting from contusions, providing ready visualization of hemorrhagic blood, as described in the following section. Treatment is generally conservative, centering on prevention of shock, control of edema, and drainage of any hematoma present.

Persistence of loss of consciousness for more than 24 hours is known as a **coma**. This is usually a serious condition and may be fatal. More than half of all comas result from trauma to the head or circulatory problems associated with hypertension, sclerosis, thrombosis, tumor or abscess formation, or insufficient flow to the brain. Other causes include metabolic reasons such as lack of insulin (i.e., diabetic coma) and uremic poisoning from disturbed kidney metabolism. Diagnosis related to a coma may involve use of CT, MRI, or both and is centered at determining, if possible, the cause of the coma. Treatment then rests on success in attacking the cause.

HEMATOMAS OF THE BRAIN

As noted, brain trauma can result in hemorrhaging of blood from a ruptured artery or vein. Although venous bleeding occurs more slowly than arterial, both types of hemorrhage and resultant edema of the brain cause an increase in the intracranial pressure. Because the skull's structure does not allow expansion, the increased pressure displaces the brain toward its opening, the foramen magnum. This trauma to the brain results in serious neurologic consequences or even death if not treated promptly. Computed tomography plays the major imaging role in diagnosis of the hemorrhaging.

A **hematoma** is a collection of blood; four primary types of cerebral hematomas have been identified. The highest mortality rate is associated with an *epidural* (extradural) *hematoma* (Fig. 11-9). Even when promptly recognized and treated, it has a mortality rate of up to 30%.

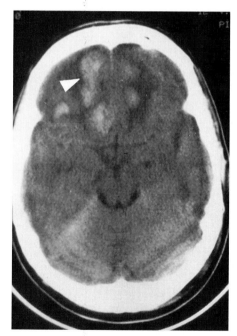

Fig. 11-8 An axial CT scan demonstrates hemorrhagic contusions of the brain as a result of a car accident for this young male. (Courtesy Riverside Methodist Hospitals, Columbus, Ohio.)

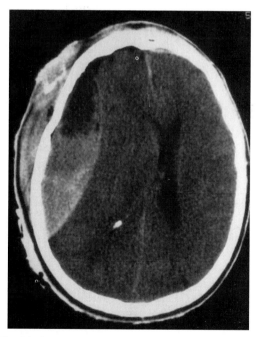

Fig. 11-9 A noncontrast axial CT view of this young male injured in an auto accident readily demonstrates a large epidural hematoma. (Courtesy Riverside Methodist Hospitals, Columbus, Ohio.)

An epidural hematoma results from a torn artery, usually the middle meningeal artery, with blood pooling between the bony skull and the dura mater. Most commonly, the artery or its branches are torn by a fracture of the thin, squamous portion of the temporal bone. In more than 80% of cases, the skull fracture is visible radiographically. As an arterial bleed, it accumulates rapidly and quickly causes neurologic symptoms, including early coma. It is seen on CT scans as an increased density, generally occupying a small area with a sharply convex appearance. Often it is accompanied by a fracture of the skull or facial bones. If not diagnosed and surgically treated quickly, the outcome is fatal as a result of brain displacement and herniation.

A *subdural hematoma* is positioned between the dura mater and the arachnoid meningeal layers (Figs. 11-10 and 11-11). It usually follows blunt trauma to the frontal or occipital lobes of the skull and results from tearing of subdural veins connecting the cerebral cortex and dural sinuses. As a venous hemorrhage, it bleeds much more slowly than an epidural hematoma. In an acute stage, it is seen on CT as a curvilinear area of increased density on portions or all of the cerebral hemispheres. It pushes the brain away from the skull and causes a mass effect (i.e., brain shift across midline), with accompanying shift of the ventricles. In a subacute stage (up to several days old), it appears on CT as a decreased or isodense fluid collection. In a chronic state (2 to 3 weeks old), the surface of the hematoma becomes concave. Delayed coma can occur with a subdural hematoma.

A *subarachnoid hematoma* accumulates between the arachnoid layer and the thin pia mater that invests the brain. It occurs most frequently at the vertex where the greatest brain movement occurs in trauma, and it results from tearing of small vessels. In most head trauma cases, a subarachnoid hemorrhage is usually limited to one or two sulci, where it has a dense appearance (Fig. 11-12). Less commonly, the rupture of a major cerebral vessel results in subarachnoid hematoma.

An *intracerebral hematoma* can result from trauma (Fig. 11-13), ruptured hemangiomas, or

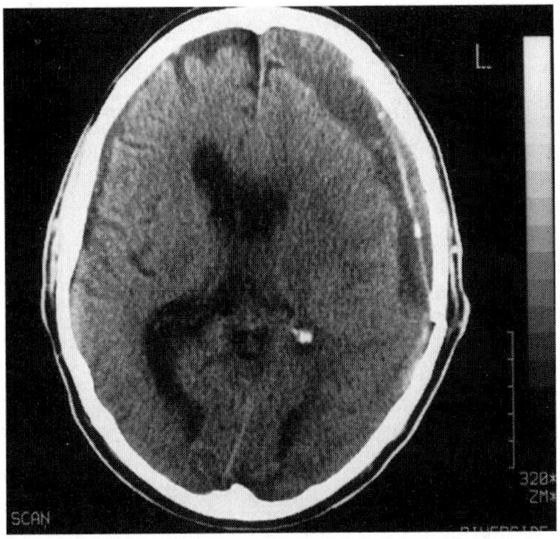

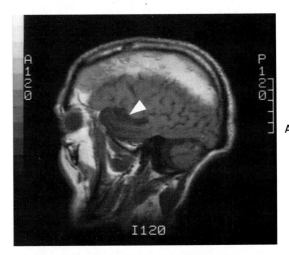

Fig. 11-10 CT demonstration of a large subdural hematoma outside the brain tissue in the left frontoparietal area of this 76-year-old man. (Courtesy Riverside Methodist Hospitals, Columbus, Ohio.)

Fig. 11-11 A, A T₁ weighted sagittal MRI view demonstrates a large subdural hematoma as well as a temporal lobe infarct *(arrow).* The white versus gray appearance of the hematoma distinguishes subacute (fresh) from older blood. (**A** Courtesy Riverside Methodist Hospitals, Columbus, Ohio.)

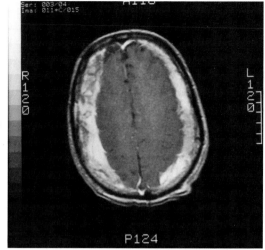

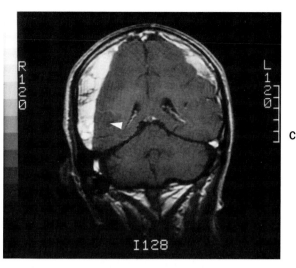

B

C

Fig. 11-11 cont'd. B, A T$_1$ weighted axial MRI view with gadolinium demonstrates a large, bilateral subdural hematoma in this 67-year-old man. **C,** A T$_1$ weighted coronal MRI view with gadolinium demonstrates the same bilateral subdural hematoma. The *arrow* indicates the right-sided temporal lobe infarct. (**B** and **C** Courtesy Riverside Methodist Hospitals, Columbus, Ohio.)

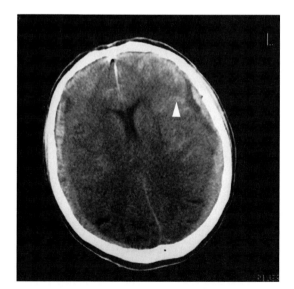

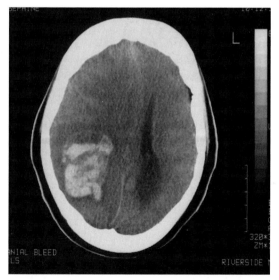

Fig. 11-12 CT demonstration of subarachnoid hematoma as indicated by the sulci opacified by blood in this 69-year-old man. Also visible is extensive bilateral subdural hematoma. (Courtesy Riverside Methodist Hospitals, Columbus, Ohio.)

Fig. 11-13 A massive intracerebral hematoma that occurred spontaneously in this 63-year-old woman. The patient expired within a few hours after the bleed began. (Courtesy Riverside Methodist Hospitals, Columbus, Ohio.)

stroke (cerebrovascular accidents) and creates bleeding within the brain. Common sites following trauma are the frontal, temporal, and occipital lobes of the brain. Small parenchymal vessels tear as a result of coup and contrecoup forces. An intracerebral hematoma is seen on CT as an increased density within the brain causing significant mass effect and may have an accompanying subarachnoid component. These hematomas develop edema around them as time passes and are slowly resorbed if the patient survives.

Diagnosis of hematomas is made primarily through clinical history and neurologic signs and symptoms. As noted, CT plays a major role in ready visualization of bleeding. Angiography may be used to visualize any defects in the cerebral vasculature. Treatment is often conservative unless active bleeding or significant mass effect is present, in which event an opening in the skull may be created surgically to allow drainage of blood and prevent complications. Prevention of infection and meningitis is important in the case of a fractured skull.

SKELETAL TRAUMA

Fractures

A **fracture** is a discontinuity of bone caused by mechanical forces either applied to the bone or transmitted directly along the line of a bone. When a fracture occurs, blood vessels are broken as a result of the break in the endosteum and periosteum. As blood and lymph and tissue fluids infiltrate this area, swelling and pain result. Such soft tissue swelling is a major clue to diagnosis.

General radiography is extremely important in the evaluation of skeletal trauma and serves several purposes. The most obvious of these is to diagnose the presence of a fracture or dislocation. If a fracture is present, for example, a determination can be made as to whether the underlying bone is normal or whether the fracture is pathologic in nature. Before the fracture is stabilized, radiographs are taken to show the position of the bone ends. Fractures are in "good

alignment" when there is no perceptible angulation or displacement in frontal and lateral projections. Postreduction films indicate the success of the fracture reduction. Finally, subsequent radiographs are taken to assess healing and any possible complications of fractures.

In any case of trauma, it is essential to have at least two projections of the part, preferably taken at right angles to one another. A minimum of two projections is also necessary to adequately determine fracture alignment. These radiographs should demonstrate the joint above and below the area of trauma because there may be dislocation and because the injury may transfer force to a point distal or proximal to the point of injury. An example is a fracture or dislocation of the fibular head concurrent with an ankle or distal tibial fracture.

Frequently, fractures are obvious by clinical examination, but radiographic changes in appearance may be subtle. Fractures usually appear as a radiolucent line, but they may be thin and easily overlooked. Occasionally a fracture appears as a radiopaque line if the fragments overlap. A step in the cortex, as indicated by a break in the normal bony contour, is a second radiographic indication. Other signs include interruption of the bony trabeculae, bulging or buckling of the cortex, soft tissue swelling, and joint effusion. Also, the relationship of the end of a bone to its shaft is an important sign, as in the loss of normal volar tilt to the distal radial articular surface with an impacted distal radial fracture.

Skeletal trauma usually causes significant soft tissue injuries, including neurovascular damage, capsular and ligamentous tears, cartilage injury, and hemarthroses. Such injury may be assessed in several ways. Stress radiographs on a joint determine ligamentous stability. Radiographs of both extremities are often used to compare epiphyseal appearance. Arteriography may also be used to assess any vascular damage as a result of skeletal trauma.

When performing radiography of the skeletal system, it is critical for the technologist to choose the appropriate exposure factors and film-screen combination to produce a radiograph demonstrating good soft tissue definition in addition to achieving good penetration of the bony anatomy. If the soft tissue is too dark or the associated bony anatomy too light (i.e., no trabecular pattern), then the radiograph is of compromised diagnostic quality. Additionally, it is often helpful to the radiologist if the technologist notes, through film markers or as written on the requisition, areas of point tenderness. This is a highly specific indication of a fracture that may be subtle. Larger body parts such as the hip, thigh, and knee are less assessable for point tenderness; instead, inability to bear weight is suggestive of a fracture. Again, an important role of the technologist is to assess the patient regarding such symptoms and signs and to provide the radiologist with as much information as possible, both on the radiographs and verbally or in writing on the requisition.

Bone tissue is unique in its ability to repair itself in that it reactivates processes that normally occur during embryogenesis. Initially, the break in the bone is filled by a large clot that temporarily bridges the fracture. Within 2 to 3 days, osteoblasts begin to slowly appear around the injured bone. Immobilization of the injured site is critical because any unnatural movement interferes with the deposition of the calcified matrix necessary for permanent union of the fracture. *Provisional callus* is mainly composed of cartilage and begins to form approximately 1 week after the fracture. As calcium continues to be deposited within the provisional callus, it is replaced by *bony callus* (Fig. 11-14), which is responsible for rigidly uniting the fracture site. Although the break is rigidly united within 4 to 6 weeks, excess bone still encircles the external fracture site, and excess bone is still found within the marrow space at this time. Remodeling of the bone and total healing require months. Weight-bearing force on the fracture site tends to guide the modeling process, so in many cases the patient may be instructed to begin using the affected limb in a limited fashion

at this point in the healing process. If everything goes well during the healing process, the bone may repair to the point that the fracture site is no longer visible on subsequent radiographs. Proper healing greatly depends on the initial immobilization (casting, splinting, pinning, or plating), proper alignment or reduction of the fracture, and proper metabolic activity, which includes good vascularity and blood supply, proper nutrition, and normal hormone levels. Bacterial infections of the fracture site may inhibit callus formation, thus complicating the healing process.

Delayed union is a term referring to a fracture that does not heal within the usual time. If a

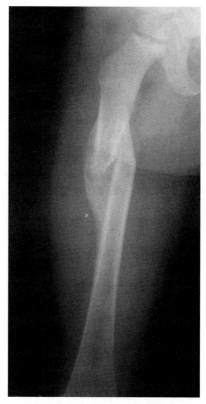

Fig. 11-14 A femoral radiograph demonstrating advanced callus formation following a transverse fracture of the femur. (Courtesy the American College of Radiology, Reston, Virginia.)

fracture is not reduced properly or is not properly immobilized, malunion may occur. *Malunion* refers to a fracture that heals in a faulty position, thus impairing the normal function or cosmetic appearance of the affected body part (Fig. 11-15). The most serious complication is nonunion. *Nonunion* refers to a fracture in which healing does not occur and the fragments do not join (Fig. 11-16). This is often due to lack of vascularization. Injuries to other soft tissue structures or organs can be associated with skeletal fractures, such as a rib fracture that penetrates the lung and results in a pneumothorax. Additional complications of skeletal fractures include muscular ossification and fat emboli occurring in bones containing yellow bone marrow.

FRACTURE CLASSIFICATIONS.

Several means of classifying fractures exist. One distinction is whether the fracture is open or closed. An **open fracture** (formerly referred to as a *compound fracture*) is one in which the bone has penetrated the skin. This type of fracture leaves an open route for bacteria to enter from outside the body, which may lead to possible infection. As described earlier, the intrusion of bacteria can alter the healing process, and pre-cautions must be taken to prevent infection from setting into the bone or surrounding soft tissue structures. A **closed fracture** (formerly referred to as a *simple fracture*) is one in which the skin is not penetrated, thus reducing the chance of infection.

Fractures may be classified according to the mechanics of stress that produce the break or the appearance of the fracture line. This includes torsion (twisting), transverse, linear, and spiral fractures. When one of the fractured bone ends is jammed into the cancellous tissue of another fragment, it is called an **impacted fracture** (Fig. 11-17).

Fractures may also be classified according to their location such as intertrochanteric (transcervical), supracondylar, or transcondylar fractures. Often they may not fit into a specific classification because they may demonstrate mixed features. The following pages discuss the appearance of common types of fractures.

COMMINUTED FRACTURES

Sometimes one or more fragments separate along the edges of the major fragment, in addition to the major line of the fracture. Such fractures are said to be **comminuted** (Fig. 11-18).

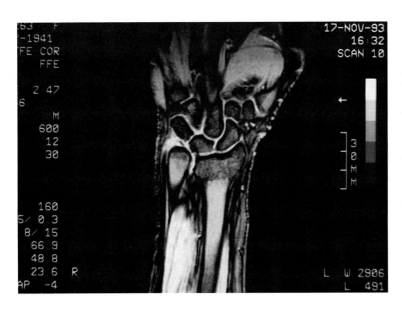

Fig. 11-15 An MRI of the wrist after fracture on a 55-year-old woman with a 2-month history of increasing pain and disability. There is malunion of the distal radial fracture with loss of palmer inclination and reversal with subsequent dorsal inclination. (Courtesy Riverside Methodist Hospitals, Columbus, Ohio.)

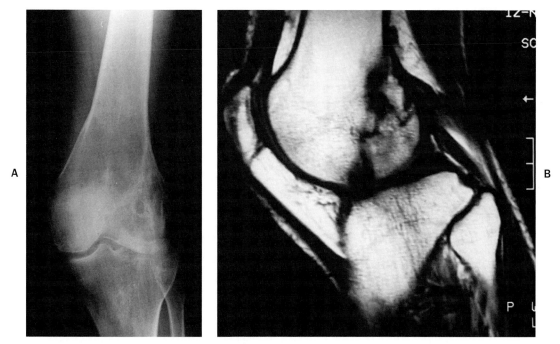

Fig. 11-16 A, A knee radiograph of a 32-year-old man who sustained a gunshot wound to the left knee 3 years prior. Nonunion of the lateral femoral condyle is demonstrated. **B,** An MRI of the same patient demonstrating nonunion of the posterior lateral femoral condyle with large subcondral defects. (**A** and **B** Courtesy Riverside Methodist Hospitals, Columbus, Ohio.)

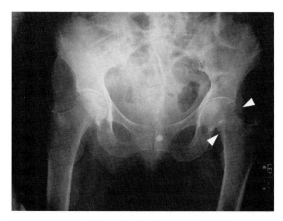

Fig. 11-17 A pelvis radiograph on an elderly woman with trauma to her left hip. The radiograph demonstrates an impacted fracture of the left hip. (Courtesy the American College of Radiology, Reston, Virginia.)

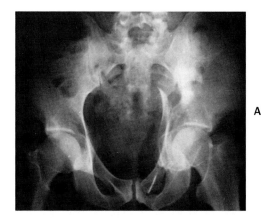

Fig. 11-18 A, A pelvic radiograph demonstrating a complex, comminuted fracture of the left hemipelvis. (Courtesy Riverside Methodist Hospitals, Columbus, Ohio.)

Continued

Comminuted fractures differ from multiple fractures as follows. In the case of a multiple fracture, each fracture is complete, leaving a fragment of intact shaft between them. Comminuted fractures do not represent a complete thickness of bone as do multiple fractures. Occasionally, the bone involved in a comminuted fracture may be extensively shattered, as might occur from a gunshot wound. Such fractures are also particularly apt to be compound.

A butterfly fracture is a comminuted fracture in which there are one or two butterfly wing or wedge-shaped fragments split off from the main fragments. A splintered fracture is a comminuted fracture with long, sharp-pointed fragments.

COMPLETE, NONCOMMINUTED FRACTURES

Complete, **noncomminuted fractures** are those in which the bone has separated into two fragments. The fractures may be recognized according to the direction of the fracture line. A spiral or oblique fracture is an example of this type. Such a fracture usually results from a rotary type of injury that twists the bone apart and is particularly common in the shafts of long bones (Fig. 11-19). A transverse fracture (Fig. 11-20)

is another type of complete, noncomminuted fracture. Demonstrated radiographically, such a fracture through normal bone is invariably ragged along the fracture line. A pathologic fracture is commonly a transverse fracture occurring in abnormal bone that is weakened by

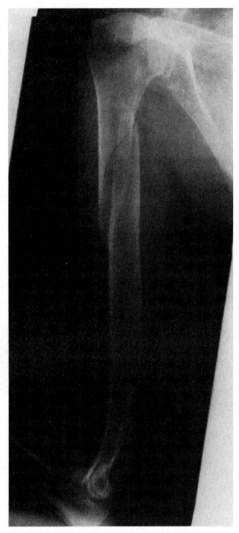

Fig. 11-19 A humerus radiograph of an individual who sustained a twisting injury of the humerus. The radiograph demonstrates a spiral fracture of the humerus. (Courtesy Riverside Methodist Hospitals, Columbus, Ohio.)

B

Fig. 11-18 cont'd. B, CT examination of the pelvis on the same patient demonstrating a major fracture plane beginning in the posterior wing of the ileum and extending just anterior to the sacroiliac joint. (Courtesy Riverside Methodist Hospitals, Columbus, Ohio.)

various diseases (Fig. 11-21). It may result from the disease process itself or from a relatively minor trauma. Often, pathologic fractures may be the first indication of the presence of pathology. Multiple fractures are another type of complete, noncomminuted fracture in which two or more complete fractures occur involving the shaft of a single bone (Fig. 11-22).

AVULSION FRACTURES

Avulsion fractures occur when a fragment of bone is pulled away from the shaft. These usually occur around joints because of ligament, tendon, and muscle tearing, as associated with a

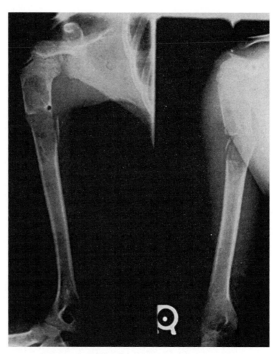

Fig. 11-21 A humerus radiograph demonstrating a pathologic fracture through a bone cyst. The patient had complained of pain and denied a history of trauma associated with this fracture. (Courtesy Riverside Methodist Hospitals, Columbus, Ohio.)

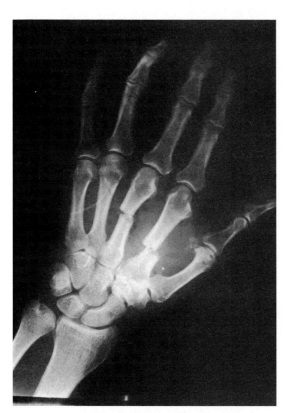

Fig. 11-20 A hand radiograph of a 32-year-old man involved in an industrial accident, demonstrating transverse fractures of the second and third metacarpals. (Courtesy Riverside Methodist Hospitals, Columbus, Ohio.)

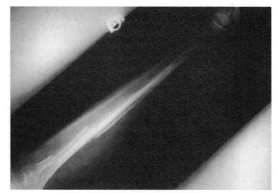

Fig. 11-22 A forearm radiograph of an individual involved in a motor vehicle accident. The radiograph revealed multiple fractures of the forearm. (Courtesy Riverside Methodist Hospitals, Columbus, Ohio.)

sprain or dislocation (Fig. 11-23). A chip fracture is an avulsion fracture of a small fragment or chip of bone from the corner of a phalynx or other long bone. These are very common in the fingers and are often tiny.

INCOMPLETE FRACTURES

Incomplete fractures are those in which only part of the bony structure gives way, with little or no displacement. A common example is the **greenstick fracture,** in which the cortex breaks on one side without separation or breaking of the opposing cortex (Fig. 11-24). The effect is similar to that of trying to break a green twig, hence its name. Greenstick fractures are found almost exclusively in infants and children under the age of 10 years because of the softness of the cancellous bone. A **torus fracture** is a greenstick fracture in which the cortex bulges outward, usually in the metaphysis, producing only a slight irregularity (Fig. 11-25).

Incomplete fractures may also occur in demineralized bone, such as occurs with osteoporo-sis. The bone in question breaks only part of the way through, resulting in a sharp angular deformity without displacement.

Penetrating fractures are a type of incomplete fracture resulting from penetration by a sharp object such as a bullet or a knife. Frequently there is a comminution at the site of the injury.

GROWTH PLATE FRACTURES

Growth plate fractures involve the end of a long bone of a child (Fig. 11-26). The fracture may be limited to growth plate cartilage and is thus not directly visible unless displacement occurs, or it may extend into the metaphysis, epiphysis, or both. Crush injuries of the growth plate can also occur. Comparison projections are often used with such fractures to compare growth plate appearances. Healed injuries of this

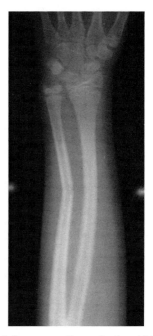

Fig. 11-24 A forearm radiograph of a child who sustained a fall. It demonstrates a greenstick fracture of the middle portion of the ulna. Notice the incomplete break of the cortex of the ulna. (Courtesy Riverside Methodist Hospitals, Columbus, Ohio.)

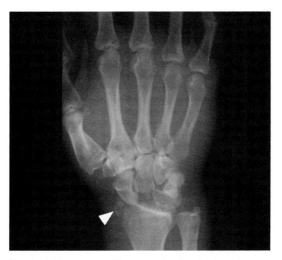

Fig. 11-23 A wrist radiograph obtained following trauma to the wrist resulting in perilunate dislocation with an associated avulsion fracture of the distal radius. (Courtesy the American College of Radiology, Reston, Virginia.)

type may result in an alteration of the length of the involved bone.

STRESS AND FATIGUE FRACTURES

Stress fractures usually occur as a result of an abnormal degree of repetitive trauma. They are generally found at the point of muscular attachments, such as in the fibula of a runner. Stress fractures may not be clearly visible on plain radiographs for up to 2 weeks but may be diagnosed with radionuclide bone scans or an MRI of the affected area (Fig. 11-27). **Fatigue fractures** occur at sites of maximal strain on a bone, usually in connection with unaccustomed activity. Most frequently, fatigue fractures are found in the metatarsals, particularly the second metatarsal—the classic "march" fracture. Other common names for fatigue fractures include *stretch* or *insufficiency* fractures.

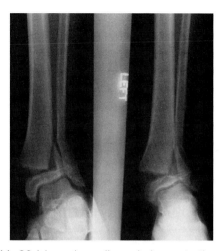

Fig. 11-26 A lower leg radiograph demonstrating an epiphyseal-metaphyseal fracture of the tibia with a transverse diaphyseal fracture of the distal fibula. (Courtesy the American College of Radiology, Reston, Virginia.)

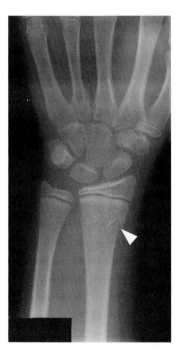

Fig. 11-25 A forearm radiograph of a 14-year-old girl who fell on her hand, resulting in a torus fracture of the distal radius. (Courtesy the American College of Radiology, Reston, Virginia.)

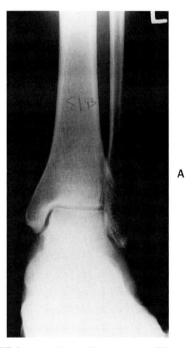

Fig. 11-27 A, An ankle radiograph on a 55-year-old woman complaining of pain in the medial aspect of the distal tibia. The radiograph appears normal with no evidence of fracture. (**A** Courtesy Riverside Methodist Hospitals, Columbus, Ohio.) *Continued*

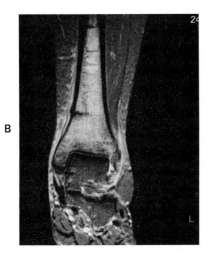

Fig. 11-27 cont'd. B, An MRI of the same patient demonstrating a stress fracture of the distal tibia.
(**B** Courtesy Riverside Methodist Hospitals, Columbus, Ohio.)

Occult Fractures and Bone Bruise

An **occult fracture** gives clinical signs of its presence without radiologic evidence. Follow-up examination within 10 days reveals bone resorption or displacement at the fracture site (Fig. 11-28). The most common sites for occult fractures are the carpal navicular and the ribs. A bruise to the bone may be revealed upon MR examination (Fig. 11-29) and is presumed to represent hemorrhage and edema, usually beneath an adjacent joint surface.

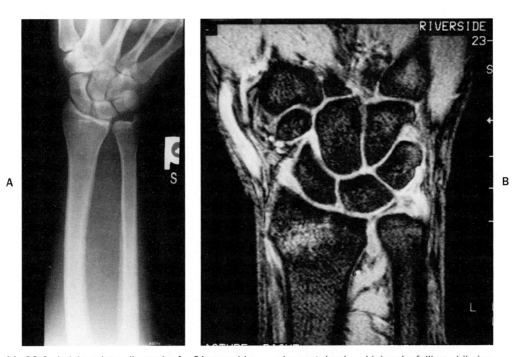

Fig. 11-28 A, A right wrist radiograph of a 31-year-old man who sustained and injury by falling while ice skating. No definite fracture or dislocation is demonstrated. **B,** An MR of the right wrist of the same patient as in "A" demonstrating an occult, oblique, intraarticular distal radial fracture beginning just proximal to the styloid and extending to the middle third of the radius. (Courtesy Riverside Methodist Hospitals, Columbus, Ohio.)

Fractures in Specific Locations

Some fractures occur in selected areas and are usually easily recognized. One of these is the *Colles' fracture* (Fig. 11-30), which is a fracture through the distal inch of the radius. The distal fragment is usually angled backward on the shaft with impaction along the dorsal aspect. An avulsion fracture of the ulnar styloid process occurs in more than half of all Colles' fractures. This is the most common wrist fracture, and it usually results from falling on an outstretched hand. The external skin contour of a Colles' fracture displays a "dinner fork" deformity. A Smith's fracture is a reverse Colles' fracture with displacement toward the palmar aspect of the hand. A direct blow or fall with the wrist in hyperflexion is the usual mechanism of injury.

A *Boxer's fracture* occurs when the fifth metacarpal (and occasionally the fourth metacarpal) fractures as a result of a blow to or with the

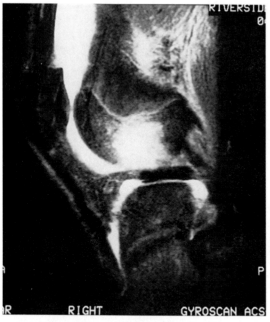

Fig. 11-29 An MRI of the right knee of a 17-year-old boy who suffered a rotary injury while playing basketball. The image demonstrates extensive bone bruising of the lateral meniscocondylar notch and femoral condyles. (Courtesy Riverside Methodist Hospitals, Columbus, Ohio.)

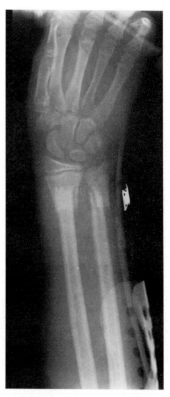

Fig. 11-30 A radiograph of a wrist on an elderly woman who fell on an outstretched hand. The radiograph demonstrates a classic Colles' fracture. (Courtesy Riverside Methodist Hospitals, Columbus, Ohio.)

hand (Fig. 11-31). A *Monteggia's fracture* is one of the proximal third of the ulnar shaft, with anterior dislocation of the radial head (Fig. 11-32). With both proximal and distal injuries to the forearm, it is important to ensure both joints are included on the radiograph.

In the ankle, the most common injuries are to the malleoli. A *Pott's fracture* involves both malleoli, with dislocation of the ankle joint (Fig. 11-33). Less common fractures may seem more like minor sprains, requiring the radiologist to examine every aspect of the bony anatomy. A *Maisonneuve fracture* (Fig. 11-34) is a less frequent ankle injury. It consists of a severe ankle sprain with a fracture of the proximal third of the fibula. This fracture may be easily overlooked because the more painful ankle injury may caused the proximal fibular injury to be missed.

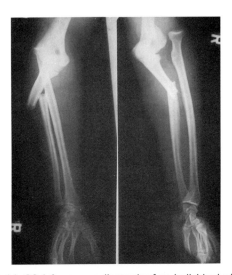

Fig. 11-32 A forearm radiograph of an individual who fell off a cliff, landing on an outstretched hand with the elbow partially flexed. The radiograph demonstrates a Monteggia's fracture of the forearm. (Courtesy the American College of Radiology, Reston, Virginia.)

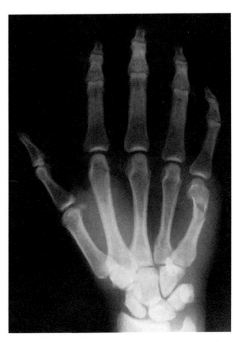

Fig. 11-31 A radiograph demonstrating a boxer's fracture of the fifth metacarpal head of the right hand. (Courtesy Riverside Methodist Hospitals, Columbus, Ohio.)

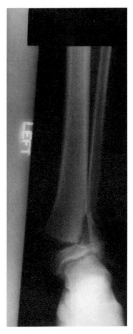

Fig. 11-33 An ankle radiograph depicting a Pott's fracture of the ankle demonstrated by a dislocation of the joint with a fracture of both malleoli. (Courtesy Riverside Methodist Hospitals, Columbus, Ohio.)

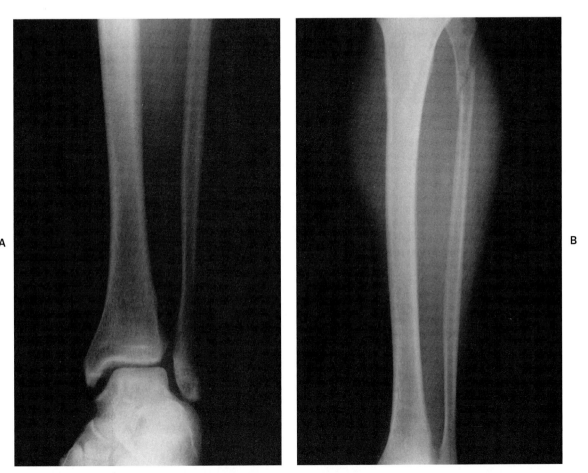

Fig. 11-34 A, A left ankle radiograph on a patient sustaining a twisting injury demonstrates a widening ankle mortise on the medial aspect with marked soft tissue swelling indicative of a Maisonneuve fracture. **B,** A left tibia-fibula radiograph on the same patient demonstrating a Maisonneuve fracture with minimal angulation and external rotation of the proximal fragment. (**A** and **B** Courtesy Riverside Methodist Hospitals, Columbus, Ohio.)

As mentioned earlier, radiographic signs of some fractures are subtle at best. Such is sometimes the case with the elbow. The elbow "fat pad sign" (Fig. 11-35) can be an indicator of a nonvisualized, underlying fracture of the bones of the elbow. In the elbow, there is normally a small accumulation of fat adjacent to the anterior surface of the distal humerus. This radiolucency is normally visible radiographically. A similar pad is found along the posterior surface but is normally not visualized radiographically. If the joint capsule is distended by fluid as a result of a fracture, the posterior fat pad becomes displaced from the bone and is visible on the lateral projection of the elbow. Visualization of a posterior fat pad is considered to be a sign of a possible underlying fracture. The anterior fat pad may also be displaced, giving a sail-shaped appearance. This is a prime example of how soft tissue demonstration can assist in making a diagnosis.

Visceral Cranial Fractures

Visceral cranial fractures refer to fractures of the facial bones and generally result from a blow to the face. More than 70% of motor vehicle accident victims sustain facial injury. As discussed earlier, facial or head trauma may also indicate a possible cervical spine fracture or injury. In addition, soft tissue injury of the eyes, nose, and mandible is often accompanied by bony fractures.

A zygomatic arch fracture may be difficult to recognize initially because of the edema. However, a fracture may be indicated by clinical signs, which include black eyes, flattening of the cheek, and a restriction of the movement of the mandible. Careful examination by palpation is performed by the physician because a fracture of the zygomatic arch may be present without accompanying facial fractures. A depressed fracture of the zygomatic arch may also be difficult to demonstrate radiographically (Fig. 11-36). An oblique submentovertical projection may be

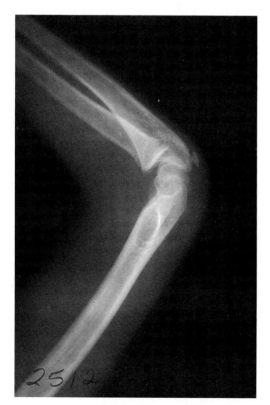

Fig. 11-35 Lateral elbow radiograph demonstrates the fat pad sign associated with a radial head fracture. (Courtesy Riverside Methodist Hospitals, Columbus, Ohio.)

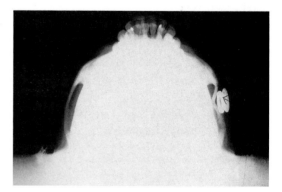

Fig. 11-36 A submentovertical projection of the zygomatic arch demonstrating a depressed fracture of the zygomatic arch resulting from a direct blow to the left cheek. (Courtesy the Ohio State University Hospitals, Columbus, Ohio.)

used to best demonstrate the extent of the fracture. A parietoacanthial (Waters' method) is also of value in examining the fractures of the zygomatic arch. A panoramic zonogram is also helpful in evaluating fractures.

The mandible is very prone to fracture because of the prominence of the chin; therefore, any patient suffering a head or face injury should be clinically examined for a mandibular fracture. Anatomically, the mandible is strongest at the center and weakest at the ends, with the most common site for fracture at the angle, followed by the condyles. Mandibular fractures (Fig. 11-37), are generally detected by the patient's inability to open the mouth and pain when moving the mandible. These fractures also cause a misalignment of the patient's teeth. Care must be taken to demonstrate all areas of the mandible (body, ramus, and symphysis) when ruling out mandibular fractures. The mandible is the slowest healing bone in the body and will show clinical union much sooner than radiographic union.

Fractures of the maxilla are serious because of the adjacent nasal cavity, paranasal sinuses, and orbit and the close proximity of the brain. The maxilla also transmits cranial nerves and major blood vessels. Maxillary fractures may be divided into three major classifications: horizontal, pyramidal, and transverse. A horizontal fracture of the maxilla (LeFort I) refers to a separation of the body of the maxilla from the base of the skull above the palate and below the zygomatic process. This type of fracture results in a freely movable jaw. A pyramidal fracture (LeFort II) involves vertical fractures through the maxilla at the malar and nasal bones, forming a triangular separation of the maxilla. A transverse fracture (LeFort III) is the most extensive and serious type of maxillary fracture; it extends across the orbits and results in separation of the visceral and cerebral cranium.

A **blow-out fracture** results from a direct blow to the front of the orbit that transfers the force to the orbital walls and floor. This fracture occurs in the thinnest, weakest portion of the orbit, the orbital floor just above the maxillary sinuses. If this condition is not diagnosed and treated, impairment of extraocular movements develops. A parietoacanthial projection (modified Waters' method) provides the most information in the radiographic diagnosis of blow-out fractures (Fig. 11-38). It demonstrates

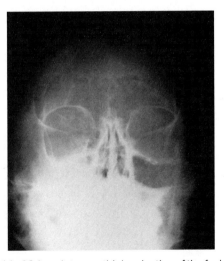

Fig. 11-38 A parietoacanthial projection of the facial bones on an individual who sustained a direct blow to the right orbit from a racquetball. The radiograph demonstrates a blow-out fracture of the left orbit. (Courtesy the Ohio State University Hospitals, Columbus, Ohio.)

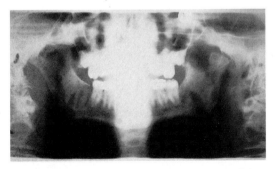

Fig. 11-37 A panoramic projection of the mandible demonstrating a fracture. (Courtesy the Ohio State University Hospitals, Columbus, Ohio.)

dense opacification of the maxillary sinus due to hemorrhage or herniated orbital contents.

A *tripod fracture* occurs when the zygomatic or malar bone is fractured at all three sutures: frontal, temporal, and maxillary (Fig. 11-39). The patient with a tripod fracture complains of restricted jaw movement because the mandible's coronoid process is trapped by the zygoma. This fracture results in a free-floating zygoma and may cause facial disfigurement if not diagnosed and properly treated.

The nasal bone is the most frequently fractured facial bone. The fracture is usually transverse and depresses the distal portion of the nasal bones. A nasal bone fracture may be accompanied by a fracture of the ascending process of the maxillae or of the nasal septum, which is composed of the vomer and the perpendicular plate of the ethmoid bone. A nosebleed, or epistaxis, is usually present with a nasal bone fracture.

Radiographs of nasal bone fractures are obtained, in addition to a clinical examination to confirm a fracture. Lateral projections demonstrate anterior or posterior displacement, whereas a parietoacanthial or intraoral projection demonstrates lateral-medial displacement of the bone fragments (Fig. 11-40).

Dislocations

Often a dislocation and a subluxation are considered synonymous. This is incorrect. A **dislocation** implies that a bone is out of its joint and not in contact with its normal articulation. A **subluxation** is a partial dislocation, often occurring with a fracture. The common sites of dislocations are the shoulder, hip, and acromioclavicular joints.

Shoulder joints most commonly dislocate anteriorly (Fig. 11-41). Such dislocations are read-

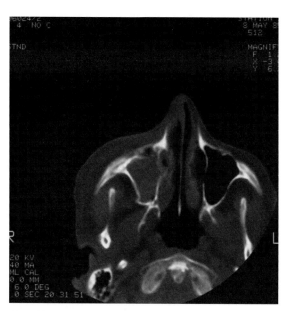

Fig. 11-39 A CT image demonstrating a tripod fracture of the right zygomatic bone. (Courtesy the Riverside Methodist Hospitals, Columbus, Ohio.)

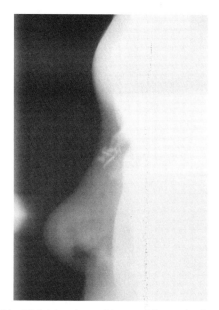

Fig. 11-40 A lateral nasal bone radiograph of a 20-year-old man who was struck in the face. The radiograph demonstrates a nasal bone fracture. (Courtesy the Ohio State University Hospitals, Columbus, Ohio.)

ily detectable radiographically because the humeral head usually locates below the glenoid fossa and coracoid process. Often an avulsed greater tuberosity is present with anterior dislocations. Posterior dislocations of the shoulder (Fig. 11-42) are more difficult to diagnose, as they may appear normal on an AP radiograph. A transscapular (Y) projection, as well as a posterior oblique projection, is useful in locating the humeral head in a suspected posterior dislocation. Other than trauma, seizure disorders and electric shock are the major causes for shoulder dislocations. In fact, a posterior dislocation may be the first sign of a seizure disorder.

With traumatic dislocation of the hip, the femoral head is most commonly displaced posteriorly to lie against the sciatic notch (Fig. 11-43). It may also displace anteriorly and lie adjacent to the pubis or obturator foramen. Congenital hip dislocations are usually unilateral and are recognized by a shortening of the extremity. If the condition is not recognized until the child begins to walk, conservative therapies may be replaced by surgical intervention.

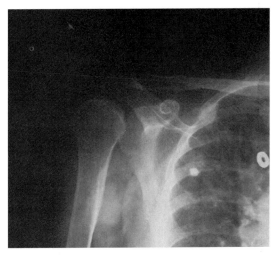

Fig. 11-42 A shoulder radiograph demonstrating a posterior dislocation of the humerus with the humeral head overlapping the rim of the glenoid fossa. The humeral head is also displaced slightly superolaterally. (Courtesy the American College of Radiology, Reston, Virginia.)

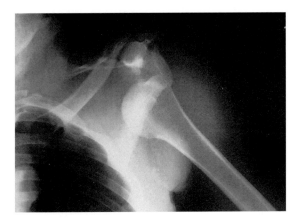

Fig. 11-41 A shoulder radiograph demonstrating an anterior dislocation of the humeral head. Note the location of the humeral head below the glenoid fossa and coracoid process. (Courtesy Riverside Methodist Hospitals, Columbus, Ohio.)

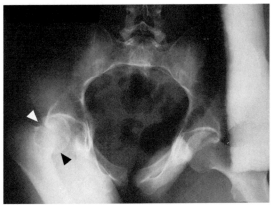

Fig. 11-43. A pelvis radiograph of a 25-year-old man whose right knee struck the dashboard in a motor vehicle accident resulting in a posterior dislocation of the right femoral head. (Courtesy the American College of Radiology, Reston, Virginia.)

Acromioclavicular joint separations (Fig. 11-44) are more common in children than adults. The typical film sequence for this diagnosis involves radiographs taken with and without weights. A joint separation is assessed by determining the alignment between the acromial end of the clavicle and the acromion process of the scapula.

Battered Child Syndrome

Battered child syndrome is a term associated with a physical form of child abuse and was first described in 1860. Physical child abuse often coexists with both emotional and sexual abuse. This syndrome affects boys and girls equally; approximately 25% of cases involve children under the age of 2 years. In addition, about 20% of the children who survive physical abuse suffer permanent injuries. An accurate incidence of child abuse is difficult to ascertain, but statistics indicate that approximately 2000 deaths per year result from child abuse.

Physical signs of battered child syndrome include bruises, burns, abrasions, and fractures in various stages of healing. In most cases, the explanation for the injury is inconsistent with the actual injury. Radiographic signs of child abuse include hematomas and single or multiple fractures of varying ages, especially in areas where it is difficult for the child to self-inflict the injury (Fig. 11-45). Often, fractures may indicate that an extremity has been twisted or turned until it breaks, or multiple rib fractures indicate repeated traumatic injuries, generally inflicted by a parent or guardian. All emergency room personnel should be familiar with signs of child abuse and are ethically required to report suspected cases of child abuse to the proper authorities.

Legg-Perthes Disease

Legg-Perthes disease is the most common form of the ischemic necrosis of bone group of diseases. Ischemia results from poor blood supply to the bone that leads to hypoxia. Ischemic

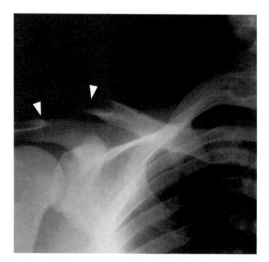

Fig. 11-44 A weight-bearing acromioclavicular radiograph demonstrating a dislocation as evidenced by uneven alignment of the acromial end of the clavicle and the acromion process of the scapula. (Courtesy the Ohio State University Hospitals, Columbus, Ohio.)

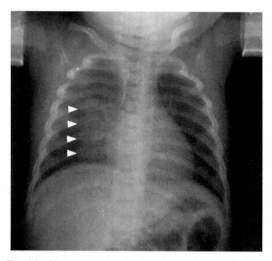

Fig. 11-45 A pediatric chest radiograph revealing numerous rib fractures with adjacent soft tissue masses resulting from hemorrhage surrounding the fracture sites. (Courtesy the American College of Radiology, Reston, Virginia.)

necrosis of the bone affects the epiphyses and may be easily mistaken for tuberculosis of the skeletal system. The etiology of this disorder is unknown, and the disease process is fairly quiet. *Perthes* refers specifically to ischemic necrosis of the head of the femur. It tends to occur in boys between the ages of 5 to 10 years and often follows injury or trauma to the affected hip. Clinically, these patients present with a limp that is accompanied by little or no pain. Radiographically, the bone in the center of the epiphysis is fragmented, and the head of the femur is flattened (Fig. 11-46). Magnetic resonance images normally demonstrate a low signal intensity from the affected hip in Legg-Perthes disease (Fig. 11-47).

TRAUMA OF THE CHEST AND THORAX

Approximately 25% of all trauma deaths occurring annually result from chest injuries. Diagnosis of the cause of the respiratory distress and the extent of the injury must be made quickly. In patients with acute respiratory distress with suspected hemothorax or pneumothorax, a chest tube may be inserted in the fourth or fifth intercostal space without waiting for a chest radiograph. A portable chest radiograph is then obtained to further evaluate the thorax following the placement of the "blind" chest tube. Bony injuries such as rib fractures, clavicular fractures, scapular fractures, and sternal fractures may penetrate the lungs and damage the heart and great vessels. Pulmonary contusion may also result from other penetrating, compressive, or decelerating trauma to the chest. Radiographically, changes in the lungs due to contusion appear 4 to 6 hours following the trauma. The radiographic appearance changes frequently during the first 24 to 48 hours, so multiple chest radiographs may be necessary to assess the damage to the lung tissue because pulmonary contusions are usually much larger than apparent on the initial chest radiograph.

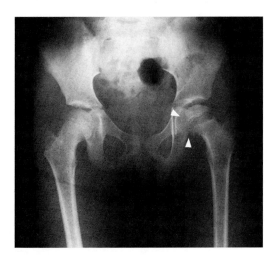

Fig. 11-46 An AP pelvis radiograph of a young man demonstrating Legg-Perthes disease of the left femoral head. Notice the asymmetry of the femoral heads. (Courtesy the American College of Radiology, Reston, Virginia.)

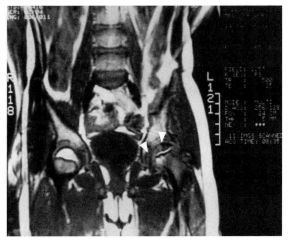

Fig. 11-47 An MRI of the patient in Fig. 11-46. The image demonstrates a low signal intensity in the left femoral epiphysis, consistent with Legg-Perthes disease. (Courtesy the American College of Radiology, Reston, Virginia.)

Pneumothorax

A **pneumothorax** occurs when free air is trapped in the pleural space and compresses the lung tissue. This air may enter the pleural space from perforation of the visceral pleura, allowing gas to enter from the lung, penetration of the chest wall, or by generation of gas by gas-forming organisms in an empyema.

Common causes of a pneumothorax include penetrating chest trauma, such as stab wounds (Fig. 11-48), gunshot wounds, fractured ribs, or a thoracocentesis needle, or a spontaneous blowout of a bleb (a flaccid vesicle, like a blister), resulting from some other pulmonary disease (Fig. 11-49). A pneumothorax may occur spontaneously from trauma or as the result of some pathologic process. The typical manifestation of a spontaneous pneumothorax is sudden, one-sided chest pain followed by dyspnea.

Radiographically, a pneumothorax appears as a strip of radiolucency devoid of vascular lung markings, with separation of the visceral and parietal pleura (Fig. 11-50). It is best demonstrated on an erect expiration chest radiograph. Occasionally, wrinkles in the patient's skin produce artifacts that can mimic a pneumothorax. Such an artifact is called a *pseudopneumothorax.*

A tension pneumothorax occurs when air enters the pleural space but cannot leave the space because of a check valve mechanism in the fistula. This results in a complete collapse of the lung and a shift of the mediastinum to the opposite side of the pneumothorax (Fig. 11-51). A tension pneumothorax requires immediate medical attention to prevent life-threatening circulatory collapse.

Treatment of a pneumothorax depends on the amount of lung collapse and the type of

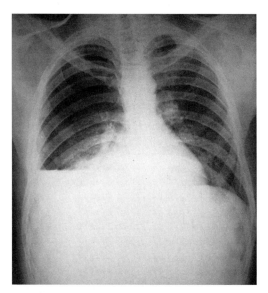

Fig. 11-48 Stab wound in the right chest of this 40-year-old man results in a pneumo-hemothorax. Fluid level in the right pleural space is blood, and the collapsed lung is outlined by its pleural margin in the upper chest. (Courtesy the American College of Radiology, Reston, Virginia.)

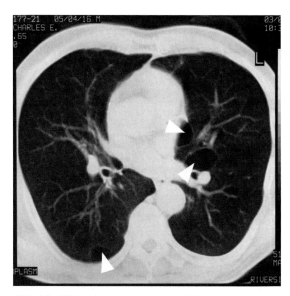

Fig. 11-49 Large emphysematous blebs as seen on CT. Spontaneous blowout of these could result in a pneumothorax. (Courtesy Riverside Methodist Hospitals, Columbus, Ohio.)

pneumothorax. A collapse of 30% or less is usually treated by bed rest. Immediate treatment of a tension pneumothorax might involve insertion of a needle into the chest wall to equalize air pressure. Otherwise, many pneumothoraces are treated through decompression by a closed tube thoracostomy attached to a water-seal drain.

Atelectasis

Atelectasis means incomplete expansion of the lung as a result of partial or total collapse. Compression atelectasis occurs when pleural effusions, pneumothoraces, or other space-occupying lesions cause collapse (Fig. 11-52). Air that is completely absorbed from alveoli beyond an obstructed bronchus results in absorption atelectasis.

   Atelectasis itself is not a disease, but it is a sign of an abnormal process. The most common

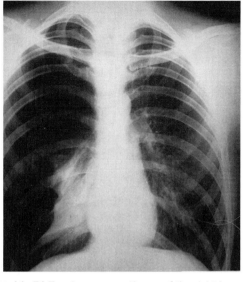

Fig. 11-51 Tension pneumothorax of the right lung following a stab wound in this 25-year-old man. The collapsed lung has almost no air in it and is seen as a soft tissue density adjacent to the heart. (Courtesy the American College of Radiology, Reston, Virginia.)

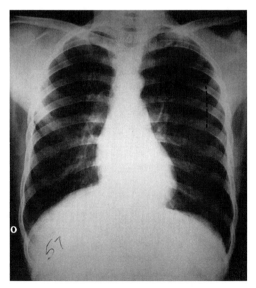

Fig. 11-50 Pneumothorax seen as thin white line around the periphery of the left lung, with an absence of lung markings in the periphery. (Courtesy the American College of Radiology, Reston, Virginia.)

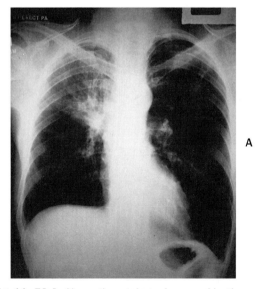

A

Fig. 11-52 A, Absorption atelectasis caused by the obstructive effects of carcinoma of the bronchus supplying the upper lobe of the right lung. (A Courtesy the American College of Radiology, Reston, Virginia.)

Continued

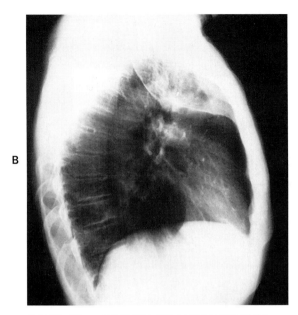

B

Fig. 11-52 cont'd. **B,** The lateral projection of the same patient clearly demonstrates atelectasis of the right upper lobe secondary to bronchogenic carcinoma. (**B** Courtesy the American College of Radiology, Reston, Virginia.)

manifestation is bibasilar atelectasis, which is seen after thoracic or abdominal surgical procedures. A chest radiograph reveals the airless area of the lung, which may be segmental or lobar. If an entire lobe is affected, the mediastinum shifts to the affected side because of loss of volume of the affected lung. The chest radiograph can also demonstrate a decrease in the intercostal interspace, elevation of the hemidiaphragm of the affected side, and depression or elevation of the hilum, depending on which lobe is affected. If the atelectasis is segmental, the radiographic shadow is triangular, with the apex of the triangle pointing toward the hilum of the affected lung.

Platelike atelectasis describes the radiographic appearance of one or more linear opacities, usually at the lung bases and parallel to the diaphragm (Fig. 11-53).

Treatment of acute atelectasis can be accomplished by appropriate respiratory therapy treat-

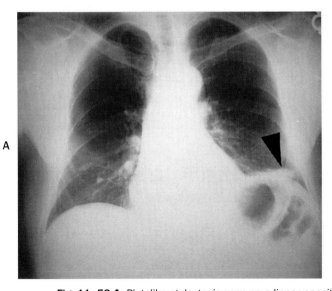

A

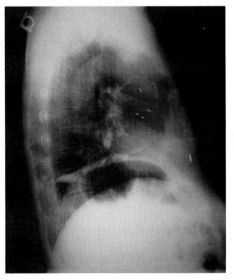

B

Fig. 11-53 **A,** Platelike atelectasis seen as a linear opacity in the base of the left lung as indicated by the *arrow* in this PA projection; **B,** a lateral projection of same patient also clearly demonstrates platelike atelectasis. (**A** and **B** Courtesy Riverside Methodist Hospitals, Columbus, Ohio.)

ments such as coughing and deep breathing. Bronchoscopy can also be used to allow suctioning of secretions that are causing an obstruction. Thoracocentesis can be used to relieve the compression caused by an effusion.

ABDOMINAL TRAUMA

Traumatic injuries to the abdomen result from gunshot wounds, stab wounds, and blunt abdominal trauma. Although abdominal injuries account for only approximately 15% of trauma deaths, most occur more than 48 hours following trauma and usually result from sepsis. Many patients with serious abdominal injuries from motor vehicle accidents initially have very minimal symptoms and physical findings. Abdominal trauma can cause serious injury not only to the GI tract but also to abdominal organs such as the liver, spleen, kidneys, and pancreas; the retroperitoneum; and the pelvic organs. Blunt trauma from steering wheel injuries often damage the liver and spleen because the energy of deceleration and compression frequently damages the parenchyma of these structures.

Supine and erect abdominal radiographs and erect chest radiographs are most desirable following abdominal injury. However, this is not always possible because of the patient's condition. Chest radiographs are important to assess diaphragmatic injury. Supine abdominal radiographs help to identify foreign objects such as bullets, separation in the bowel loops or loss of the psoas muscle shadow due to fluid or blood within the peritoneum, and air around the right kidney or psoas muscle margins. The initial inspection of the abdominal trauma may be followed by specific studies involving the urinary tract (Fig. 11-54). Intravenous urograms may be indicated if injury to the urinary system is suspected, however, CT examination of the abdomen following an injection of an iodinated contrast agent provides a much clearer view of renal anatomy and organ injury.

Computed tomography has also proven to be the best means of diagnosing GI trauma

and is capable of visualizing lacerations, hematomas, and ruptures. Even small amounts of intraabdominal hemorrhage can be readily detected. The duodenum is the portion of the GI tract most often damaged by blunt trauma. Because of its relationship to the spine, the duodenum can be compressed between the abdominal wall and the spine, resulting in a duodenal hematoma. Often CT evaluation of liver and spleen injuries help in evaluating operative versus nonoperative management of these injuries.

Penetrating abdominal wounds, as occur with a gunshot, may produce free air if the bowel has been injured. Some of the common conditions seen radiographically after trauma are fractures of the spine, pelvis, or ribs; obliteration of normal fat planes and visceral margins; accumulation of peritoneal fluid such as

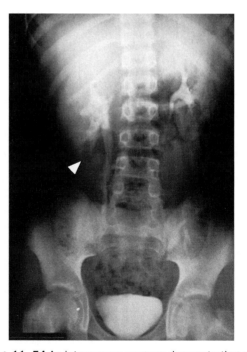

Fig. 11-54 An intravenous urogram demonstrating a fractured right kidney following a football injury. (Courtesy Riverside Methodist Hospitals, Columbus, Ohio.)

blood; and the presence of free peritoneal air (Fig. 11-55).

Intraperitoneal Air

In the normal patient, the peritoneum is a closed cavity (except for the female reproductive system), containing only small amounts of serous fluid. The presence of free air in this cavity, a **pneumoperitoneum,** is usually abnormal and can indicate perforation of the GI tract. Large amounts of air are likely due to colon perforation, whereas small amounts of air are more indicative of duodenal perforation.

The common causes of a pneumoperitoneum (Fig. 11-56) include the perforation of a peptic ulcer (either gastric or duodenal), carcinoma of the stomach or colon, cecum perforation from distal colon obstruction, colonic diverticula perforation, or traumatic rupturing of the stomach or intestines. In response to perforation, an intense inflammatory response develops and may eventually wall off the perforation into an abscess.

Free air is best demonstrated radiographically with the patient in an erect position. Often, it is well seen on a chest radiograph because of the proximity of the central ray to the diaphragms. Free air ascends and accumulates under the diaphragm on one or both sides. Amounts as small as 1 cc of air can be demonstrated on an erect projection. Much larger amounts of air must be present to be visualized on a supine radiograph. Left lateral decubitus radiographs can be substituted for the erect projection, with any free air present accumulating over the lateral aspect of the liver and the lateral aspect of the pelvis. The patient should remain on the left side for approximately 10 minutes before the exposure to allow sufficient time for the air to ascend.

In the supine position, the football sign may be demonstrated as an indicator of a pneu-

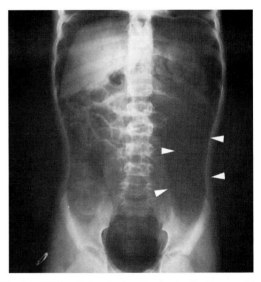

Fig. 11-56 An abdominal radiograph of a 5-year-old child with a passive pneumoperitoneum resulting from perforation of the stomach during anesthesia. Note how the free air outlines the outer border of the bowel, liver, and spleen. (Courtesy the American College of Radiology, Reston, Virginia.)

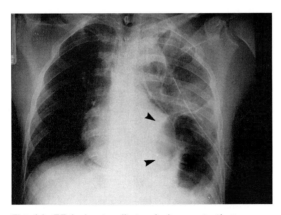

Fig. 11-55 A chest radiograph demonstrating a traumatic diaphragmatic hernia resulting from a motor vehicle accident. (Courtesy the Ohio State University Hospitals, Columbus, Ohio.)

moperitoneum. This is a lucent, oval gas collection that corresponds to the anterior peritoneal cavity. The pattern of gas resembles the shape of a football with the seam of the football being the falciform ligament outlined by free air. Visualization of this sign requires a relatively large amount of free air to demonstrate such a pattern.

QUESTIONS

1. A contusion formed on the side of the head where trauma occurs is called a:
   a. concussion
   b. contrecoup lesion
   c. coup lesion
   d. spondylosis

2. Demonstration of acute cerebral bleeding leading to a hematoma is best done by:
   a. angiography
   b. CT
   c. MRI
   d. plain films

3. A fracture of the skeletal system in which the bone has penetrated the skin is termed:
   a. closed
   b. comminuted
   c. noncomminuted
   d. open

4. Fractures that occur at sites of maximal strain on a bone, usually in connection with unaccustomed activity, are classified as _____ fractures.
   a. avulsion
   b. fatigue
   c. growth plate
   d. stress

5. A fracture that heals in a faulty position is termed:
   a. callus
   b. delayed union
   c. malunion
   d. nonunion

6. Shoulder dislocations are most commonly displaced:
   a. anteriorly
   b. posteriorly

7. Incomplete expansion of a lung as a result of partial or total collapse defines:
   a. atelectasis
   b. empyema
   c. pleurisy
   d. pneumothorax

8. Spontaneous blowout of a bleb could lead to a(n):
   a. atelectasis
   b. emphysematous lesion
   c. pleurisy
   d. pneumothorax

9. Demonstration of a pneumothorax is best accomplished by making the exposure:
   a. in an erect, lateral position
   b. in a lateral decubitus position
   c. in an erect PA position on expiration
   d. in an erect PA position on inspiration

10. Which portion of the GI system is most frequently damaged by blunt trauma of the abdomen?
    a. cecum
    b. duodenum
    c. ileum
    d. jejunum

11. Describe the differences among level I, II, and III trauma centers.

12. Spinal cord compression results in neurologic dysfunction, which may be temporary or permanent. Explain the mechanism for each type of dysfunction described in the text.

13. Differentiate between the four types of hematomas to the brain, and specify which type has the highest mortality rate. Why?

14. What imaging modality or modalities best demonstrate stress or fatigue fractures? Why?

15. Describe the difference between comminuted and noncomminuted fractures of the skeletal system.

Answer Key

CHAPTER 1
1. C
2. B
3. B
4. B
5. B
6. C
7. B
8. A
9. D
10. D

CHAPTER 2
1. B
2. B
3. B
4. A
5. D
6. A
7. C
8. B
9. B
10. C
11. C
12. D
13. B
14. C
15. D

CHAPTER 3
1. C
2. C
3. C
4. B
5. C
6. D
7. A
8. D
9. B
10. B

CHAPTER 4
1. A
2. C
3. C
4. C
5. C
6. C
7. D
8. A
9. D
10. A

CHAPTER 5
1. B
2. B
3. B
4. D
5. D
6. B
7. D
8. D
9. A
10. B

CHAPTER 6
1. D
2. A
3. C
4. A
5. B
6. C
7. D
8. E
9. D
10. B
11. D
12. D
13. C
14. A
15. B

CHAPTER 7
1. D
2. D
3. D
4. B
5. A
6. A
7. B
8. D
9. D
10. D
11. D
12. C
13. A
14. B
15. C

CHAPTER 8
1. D
2. A
3. B
4. B
5. B
6. E
7. A
8. B
9. C
10. C
11. B
12. D
13. C
14. B
15. E

CHAPTER 9
1. C
2. A
3. D
4. B
5. B
6. D
7. D
8. A
9. B
10. B

CHAPTER 10
1. A
2. B
3. B
4. C
5. B
6. A
7. B
8. B
9. B
10. D

CHAPTER 11
1. C
2. B
3. D
4. B
5. C
6. A
7. A
8. D
9. C
10. B

Glossary

Abruptio Placentae—Condition in which a normally implanted placenta prematurely separates from the uterus.

Absorption Atelectasis—Type of atelectasis that occurs when air is completely absorbed from alveoli beyond an obstructed bronchus.

Achalasia—A neuromuscular abnormality of the esophagus which results in failure of the lower esophageal sphincter to relax.

Achondroplasia—A hereditary, congenital disturbance which causes inadequate bone formation and results in a peculiar form of dwarfism.

Acquired Immune Deficiency Syndrome (AIDS)—An acquired viral infection which paralyzes normal human immune mechanisms.

Acromegaly—A disease marked by progressive enlargement of the head, hands, and feet caused by abnormal secretion of growth hormone.

Acute—Having a quick onset and lasting a short period of time with a relatively severe course.

Additive Pathologies—A radiographic term used to describe diseases that are more difficult than normal to penetrate.

Adenocarcinoma—Carcinoma derived from glandular tissue.

Adenomatous Polyp—A saccular projection into the bowel lumen.

Air-bronchogram Sign—Radiographic sign seen in various respiratory diseases where air-filled bronchi become visible when surrounded by non-aerated alveoli.

Albers Schönberg Disease—A form of osteosclerotic osteopetrosis, this is a benign skeletal anomaly that involves increased bone density in conjunction with fairly normal bone contour.

Alimentary Tract—Extending from the mouth to the anus, the major portion consists of the gastrointestinal system, which digests and absorbs food.

Anemic—Condition in which level of hemoglobin in blood is less than 12 g per 100 ml.

Anencephaly—Congenital absence of the cranial vault.

Aneurysm—A localized ballooning or outpouching of a vessel wall as a result of weakening due to atherosclerotic disease, trauma, infection, or congenital defects.

Ankylosing Spondylitis—A form of rheumatoid arthritis of unknown etiology that affects the spine in a progressive fashion, eventually fusing the spine into a rigid block of bone.

Anomaly—Any marked deviation from the norm, especially as a result of congenital or hereditary defects.

Anthracosis—Pneumoconiosis caused by inhalation and deposition of coal dust.

Appendicitis—An inflammation of the appendix.

Arthritis—Inflammation in which lesions are confined to the joints.

Asbestosis—Pneumoconiosis caused by inhalation and deposition of asbestos dust.

Ascites—An accumulation of fluid in the peritoneal cavity.

Aspiration Pneumonia—Pneumonia caused by entrance of foreign particles (e.g., vomitus) aspirated into the lower respiratory tract.

Astrocytoma—A glioma composed of astrocytes, which are star-shaped neuroglial cells with many branching processes.

Asymptomatic—Showing or causing no identifiable symptoms.

Atelectasis—Loss of air in a lung resulting from a partial or total collapse of a lung.

Atheroma—A mass of plaque occurring in atherosclerosis.

Atherosclerosis—A common form of arteriosclerosis in which deposits of fibro-fatty plaque or thickenings form within the intima or intermedia of large and medium-sized arteries.

Autoimmune Disorder—Diseases in which antibodies form against and injure the patient's own tissues, in contrast to the normal process in which antibodies form in response to foreign antigens.

Autosome—The 22 pairs of chromosomes found in a typical cell, other than the sex chromosomes.

Avulsion Fracture—A fracture in which a fragmented bone is pulled away from the shaft, usually occurring around a ligament or tendon, and often with muscle-tearing, as is associated with a sprain or dislocation.

Benign—Refers to a localized and generally noninvasive lesion.

Bicornuate Uterus—A uterus with paired uterine horns extending to the uterine tubes.

Bleb—A flaccid vesicle.

Blood-brain Barrier—The special functioning of the cerebral capillaries that prevents the passage of unwanted substances into the brain.

Blow-out Fracture—A fracture of the orbital floor resulting from a direct blow to the front of the orbit, with the force of the blow transferred to the orbital walls and floor.

Bone Bruise—An indication of an occult fracture, revealed by MRI, and presumed to represent hemorrhage and edema, usually beneath an adjacent joint surface.

Bone Cyst—A benign lesion consisting of a wall of fibrous tissue filled with fluid.

Bowel Sounds—The normal sounds of the bowel in motion as heard on auscultation.

Boxer's Fracture—A fracture of the fifth metacarpal bone as a result of a blow to or with the hand.

Bradycardia—A very slow heart rate.

Bronchial Adenoma—A glandular tumor, either benign or malignant, situated in the submucosal tissues of large bronchi.

Bronchiectasis—Chronic dilatation of the bronchi, with inflammation and destruction of bronchial walls and cilia.

Bronchitis—Inflammation of one or more bronchi.

Bronchogenic Carcinoma—Carcinoma of the lung that arises from the epithelium of the bronchial tree.

Bruise—Bleeding into the tissue spaces as a result of capillary rupture; also known as a contusion.

Bulla—A large vesicle, usually 2 cm or more in diameter, filled with air.

Bursitis—Inflammation of the bursae of the tendons, with the subdeltoid bursa as the most common site.

CAD—Coronary artery disease, resulting from deposition of atheromas in the arteries supplying blood to the heart muscle.

CVA—Cerebrovascular accident, generally resulting from a loss of blood supply to the brain or from a cerebral bleed.

Callus—An unorganized meshwork of wovenbone formed following a fracture, ultimately replaced by hard, adult bone.

Cancellous—Refers to the spongy, latticelike structure of bone filled by bone marrow.

Cancer—A general term used to denote various types of malignant neoplasms.

Cantor Tube—A single-lumen, mercury-weighted gastric tube used for intestinal intubation and decompression.

Carcinoma—A malignant growth comprised of epithelial cells that tends to invade surrounding tissues and give rise to metastases.

Cardiac Series—Radiographic procedure used to visualize the borders of the heart; esophagus is filled with barium sulfate, and a 45-degree RAO and a 60-degree LAO radiographs are exposed.

Cardiomegaly—The appearance of an enlarged heart, as indicative of many cardiovascular disorders.

Celiac Disease—A malabsorption syndrome that occurs as a result of sensitivity to gluten, an agent found in wheat products.

Cervical Spondylosis—Degenerative joint disease affecting the cervical vertebrae, vertebral discs, and surrounding ligaments and connective tissue.

Chest Tube—Tube inserted through the chest wall between the ribs to allow for drainage of air and/or fluid from the thoracic cavity.

Chip Fracture—An avulsion fracture consisting of a small fragment or chip of bone from the corner of a phalanx or other long bone.

Cholecystitis—An acute inflammation of the gallbladder most frequently caused by obstruction.

Cholelithiasis—The presence of gallstones.

Chondrosarcoma—A malignant bone tumor composed of atypical cartilage.

Chronic—Presenting slowly and persisting over a long period of time.

Chronic Obstructive Pulmonary Disease (COPD)—Designation applied to conditions which result in pulmonary obstruction, most commonly chronic bronchitis and pulmonary emphysema.

Cirrhosis—Liver condition in which the parenchyma and architecture are destroyed and replaced by fibrous tissue and regenerative nodules.

Closed Fracture—A fracture that does not produce an open wound.

Clubfoot—Deformity of the foot involving the talus.

Coarctation—A narrowing or compression.

Coccidiomycosis—Systemic, fungal infection caused by a fungus that thrives in semi-arid soil and is particularly endemic in the southwestern United States and northern Mexico.

Colles' Fracture—A fracture through the distal 1 inch of the radius in which the distal fragment is displaced posteriorly.

Colonic Atresia—Congenital failure of development of the distal rectum and anus to a variable extent, frequently accompanied by fistula formation to the genitourinary system.

Coma—A state of unconsciousness from which the patient cannot be aroused.

Comminuted Fracture—A fracture in which the bone is splintered or crushed.

Communicating (External) Hydrocephalus—Type of hydrocephalus caused by poor resorption of cerebrospinal fluid (for a variety of reasons) by the arachnoid villi.

Compact—Refers to the dense, outer portion of bone.

Complete Noncomminuted Fracture—A fracture in which the bone separates into two fragments.

Compound Fracture—A fracture in which the bone ends penetrate the soft tissue and skin; also termed open fracture.

Compression Atelectasis—Type of atelectasis that occurs when pleural effusions, pneumothoraces, or other space-occupying lesions cause collapse.

Compression Fracture—A fracture produced by compression.

Concussion—Brief loss of consciousness as a result of a blow to the head.

Congenital—Existing at, and usually before, birth and resulting from genetic or environmental factors.

Congenital Megacolon—Hirschprung's disease, consisting of an absence of neurons in the bowel wall, typically in the sigmoid colon.

Congestive Heart Failure—Condition existing when the heart is unable to propel blood at a sufficient rate and volume to prevent congestion of subcirculatory systems.

Consolidation—The process of tissue or fluid accumulation.

Contre Coup Lesion—A contusion formed on the opposite side of the skull in reference to a trauma site.

Contusion—An injury in which the tissue is bruised but not broken.

Corpus Luteum Cyst—A cyst that develops in the yellow endocrine body formed in the ovary in the site of a ruptured ovarian follicle.

Coup Lesion—A contusion formed on the side of the head in which trauma occurs.

Craniopharyngioma—A cystic, benign tumor that usually grows above the sella and upward into the third ventricle of the brain.

Craniosynostosis—Premature or early closure of the sutures of the skull.

Crohn's Disease—A chronic granulomatous inflammatory disease of unknown etiology involving any part of the gastrointestinal tract, but commonly involving the terminal ileum.

Crossed Ectopy—A condition in which one kidney lies across the body midline and is fused to the other kidney.

Cryptococci—Yeastlike organisms of a fungal origin.

CVP Line—Specialized catheter inserted usually via the subclavian vein to the level of the right atrium to compensate for loss of peripheral infusion sites or to allow for fluid infusion in significant amounts.

Cystadenoma—Adenoma associated with cystoma.

Cystadenocarcinoma—Malignant neoplasm of the ovary; generally occurs in females over the age of 40 years.

Cystic Fibrosis—Congenital disorder affecting exocrine gland function, with respiratory effects including excessive secretions, obstruction of the bronchial system, infection, and tissue damage.

Cystitis—Inflammation of the bladder as a result of its infection.

Degenerative—Refers to deterioration of the body usually associated with the aging process.

Degenerative Disk Disease—The gradual, degenerative changes to the spine associated with aging.

Delayed Union—Refers to a fracture that does not heal in the usual amount of time.

Depressed Fracture—A fracture of the skull in which a fragment is depressed inward.

Dermoid Cysts (Cystic Teratomas)—Cystic masses arising from unfertilized ova, containing hair, fat, or bone, and located in an ovary.

Diagnosis—The name of a disease an individual is believed to have.

Diastole—The phase of the heart cycle in which the myocardium is relaxing.

Diploe—The spongy bone tissue found between the two tables of the cranial bones.

Disease—Any abnormal disturbance of the normal function or structure of a body part, organ, or system that may display a variety of manifestations.

Dislocation—The displacement of any part out of contact with its normal articulation.

Dissecting Aneurysm—An aneurysm resulting from hemorrhage that causes longitudinal splitting of the arterial wall.

Diverticula—A pouch or sac of variable size occurring normally or created by herniation of a mucous membrane through a defect in its muscular coat.

Diverticulitis—Inflammation of a diverticula.

Diverticulosis—The presence of diverticula in the absence of inflammation.

Dobhoff Tube—An enteral tube used to deliver a liquid diet directly to the duodenum.

Dominant—In relation to hereditary diseases, refers to a disease transmitted by a single gene from either parent.

Dysphagia—Difficulty in swallowing.

Ectopic Kidney—A kidney that is out of its normal position, usually found lower than normal.

Embolus—A mass of undissolved matter (solid, liquid, or gas) present in a blood vessel brought there by blood current. Vessel occlusion by an embolus usually results in development of an infarct.

Embolization—Interventional angiography procedure in which devices such as coils are used to intentionally clot off vessels, often before surgery to prevent excessive bleeding.

Emphysema—A lung condition characterized by an increase in the air spaces distal to the terminal bronchioles and with destruction of alveolar walls.

Empyema—An accumulation of pus in the pleural cavity.

Emergency Medical System (EMS)—A system for trauma care that provides prehospital care, acute hospital care, and rehabilitative care.

Encephalitis—Inflammation of the brain.

Enchondroma—A benign growth of cartilage arising in the metaphysis of a bone.

Endemic—Term given to disease of high prevalence in an area where the causative organism is commonly found.

Endometriosis—A condition in which endometrial tissue implants in aberrant pelvic locations.

Endoscopy—The use of lighted instruments with optic connections to visualize disease of the esophagus and stomach, or rectum and distal colon (e.g., sigmoidoscopy).

Endotracheal Tube—Tube inserted via the nose or mouth into the trachea for purposes of airway management, suctioning, or mechanical ventilation.

En Face—A radiographic descriptor referring to visualization of a pathology in a "head-on" or "straight-on" fashion, as compared to a profile-like image.

Ependymoma—A glial tumor that is firm and whitish and arises from the ependyma, the ventricle lining.

Epidemiology—The investigation of disease in large groups.

Epidural Hematoma—A hematoma positioned between the bony skull and the dura mater.

Epididymoorchitis—A testicular condition that may result in benign masses of the testes.

Epiphrenic Diverticulum—A pulsion diverticulum of the distal esophagus just above the hemidiaphragm.

Erythrocytes—Red blood cells.

Esophageal Atresia—Congenital lack of esophageal development past some point, commonly associated with tracheoesophageal fistula.

Esophageal Varices—Varicose veins of the esophagus that occur in patients with portal hypertension.

Etiology—The study of the cause and origin of disease.

Ewald/Edlich tube—A large bore gastric tube used to evacuate the contents of the stomach.

Ewing's Sarcoma—A primary malignant bone tumor arising in medullary tissue, occurring more often in cylindrical bones.

Exostosis—A benign bone growth, projecting outward from the bony cortex.

Expectoration—Expulsion of mucus or phlegm from the throat.

Fat Pad Sign—A radiographic indicator of a nonvisualized, underlying fracture of the bones of the elbow that displays as a tear-shaped radiolucency adjacent to the anterior and sometimes posterior surface of the distal humerus.

Fecalith—A hardened ball of stool that forms in the intestine.

Fibroadenoma—Adenoma containing fibrous tissue.

Fibrocystic Disease—A benign, generally bilateral breast condition characterized by various-sized cysts located throughout the breasts.

Filling Defect—An area of total or relative radiolucency within a column of barium.

Fistula—An abnormal, tubelike passage from one structure to another.

Foley Catheter—A catheter that is placed through the urethra and retained in the urinary bladder by a balloon which is inflated with air or fluid.

Follicular Cyst—A cyst arising from the ovum.

Fracture—The breaking or rupturing of bone caused by mechanical forces either applied to the bone or transmitted directly along the line of a bone.

Fusiform Aneurysm—An arterial aneurysm in which the entire circumference of the vessel wall is affected.

Gallstone Ileus—A condition in which gallstones erode from the gallbladder, creating a fistula to the small bowel that may cause a bowel obstruction.

Ganglion—Cystic swelling that develops in connection with a tendon sheath, usually on the back of the wrist.

Gastritis—Inflammation of the stomach mucosa.

Gastroenteritis—General grouping of a number of inflammatory disorders of the stomach and intestines.

Glioma—A tumor composed of tissue that represents neuroglia, commonly occurring in the cerebral hemispheres of the posterior fossa.

Glomerulonephritis—An inflammatory reaction of the renal parenchyma caused by streptococcal infection.

Gouty Arthritis—An inherited, metabolic disorder with excess amounts of uric acid produced and deposited in the joint and adjacent bone, most commonly in the metatarsophalangeal joint of the great toe.

Greenfield Filter—A specialized basket placed in the inferior vena cava during interventional angiography to catch clots before they enter the heart.

Greenstick Fracture—A fracture in which the cortex breaks on one side without separation or breaking of the opposing cortex.

Growth-plate Fracture—A fracture that involves the end of a long bone of a child, and that may be limited to growth-plate cartilage or extend into the metaphysis, epiphysis, or both.

Hangman's Fracture—A fracture of the arch of the second cervical vertebra, usually accompanied by anterior subluxation of the second cervical vertebra on the third cervical vertebra; also known as atraumatic spondylosis, these usually result from acute hyperextension of the head.

Harris Tube—A single lumen gastric tube using mercury as a weight that is used as a decompression and diagnostic aid.

Heartburn—Burning symptoms experienced substernally as a result of the reflux of gastric acids into the esophagus.

Hematocrit—A common laboratory test that determines the body's total number of red blood cells.

Hemangioma—A benign tumor of dilated blood vessels.

Hematoma—A localized collection of blood in an organ, space, or tissue due to a break in the wall of a blood vessel.

Hemorrhagic Stroke—A stroke in which a blood vessel in the brain breaks or ruptures.

Hemothorax—Pleural effusion containing blood.

Hepatitis—An inflammation of the liver resulting from a variety of causes.

Hepatoma—A primary malignant tumor of the liver.

Hepatomegaly—Enlargement of the liver as might be seen with viral hepatitis.

Hereditary—Genetically transferred from either parent to child and derived from ancestors.

Hernia—The protrusion of a part of an organ (e.g., bowel loop) through a small opening in the wall of a cavity.

Herniated Nucleus Pulposus—Herniation of the nucleus pulposus of the disc through a rupture in the anulus fibrosus.

Herpes—An inflammatory skin disease caused by a virus.

Hiatal Hernia—Protrusion of any structure, especially some portion of the stomach, into the thoracic cavity through the esophageal hiatus of the diaphragm.

Hickman Catheter—Specialized catheter inserted via the subclavian vein to allow for multiple tapping for injection of various agents, especially tissue-toxic chemotherapeutic agents.

Hirschprung's Disease—An absence of neurons in the bowel wall, typically in the sigmoid, preventing relaxation of the colon and normal peristalsis; congenital megacolon.

Histoplasmosis—Systemic, fungal infection caused by a fungus that thrives in soil, especially that fueled by bird or bat excreta; especially endemic to the Ohio and Mississippi River valleys.

Hodgkin's Disease—A malignant condition of lymphoid tissue associated with Reed Sternberg cells.

Homeostasis—The body's normal, internal resting state of equilibrium.

Horseshoe Kidney—A condition where the lower poles of the kidney are joined across midline by a band of soft tissues, resulting in a rotation anomaly on one or both sides.

Human Immunodeficiency Virus (HIV)—The virus associated with acquired immune deficiency syndrome.

Hyaline Membrane Disease—Also known as respiratory distress syndrome, it is a disorder of prematurity caused by incomplete maturation of the alveoli that makes proper gas exchange difficult.

Hydatiform Mole—Represents an abnormal conception where there is usually no fetus, the uterus is filled with cystically dilated chorionic villi that resemble a bunch of grapes.

Hydrocele—A benign testicular mass consisting of a collection of fluid in the testis or along the spermatic cord.

Hydrocephalus—A congenital or acquired condition resulting from accumulation of cerebrospinal fluids in the ventricles of the brain and leading to ventricular enlargement, compression of brain tissue, and increased intracranial pressure.

Hydronephrosis—An obstructive disease of the urinary system that causes a dilatation of the renal pelvis and calyces with urine.

Hypernephroma—The most common malignant tumor of the kidney.

Hyperparathyroidism—Abnormally increased activity of the parathyroid glands, causing excess hormone production, which overstimulates osteoclasts, which are responsible for bone removal.

Hyperplasia—Overdevelopment.

Hypertrophic Pyloric Stenosis—A congenital anomaly of the stomach in which the pyloric canal is greatly narrowed because of hypertrophy of the pyloric sphincter.

Hypoplasia—Less than normal development.

Hysterosalpingogram—A radiographic examination for screening of the nongravid female; injection of contrast into the uterus and the flow into the uterine tubes reveals their patency which may affect the ability to become pregnant.

Iatrogenic—Pertains to any adverse condition in a patient occurring as a result of medical treatment.

Idiopathic—No identifiable causative factor.

Ileal Atresia—A congenital absence of the ileum portion of the small intestines.

Imperforate Anus—Congenital disorder characterized by lack of an anal opening to the exterior.

Incarcerated Hernia—A hernia in which the bowel is trapped by tissues that prevent it from being reduced, possibly causing an obstruction.

Incidence—A statistical measure that refers to the number of new cases of a disease found in a given time period.

Incompetency (Valvular)—Regurgitation of blood through the heart valves as a result of improper closure.

Incomplete Fracture—A fracture in which only part of the bony structure gives way, with little or no displacement.

Infarct—An area of ischemic necrosis.

Infection—An inflammatory process caused by exposure to some disease-causing organism.

Inflammatory—Refers to the body process of destroying, diluting, or walling off a localized injurious agent.

Inguinal Hernia—Hernia in which a bowel loop protrudes through a weakness in the inguinal ring, with descension into the scrotum.

Insufficiency (Valvular)—Regurgitation of blood through the heart valves.

Intraaortic Balloon Pump—Specialized catheter with a balloon at its distal end; inflation and deflation from a pump provides mechanical support of the left ventricle and the systemic circulation.

Intracerebral Hematoma—Bleeding within the brain tissue, commonly in the frontal lobe, which results from trauma or a ruptured hemangioma.

Intrathoracic Stomach—Condition in which all of the stomach slides above the diaphragm into the thoracic cavity.

Intussusception—The prolapse of a segment of bowel into a distal segment.

Involucrum—A shell or sheath of new supporting bone laid down by periosteum around a sequestrum of necrosed bone.

Ischemia—A local and temporary impairment of circulation caused by obstruction of circulation.

Ischemic Stroke—A stroke in which a blood clot blocks a blood vessel in the brain.

Jaundice—Yellowish discoloration of the skin and whites of the eyes caused by bilirubin accumulation in the body tissues.

Kaposi's Sarcoma—A sarcoma present in the connective tissues of about one fourth of all AIDS patients.

Lacunar Infarction—Small vessel disease that results in a thrombotic stroke.

Le Fort Fracture—Bilateral, horizontal fractures of the maxillae, subcategorized as Le Fort I, II, or III fractures, depending on the extent of injury.

Left Ventricular Failure—Congestive heart failure that results when the left ventricle cannot pump an amount of blood equal to the venous return in the right ventricle.

Legionnaire's Disease—Severe, bacterial pneumonia named for its outbreak at an American Legion Convention in Pennsylvania in 1976.

Leiomyoma—A benign tumor derived from smooth muscle.

Lesion—General term used to describe the various types of cellular change that can occur in response to a disease.

Leukemia—A malignant disease of the leukocytes and their precursor cells in the blood and bone marrow.

Leukocytes—White blood cells.

Levacuator Tube—A wide double-lumen tube used for evacuation of gastric contents and irrigation of stomach.

Levin Tube—A gastroduodenal catheter of a small enough caliber to allow transnasal passage, often termed a nasogastric tube.

Linear Fracture—A fracture that extends lengthwise through a bone.

Maisonneuve Fracture—An infrequent ankle injury consisting of a severe ankle sprain with a fracture of the proximal one third of the fibula.

Malabsorption Syndrome—Group of diseases of various causes in which there is interference with normal digestion and absorption of food to the small bowel.

Malignant—Refers to a lesion that grows, spreads, and invades other tissues.

Malrotation—Unnatural position of the intestines caused by failure of normal rotation during embryologic development.

Malunion—Union of fragments of a fractured bone in a faulty position, impairing normal function or cosmetic appearance.

Manifestation—Observable changes resulting from cellular changes in the disease process.

Mantoux Text—Injection of purified protein derivative (PPD) under the skin for purposes of diagnosing tuberculosis.

Mastitis—Inflammation of the breast, most often caused by staphylococcus bacteria.

Mechanical Obstruction—Refers to a bowel obstruction that occurs as a result of blockage of the bowel lumen.

Mediastinal Emphysema (Pneumomediastinum)—The presence of air or gas in the mediastinum as a result of leakage of air from the bronchial tree.

Medical Jaundice—Jaundice that occurs due to hemolytic disease, in which excessive amounts of red blood cells are destroyed, or when the liver is damaged as a result of cirrhosis or hepatitis.

Medullary Sponge Kidney—A congenital anomaly of the urinary system in which the only visible abnormality is the dilatation of the medullary and papillary portions of the collecting ducts, usually bilaterally.

Medulloblastoma—Soft, infiltrating tumors of neuroepithelial tissue that are highly malignant.

Meningioma—A hard, usually vascular tumor that occurs mainly along meningeal vessels and the superior longitudinal sinus.

Meningitis—Inflammation of the meninges caused by bacteria or virus.

Meningocele—Hernial protrusion of the meninges through a defect of the skull or vertebral column.

Meningomyelocele—Protrusion of the spinal cord and meninges through a defect of the vertebral column, as is commonly associated with spina bifida.

Metabolic—Pertaining to the normal physiologic function of the body.

Metastasis—The spread of cancer cells.

Miliary Tuberculosis—Type of tuberculosis caused by hematogenous spread of the disease, with a characteristic appearance similar to millet seeds, which are small, white grains.

Milk of Calcium—A semiliquid sludge seen radiographically in the gallbladder; it results from the settling of bile caused by an obstruction at the neck of the gallbladder.

Miller-Abbott Tube—A double-lumen intestinal tube with an inflatable balloon at the distal end, used in the treatment of bowel obstructions.

Monteggia Fracture—A fracture in the proximal third of the ulnar shaft with dislocation of the radius.

Morbidity Rate—The incidence of illness in the population sufficient to interfere with an individual's normal daily routine.

Morphology—The form and structure of disease.

Mortality Rate—The number of deaths from a particular disease averaged over a population.

Multiple Myeloma—A malignant neoplasm of plasma cells characterized by skeletal destruction, pathologic fractures, and bone pain.

Multiple Sclerosis—A chronic, slowly progressive disease of the central nervous system, characterized by demyelination of the nerve sheath.

Mycoplasma Pneumonia—The most common form of primary atypical pneumonia, occurring most frequently in young adults.

Myelocele—Protrusion of the spinal cord through the normally closed bony neural arch of the spine.

Mycobacterium Avium—A type of tubercle bacillis that may cause tuberculosis; rare in humans, but most common in chickens and swine.

Necrosis—Tissue death.

Neoplastic—Pertaining to new, abnormal tissue growth.

Nephroblastoma (Wilm's Tumor)—A rapidly developing malignancy of the kidneys, usually affecting children before age 5.

Nephrocalcinosis—A condition characterized by precipitation of calcium in the tubules of the kidney, resulting in renal deficiency.

Nephroptosis—Prolapse of a kidney.

Nephrosclerosis—Intimal thickening of predominantly the small vessels of the kidney as a result of reduced blood flow through arteriosclerotic renal vasculature.

Nephrostomy Tube—A tube inserted through the abdominal wall into the renal; pelvis to drain urine.

Neurofibroma—A tumor of peripheral nerves caused by abnormal proliferation of Schwann cells.

Neurogenic Bladder—A bladder dysfunction caused by interference with the nerve impulses concerned with urination.

Nidus—An area of sclerosis with a radiolucent center associated with an osteoid osteoma.

Noncommunicating (Internal) Hydrocephalus—Type of hydrocephalus where obstruction occurs congenitally, from tumor growth, trauma and inflammation; interferes or blocks normal CSF circulation.

Nonunion—Complication of a fracture when healing does not occur and fragments do not join.

Nosocomial—Refers to diseases acquired in or from a health care environment.

Occult Fracture—A fracture that gives clinical signs of its presence without radiologic evidence; followup within ten days reveals bone resorption or displacement at the fracture site.

Oligodendroglioma—A glioma, it is a slow-growing astrocytic tumor that is usually relatively benign.

Oligohydramnios—The presence of too little (less than 300 ml) amniotic fluid at term, generally associated with renal disorders in the fetus.

Osteoarthritis—Noninflammatory degenerative joint disease occurring mainly in older persons, producing gradual deterioration of the joint cartilage.

Osteoblasts—The bone-forming cells responsible for bone growth, ossification, and regeneration.

Osteochondroma—A benign tumor of adult bone capped by cartilage.

Osteoclastoma (Giant Cell Tumor)—A tumor that is usually benign and characterized by osteolytic areas, most commonly found around the knee and wrist of young adults.

Osteoclasts—Cells which are associated with absorption and removal of bone.

Osteogenesis Imperfecta—A congenital disease in which the bones are abnormally brittle and subject to fractures.

Osteoid Osteoma—A benign tumor of bonelike structure developing on a bone and sometimes other structures.

Osteomalacia—A condition marked by softening of the bones, caused by lack of calcium in the tissues and a failure of bone tissue to calcify.

Osteomyelitis—Infection of bone, most often caused by staphylococcus, which may localize or spread to the bone to involve the marrow and other bone tissues.

Osteopetrosis—A hereditary disease characterized by abnormally dense bone, likely as a result of faulty bone resorption.

Osteophytes—An osseous outgrowth (spur).

Osteoporosis—Metabolic bone disorder resulting in demineralization of bone, most commonly seen in women past menopause.

Osteosarcoma—A primary malignancy of bone usually arising in the metaphysis, most commonly around the knee.

Paget's Disease—A metabolic disorder of unknown etiology, most common in the elderly, characterized by an early, osteolytic stage and a late, osteoblastic stage.

Pancreatitis—Acute or chronic, asymptomatic or symptomatic, inflammation of the pancreas caused by autodigestion by pancreatic enzymes.

Paraesophageal Hiatal Hernia—A hiatal hernia in which the stomach or adjacent structures herniate above the diaphragm, while the gastroesophageal junction remains below the diaphragm.

Paralytic Ileus—A failure of bowel peristalsis, often seen following abdominal surgery, that may result in bowel obstruction.

Patent Ductus Arteriosis—Abnormal persistence of an open ductus arteriosis after birth, resulting in recirculation of arterial blood through the lungs.

Pathologic Fracture—A fracture which occurs in abnormal bone weakened by a disease process.

Pathology—The study of structural and functional manifestations of disease.

Palliative—Treatment designed to relieve pain without the goal of curing the disease.

Peau d'Orange Appearance—Appearance of multiple small depressions on the skin surface as a result of hair follicles becoming visible from skin edema, as might occur with breast cancer.

Pedunculated Polyp—A polyp attached to the bowel wall by a narrow stalk.

Pelvic Inflammatory Disease (PID)—A bacterial infection of the female genital system, most often caused by bacteria.

Penetrating Fracture—A type of incomplete fracture resulting from penetration by a sharp object, frequently with comminution at the site of injury.

Peptic Ulcer—Ulceration of the mucous membrane of the esophagus, stomach, or duodenum by action of acidic gastric juice.

Percutaneous Transluminal Angioplasty (PTA)—Use of a specialized catheter, typically equipped with an inflatable balloon, to perform vessel repair from within the artery or vein during angiography.

Permanent Catheterization—Interventional angiography procedure in which a catheter is placed in the subclavian or jugular vein, and tunneled under the skin to allow for improved dialysis access.

Pessary—A device inserted into the vagina to provide proper support to a uterus that lacks proper support.

Phlebitis—Inflammation of a vein, often associated with venous thrombosis.

Placental Accreta—An abnormal adhesion of the placenta to the uterine wall.

Placenta Previa—The condition in which the placenta develops in the lower half of the uterus, encroaching or on, and completely or partially covering, the internal cervical os.

Platelike Atelectasis—Radiographic appearance seen in atelectasis in which one or more linear opacities are seen, usually at the lung bases and parallel to the diaphragm.

Pleural Effusion—A collection of excess fluid in the pleural cavity.

Pleurisy—Inflammation of the pleura with exudation into the pleural cavity and on its surface.

Pneumatocele—A thin-walled, air-containing cyst that is a characteristic radiographic lesion seen in staphylococcal pneumonia.

Pneumococcal Pneumonia—The most common bacterial pneumonia, generally affecting an entire lobe of a lung.

Pneumoconioses—A group of occupational diseases characterized by permanent deposits of particulate matter in the lungs and by resultant pulmonary fibrosis.

Pneumocystitis Carinii Pneumonia—Life-threatening infection of the lungs most commonly associated with AIDS.

Pneumonia—The most frequent type of lung infection, resulting in an inflammation of the lung with compromised pulmonary function.

Pneumoperitoneum—The presence of air or gas in the peritoneal cavity.

Pneumothorax—An accumulation of free air or gas in the pleural space that compresses the lung tissue.

Polycystic Kidney Disease—A familial kidney disorder in which innumerable tiny cysts that are present congenitally gradually enlarge during aging to compress and eventually destroy normal tissues.

Polycystic Ovaries—Ovaries that contain multiple small cysts.

Polydactyly—The presence of more than five digits.

Polyhydramnios—An excess of amniotic fluid; it may be associated with anencephaly or gastrointestinal disturbances in the fetus.

Polyp—A small mass of tissue arising from mucous membrane to project inward into the lumen of the bowel.

Pott's Fracture—A fracture of the lower part of the fibula involving both malleoli with dislocation of the ankle joint.

Prevalence—A statistical measure that refers to the number of cases of a disease found in a given population.

Prognosis—The prediction of course and outcome for a given disease.

Provisional Callus—An early indication of fracture healing, mainly composed of cartilage that begins to form approximately one week after a fracture.

Pseudocyst—An abnormal or displaced space resembling a cyst.

Pseudopneumothorax—A radiographic artifact produced by a wrinkle in the skin that mimics a pneumothorax.

Pseudopolyps—Islands of unaffected mucosa that are visible when surrounded by the affected mucosa of ulcerative colitis.

Pulsion Diverticulum—A diverticulum created by herniation of the mucous membrane through the muscular coat of the esophagus as a result of pressure from within.

Punctate—Pinpoint punctures or depressions; commonly used in reference to the appearance of a type of hemorrhaging.

Pyelonephritis—Bacterial infection of the kidney and its pelvis.

Pyogenic Arthritis—Joint inflammation that occurs secondary to other infections.

Pyuria—The presence of pus in the urine created by its drainage from renal abscesses into the kidney's collecting tubules.

Rales—An abnormal sound heard on auscultation of the chest.

Recessive—In relation to hereditary disease, refers to a disease transmitted by both parents to an offspring.

Reed-Sternberg Cells—A specific cell type that helps differentiate Hodgkin's lymphomas from other types of lymphatic disease.

Reflux Esophagitis—The backward flow of gastric acids into the esophagus.

Regeneration—Process in which damaged tissues are replaced by new tissues that are essentially identical to those replaced.

Regional Enteritis—A chronic granulomatous inflammatory disease of unknown etiology involving any part of the gastrointestinal tract, but commonly involving the terminal ileum.

Renal Agenesis—The absence of the kidney on one side, with an unusually large kidney on the other side.

Renal Colic—Severe, agonizing pain that refers along the course of a ureter toward the genital and loin regions in response to the movement of a renal calculus.

Renal Failure—The end result of a chronic process that gradually results in lost kidney function.

Reticuloendothelial System—Specialized cells found in the liver, bone marrow, and spleen, whose function is phagocytosis.

Rheumatoid Arthritis—A chronic, systemic disease primarily of joints, characterized by an overgrowth of synovial tissues and articular structures, and progressive destruction of cartilage, bone, and supporting structures.

Rh Factor—Blood factor first discovered in the blood of the rhesus monkey; contained by approximately 85% of the population who are said to be "Rh positive."

Rickets—Osteomalacia that occurs before growth-plate closure, caused by deficiency of vitamin D, especially in infants and children.

Right Ventricular Failure—Congestive heart failure that results when the right ventricle cannot pump as much blood as it receives from the right atrium, slowing venous blood flow.

Saccular Aneurysm—A localized sac affecting only a part of the circumference of an arterial wall.

Sail sign—Radiographic appearance of an enlarged thymus in an infant, so described because of its characteristic sail-like appearance.

Sarcoma—A type of tumor, often highly malignant, composed of a substance like embryonic connective tissue.

Schatzki's Ring—A ring of mucosa that protrudes into the lumen of the esophagus, thought to develop as a defense mechanism against gastric reflux.

Scoliosis—Abnormal lateral curvature of the spine.

Seminoma—A malignant neoplasm of the testis, usually occurring in males between the ages of 30 and 40 years.

Sequestrum—A piece of dead, devascularized bone that separates from living bone during the process of necrosis.

Sessile Polyp—A polyp with a wide base attached directly to the bowel wall.

Shunt—An artificial passageway used to drain excess fluids (e.g., from the ventricles into the internal jugular vein, the heart, or the peritoneum in the case of excess CSF).

Sign—An objective manifestation of disease perceptible to the managing physician, as opposed to subjective symptoms perceived by the patient.

Silicosis—Pneumoconiosis caused by inhalation of silica dust, as is common among miners, grinders, and sand blasters.

Sinoatrial (SA) node—The heart's "pacemaker", this is a bundle of nerve fibers located in the upper portion of the right atrium near the superior vena cava. From this node, an electrical current is transmitted through the myocardium, resulting in a heartbeat.

Sinusitis—Inflammation of a sinus, which may be purulent or nonpurulent, acute or chronic.

Situs Inversus—Complete reversal of the viscera of the thorax and abdomen.

Sliding Hiatal Hernia—A hiatal hernia in which a portion of the stomach and gastroesophageal junction are both situated above the diaphragm.

Somatic Cells—Those body cells other than the germ cells of the egg in the female and spermatozoa in the male.

Spermatocele—A cystic dilatation of the epididymis

Spina Bifida—A developmental anomaly characterized by incomplete closure of the vertebral canal, through which the choriomeninges may or may not protrude.

Spiral (Oblique) Fracture—A fracture in which the bone has been twisted apart, usually resulting from a rotary-type injury.

Spondylolisthesis—Forward displacement of one vertebra over another (commonly occurring at the L5/S1 junction), usually caused by a developmental defect in the pars interarticularis.

Spondylolysis—A condition marked by a cleft or breaking down of the body of a vertebra between the superior and inferior articular processes.

Staghorn Calculus—A large renal calculus that assumes the shape of the pelvicalyceal junction, resembling the horn of a stag.

Staphylococcal Pneumonia—Pneumonia caused by infection with staphylococcus that localizes in and/or around the bronchi.

Stent—A specialized device placed to provide patency, usually in a vessel or duct.

Strangulated Hernia—Herniation in which the bowel loop passes through a constriction tight enough to cut off its blood supply, leading to necrosis of that portion of the bowel without prompt surgical intervention.

Strangulation—A constriction that cuts off blood supply.

Stress Echocardiography—Echocardiography combines an exercise test with an echocardiogram to check the heart's contraction ability and its pumping efficiency; in patients where exercise is not possible, certain drugs may be given to create the effect of exercise on the heart.

Stress Fracture—A fracture that occurs at a site of maximal strain on a bone, usually connected with some unaccustomed activity (also known as march, stress, or insufficiency fractures).

Subarachnoid Hematoma—A hematoma that accumulates between the brain's arachnoid layer and its pia mater.

Subcutaneous Emphysema—The presence of air or gas in the subcutaneous tissues of the body.

Subdural Hematoma—A hematoma positioned between the dura mater and the arachnoid meningeal layer.

Subluxation—An incomplete or partial dislocation.

Subtractive Pathology—A radiographic term used to describe diseases that are easier than normal to penetrate.

Supernumerary Kidney—A relatively rare anomaly consisting of the presence of a third, small rudimentary kidney.

Surgical Jaundice—Jaundice that occurs as a result of biliary system blockage, which prevents bile from entering the duodenum.

Swan-Ganz Catheter—Specialized, multilumen catheter inserted usually via the subclavian vein for positioning outside the pulmonary artery for purposes of evaluating cardiac function.

Sylvian Triangle—An anatomic landmark in cerebral angiography, created by the middle cerebral artery and its branches.

Symptom—Any subjective evidence of a disease as perceived by a patient.

Syndactyly—A webbing or fusion of digits.

Syndrome—A group of signs and symptoms that occur together and characterize a specific abnormal disturbance.

Systole—The phase of the heart cycle in which the myocardium is contracting.

Tendinitis—Inflammation of a tendon.

Tenosynovitis—Inflammation of a tendon and its sheath.

Tension Pneumothorax—A pneumothorax in which air enters the pleural space but cannot leave because the tissues surrounding the opening into the pleural cavity act as valves; it results in a complete lung collapse and a mediastinal shift to the opposite side of the pneumothorax.

Teratoma—A neoplasm comprised of different types of tissue, none of which is native to the area where it occurs, commonly found in the ovary or testis.

Tetrology of Fallot—A combination of four congenital cardiac defects: pulmonary stenosis, ventricular central defect, overriding aorta, and hypertrophy of the right ventricle.

Thrombocytes—Platelets.

Thrombolysis—An interventional angiography procedure where urokinase, a high intensity anticoagulant, is dripped over a period of hours directly onto a clot to dissolve it.

Thrombophlebitis—The presence of inflammation and blood clots within a vein.

Thrombus—A blood clot that obstructs a blood vessel.

TNM System—A recognized, standard system for clinical classification of cancer.

Torus Fracture—A fracture in which the cortex folds back upon itself, with little or no displacement of the lower end of the bone.

Toxic Megacolon—An acute dilatation of the colon from paralytic ileus, particularly susceptible to rupture.

Toxoplasma Gondii—intracellular parasites of sporozoa origin which affect tissue and organs of mammals and birds.

Trabecula—The spongy substance found within a bone; it gives a characteristic appearance to bony detail.

Traction Diverticulum—A localized bulging of the full thickness of the esophageal wall, caused by adhesions from an external lesion.

Transesophageal Echocardiography (TEE)—A newer type of echocardiography procedure in which the patient swallows a mobile, flexible probe. The heart's structure can then be readily visualized without having structures such as the skin, rib cage, and chest muscles interfere.

Transjugular Intrahepatic Portosystemic Stent (TIPS)—An interventional angiography procedure in which a catheter is used to connect the jugular vein to the portal vein to reduce the flow of blood through a diseased liver.

Transient Ischemic Anemia (TIA)—A temporary episode of neurologic dysfunction that can precede a cerebrovascular accident.

Transitional Vertebra—A vertebra that assumes the characteristics of the vertebrae on each side of a major spine division.

Transposition—Displacement of a viscus to the opposite side.

Transposition of Great Vessels—Congenital malformation of the cardiovascular system in which the aorta arises from the right ventricle and the pulmonary artery from the left ventricle.

Transverse Fracture—A type of complete, noncomminuted fracture that occurs at right angles to the axis of the bone.

Traumatic—Pertaining to the effects of a wound or injury, whether physical or psychic.

Tripod Fracture—A fracture of the zygoma at its three sutures: frontal, temporal, and maxillary.

Tuberculosis—Any of the infectious diseases of man and animals caused by mycobacterium tuberculosis, generally affecting the lungs in the human body.

Ulcerative Colitis—A chronic, recurrent ulceration of the colon mucosa of unknown etiology.

Unicornuate Uterus—A uterus whose uterine cavity is elongated and has a single uterine tube emerging from it.

Ultrafast C.T.—A newer technique being used to examine the heart, particularly as related to coronary artery calcifications. This specialized C.T. unit uses a scanning focused x-ray beam to provide complete cardiac imaging in 50 msec without the need for ECG gating.

Uremia—The retention of urea in the blood, as characteristic of renal failure.

Ureteral Stent—A tube used to maintain patency of the ureter with the proximal end placed in the renal pelvis and the distal end placed in the urinary bladder.

Ureterocele—Cystlike dilatation of the terminal portion of the ureter as a result of stenosis of the ureteral meatus.

Urethral Valves—Congenital presence of mucosal folds that protrude into the posterior urethra, which may cause significant obstruction to urine flow.

Urinary tract infection (UTI)—The most common of all bacterial infections, a UTI is an infection in the urinary tract usually caused by a gram-negative bacillus that invades by an ascending route through the urethra to the bladder to the kidney.

Urokinase—A high intensity anticoagulant used, among other things, for thrombolysis to dissolve clots.

Uterus Didelphys—Complete duplication of the uterus, cervix, and vagina.

Venous Thrombosis—The formation of blood clots within a vein.

Ventricular Pacing Electrodes—Either temporary or permanent, they provide electrical pacing of the heart in situations in which the normal electrical system of the heart is misfiring.

Vesicoureteral Reflux—The backward flow of urine out of the bladder and into the ureters.

Viral Pneumonia—Pneumonia caused by a virus, spread by an infected person to a nonimmune individual.

Virulence—The ease with which an organism overcomes body defenses.

Volvulus—An intestinal obstruction caused by a twisting of the bowel about its mesenteric base.

Whiplash—Hyperextension-flexion injury of the spine.

Wound—An injury of soft body parts associated with rupture of the skin.

Zenker's Diverticulum—A pulsion diverticulum located at the pharyngoesophageal junction.

Bibliography

American College of Radiology: *Index for radiological diagnoses,* ed 3, Reston, Virginia, 1986, The American College of Radiology.

Ameican Joint Committee on Cancer: *Manual for staging of cancer,* ed 3, New York, 1988, JB Lippincott.

Atlas: *Magnetic resonance imaging of the brain and spine,* New York, 1991, Raven Press.

Benson, Ralph, M.D. and Peronll, Martin, M.D.: *Handbook of obstetrics and gynecology,* New York, 1994, McGraw-Hill.

Black, Robert M, M.D.: *Rose and Black's clinical problems in nephrology,* Boston, 1996, Little, Brown, and Company.

Bontrager, KL: *Textbook of radiographic positioning and related anatomy,* ed 3, St Louis, 1993, Mosby.

Bradley W and Brant-Zawadzki M: *The Raven MRI teaching,* Vols. I-III, New York, 1991, Raven Press.

Braunwald, Eugene, M.D.: *Heart disease,* ed 5, Philadelphia, 1997, W.B. Saunders Company.

Brenner, Barry M, M.D.: *Brenner and Rector's the kidney,* ed 5, Vols. 1 and 2, Philadelphia, 1996, W.B. Saunders.

Bullock, Barbara: *Pathophysiology: adaptations and alterations in function,* ed 4, Philadelphia, 1996, Lippincott-Raven.

Cawson RA et al: *Pathology: the mechanisms of disease,* ed 2, St Louis, 1989, Mosby.

Chey WY: *Functional disorders of the digestive tract,* New York, 1983, Raven Press.

Chopra S and May R: *Pathophysiology of gastrointestinal diseases,* Boston, 1989, Little, Brown, and Co.

Crowley LV: *Introductory concepts in pathology,* Chicago, 1972, Mosby.

Crowley LV: *Introduction to human disease,* ed 4, Boston, 1997, Bartlett.

Gitnick G: *Gastroenterology,* New York, 1983, John Wiley and Sons.

Gore R, et al: *Textbook of gastrointestinal radiology,* Philadelphia, 1996, W.B. Saunders.

Greenberger N: *Gastrointestinal disorders: a pathophysiologic approach,* ed 3, Chicago, 1986, Mosby.

Hatfield P and Wise R: *Radiology of the gallbladder and bile ducts, In Golden's Diagnostic Radiology,* Baltimore, 1976, Williams and Wilkins.

Heptinstall R: *Pathology of the kidney,* ed 3, Volumes I-III, Boston, 1983, Little, Brown and Co.

Hinshaw HC and Murray J: *Diseases of the chest,* ed 4, Philadelphia, 1980, WB Saunders.

Hudson L, et al: *Respiratory infections,* New York, 1986, Churchill Livingstone.

Hurst, J. Willis: *Current therapy in cardiovascular disease,* Vols. 1 and 2, Philadelphia, 1991, B.C. Decker, Inc.

Jacobson, Harry R., M.D., Striker, Gary E., M.D., and Klahr, Saulo, M.D.: *The principles and practice of nephrology,* St Louis, 1995, Mosby.

Jaffe, Richard, M.D., Pierson, Roger A., M.S., and Abramowicz, Jacques M.D.: *Imaging in infertility and reproductive endocrinology,* Philadelphia, 1994, J.B. Lippincott Company.

Jariwalla G and Fry J: *Respiratory diseases,* Lancashire, UK, 1985, MTP Press Limited.

Lapides J: *Fundamentals of urology,* Philadelphia, 1976, WB Saunders.

Lieberman J: *Inherited diseases of the lung,* Philadelphia, 1988, WB Saunders.

Latchaw R: *MR and CT imaging of the head, neck, and spine,* vols 1 and 2, St Louis, 1991, Mosby.

Levine D: *Care of the renal patient,* ed 2, Philadelphia, 1991, WB Saunders.

Marcove A, Ralph C., and Myron Arlen: *Atlas of bone pathology with clinical and radiographic correlations (based on Henry L. Jaffe's course),* Philadelphia, 1992, J.B. Lippincott.

Margulis, A and Burhenne I, *Alimentary tract radiology,* ed 4, Vols 1 and 2, Philadelphia, 1994, W.B. Saunders.

Mulvihill M: *Human diseases: a systemic approach,* ed 3, East Norwalk, Connecticut, 1991, Appleton and Lange.

National Center for Health Statistics, Health: U.S., 1994, Hyattsville, Maryland, Public Health Service.

Norris H: *Pathology of the colon, small intestine, and anus,* ed 2, New York, 1991, Churchill Livingstone.

Pomeranz, S: *Craniospinal MRI,* Philadelphia, 1991, WB Saunders.

Purtilo D and Purtilo R: *A survey of human diseases,* ed 2, Boston, 1989, Little, Brown, and Co.

Resnick, Donald, M.D., and Holger Pettersson, M.D.: *Skeletal radiology,* Coconut Creek, Florida, Merit Communications.

Robbins, Stanley L., M.D., Ramzi S., Cotran, M.D., and Vinay Kumar, M.D.: *Pathologic basis of disease,* ed 5, Philadelphia, 1994, W.B. Saunders Company.

Scheld WM, Whitley, RJ, and Durack D: *Infections of the central nervous system,* New York, 1991, Raven Press.

Sheldon, Huntington: *Boyd's introduction to the study of disease,* ed 11, Philadelphia, 1992, Lea and Febiger.

Sherlock S: *Diseases of the liver and biliary system,* ed 8, Boston, 1989, Blackwell Scientific Publications.

Silver, Malcom: *Cardiovascular pathology,* New York, 1991, Churchill Livingstone.

Sleisenger M and Fordtran J: *Gastrointestinal disease: pathophysiology, diagnosis, management,* ed 3, vols I and II, Philadelphia, 1983, WB Saunders.

Snively WD and Beshear D: *Textbook of pathophysiology* Philadelphia, 1972, JB Lippincott.

Sutton, D: *A textbook of radiology and imaging,* ed 4, London, 1987, Churchill-Livingstone.

Swash M and Kennard C: *Scientific basis of clinical neurology,* New York, 1985, Churchill Livingstone.

Taussig MJ: *Processes in pathology,* Oxford, 1979, Blackwell Scientific Publications.

Tattersfield AE and McNicol M: *Respiratory disease,* New York, 1987, Springer-Verlag.

Wallach, Edward, M.D., and Zacur, Howard, M.D., Ph.D., *Reproductive medicine and surgery,* St Louis, 1995, Mosby.

Walton J: *Brain's diseases of the nervous system,* ed 9, New York, 1985, Oxford University Press.

Wilson, R and Alexander, J: *Management of trauma-pitfalls and practice,* ed 2, Baltimore, 1996, Williams and Wilkins.

Yochum, Terry R and Rowe, Lindsay J: *Essentials of skeletal radiology,* ed 2, Vols. 1 and 2, Baltimore, 1996, Williams and Wilkins.

Index

A

Abdomen. *See also* Gastrointestinal system
  anatomy and physiology review, 79-82
  computed tomography of, 87
  congenital/hereditary anomalies of, 91-94
  degenerative diseases of, 104-107
  imaging considerations, 82-83
  magnetic resonance imaging, 87-88
  neoplastic diseases of, 114-118
  traumatic disease of, 287-289
    intraperitoneal air, 288-289
  tubes and catheters, 88-91
Abscess, lung, 71-72
Achalasia, 110
Achondroplasia, 17-18
Acoustic neurilemoma, 250-251
Acoustic neuroma, 250-251
Acquired immune deficiency syndrome, 222-223
Acromegaly, 33-34, 248
Acromioclavicular joint separations, 282
Acute diseases, 2
Adenocarcinoma, 115-116, 161-162
  of endometrium, 175-176
Adenomatous polyps, 116
Agglutination, 219
Albers-Schönberg disease, 18-19
Alimentary tract, 81
Alveoli, 48
Ambulatory care center, 3
American Joint Committee on Cancer, 10
Amniocentesis, 7
Amniotic fluid, disorders of, 179-180

Anemia, 218
Anencephaly, 22
Aneurysms, 213-214
  dissecting, 213
  saccular, 213
Angiography
  for cardiovascular disease, 199-203
  central nervous system, 234
Ankylosing spondylitis, 26-27
Annulus fibrosus, 231
Anthracosis, 70
Appendicitis, 101
Arteries, 192-193
  stents, 201
Arthritis, 24-26
  acute, 25
  ankylosing spondylitis, 26-27
  degenerative joint disease, 27-28
  gouty, 30-31
  juvenile, 26
  osteoarthritis, 27-28
  pyogenic, 25
  rheumatoid, 7, 25-26
  types of, 25
Asbestosis, 70
Ascites, 128-129
Aspiration pneumonia, 64
Astrocytomas, 244-246
Asymptomatic, 2
Atelectasis, 285-287
Atheroma formation, 208
Atherosclerosis, 9, 208-209

Atherothrombic brain infarction, 212
Atresia, 91-93
  bowel, 92-93
  esophageal, 91-92
Atria, right/left, 190-191
Atrial septal defects, 204
Autoimmune disorders, 7
Avulsion fracture, 271-272

B

Barium enema, 86
Barrett's esophagus, 114-115
Basilar skull fracture, 261-262
Battered child syndrome, 282
Benign neoplasm, 10
Bicornuate uterus, 171-172
Biliary tree, 122
Black lung disease, 70
Bladder, 139-140. *See also* Urinary system
  carcinoma, 163
  cystitis, 154
  diverticula of, 150
  neurogenic, 154
  trabeculated, 154-155
  vesicoureteral reflux, 154
Blood, 218-220
  types of, 219-220
Blood-brain barrier, 230-231
Blow-out fracture, 279-280
Bone(s), 13-15. *See also* Skeletal system
  cartilaginous growth plate, 15
  cellous, 14
  classification of, 15, 16
  compact, 14
  composition of, 14, 15
  involucrum, 23
  sequestrum, 23
Bone bruise, 274
Bone cyst, simple, 37
Bone densitometry units, 17
Bone marrow, 14
Bowel
  atresia, 92-93
  imaging considerations, 85-87
  large, 82
  obstruction of, 107-110
    mechanical, 108-109
    paralytic ileus, 109-110
  small, 82
    neoplasms, 116

Boxer's fracture, 275
Brain. *See also* Central nervous system
  anatomy/physiology review, 228-231
  hematomas of, 263-266
  traumatic disease and, 260-266
  tumors, 243-250
Breast(s), 168-169
  carcinoma of, 178-179
  fibroadenoma, 176
  fibrocystic, 176-178
  imaging considerations, 171
  mastitis, 173
Bright's disease, 154
Bronchi, 47, 48
Bronchial adenomas, 74
Bronchiectasis, 64
Bronchitis, chronic, 67
Bronchogenic carcinoma, 74-75
Burn, 9
Bursitis, 28
Butterfly fracture, 270

C

Calcifications, urinary tract, 156-159
Calcium, 15
Calculi
  renal, 141-142, 156-158
  staghorn, 157
Cancer. *See also* Carcinoma
  vs. carcinoma, 10
  defined, 10
  staging of, 10
Cantor tube, 90
Capillaries, 192-193
Carcinoma. *See also* Neoplastic disease
  adenocarcinomas, 115-116
  bladder, 163
  breast, 178-179
  bronchogenic, 74-75
  vs. cancer, 10
  cervical, 175
  colon, 116
  defined, 10
  esophageal, 114-115
  gallbladder, 135-136
  pancreatic, 136-137
  prostate, 183-184
  renal, 134-135, 161-163
  testicular, 184-187
  uterus, 175-176

Cardiac series, 195-196
Cardiomegaly, 195
Cardiovascular system
    anatomy and physiology review, 190-192
        cardiac cycle, 192
        circulatory vessels, 192
    congenital/hereditary diseases, 203-206
        coarctation of aorta, 204-205
        patent ductus arteriosus, 204
        septal defects, 204
        tetralogy of Fallot, 206
        transposition of great vessels, 204-206
    congestive heart failure, 207-208
    degenerative diseases, 208-213
        aneurysms, 213-214
        atherosclerosis, 208-209
        cerebrovascular accident, 210-213
        coronary artery disease, 209-210
        myocardial infarction, 210
        venous thrombosis, 214
    imaging considerations
        angiography, 199-203
        cardiac series, 195-196
        controllable factors, 193-195
        Doppler sonography, 196-198
        echocardiography, 196-197
        fluoroscopy, 196
        gated cardiac blood pool scans, 199
        myocardial perfusion scan, 198-199
        ultrafast CT, 203
        uncontrollable factors, 195
    valvular disease, 206-207
        rheumatic fever, 206
        valvular stenosis, 206-207
Cartilaginous joints, 16
Catheter
    Foley, 90-91, 146
    Hickman, 59-60
    intra-aortic balloon pump, 60
    permanent, 202
    pulmonary artery, 59
    Swan-Ganz, 59
Celiac disease, 98-99
Cell necrosis, local and systemic effects of, 8
Cellous bone, 14
Center for Disease Control, 3
Central nervous system
    anatomy/physiology review, 228-231
    congenital/hereditary disease,
        hydrocephalus, 236

Central nervous system—cont'd
    congenital/hereditary disease—cont'd
        meningomyelocele, 235-236
    degenerative diseases
        cervical spondylosis, 242
        degenerative disk disease, 240-242
        herniated nucleus pulposus, 240-242
        multiple sclerosis, 242-243
    imaging considerations, 231-235
        computed tomography, 234
        MRI, 233-234
        plain skull films, 231-233
    inflammatory disease
        encephalitis, 239-240
        meningitis, 238-239
    neoplastic diseases, 243-253
        craniopharyngioma, 250
        gilomas, 243-246
        medulloblastoma, 246
        meningloma, 246-248
        metastases from other sites, 252
        pituitary adenoma, 248-249
        spinal tumors, 252-253
        tumors of central nerve sheath cells, 250-251
    traumatic disease and, 260-266
        brain trauma, 262-263
        cerebral cranial fractures, 261-262
        hematomas of brain, 263-266
Central venous pressure lines, 58-59
Cerebrovascular accident, 210-213
Cervical spondylosis, 242
Cervix, carcinoma of, 175
Chest radiograph. *See* Respiratory system
Chest tube, 57-58
Child abuse, 282
Chip fracture, 272
Cholecystitis, 131
Cholelithiasis, 130-132
Chondrosarcoma, 42
Choriocarcinomas, testicular, 184, 187
Chromosomes, 6
Chronic diseases, 2
Chronic obstructive pulmonary disease, 67-68
    chronic bronchitis, 67
    emphysema, 67-68
Cirrhosis, 128-129
    ascites, 128-129
Closed fracture, 268
Closed head injury, 262
Clubfoot, 19-20

Coarctation of aorta, 204-205
Coccidioidomycosis, 71
Colic, renal, 157-158
Colles' fracture, 275
Colon, 82
    atresia of, 93
    cancer of, 117-118
    diverticula of, 113
    polyps of, 116-117
Colonoscopy, 102
Colostomy, 86
Coma, 263
Comminuted fractures, 268-270
Compact bone, 14
Compensatory hypertrophy, 146
Complete fracture, 270-271
Compound fracture, 268
Compression fractures, 258-259
Computed tomography
    central nervous system, 234
    of gastrointestinal system, 87
    hepatobiliary system, 126
    respiratory system, 51-52
    skeletal system, 16-17
    urinary system, 144
Concussion, 262
Congenital/hereditary disorders
    of cardiovascular system, 203-206
    central nervous system, 235-238
    defined, 6
    of female reproductive system, 171-172
    of gastrointestinal system, 91-94
    of male reproductive system, 183
    megacolon, 111
    of respiratory system, 60-61
    of skeletal system, 17-22
    urinary system, 146-152
Congestive heart failure, 207-208
Contrecoup lesions, 262
Contusion, 9, 262
Coronary artery disease, 209-210
Corpus luteum ovarian cysts, 173
Coup lesion, 262
Craniopharyngioma, 250
Craniosynostoses, 21-22
Craniotubular dysplasias, 19
Crohn's disease, 99-100
Crossed ectopy of kidneys, 147-148
Cyst(s)
    ovarian, 173-174

Cyst(s)—cont'd
    renal, 150-151, 159-161
    simple bone, 37
Cystadenocarcinoma, 174
Cystic fibrosis, 60-61
Cystic teratomas, 174
Cystitis, 154
Cystogram, urinary system, 144

D

Death rates, age and cause of death, 4-6, 257
Debridement, 7-8
Degenerative disease, 9
    central nervous system, 240-243
    urinary system, 155-159
Degenerative joint disease, 27-28
Dehydration, 9
Depressed fracture, 261
Dermoid cysts, 174
Diabetes, 9
Diagnosis, defined, 3
Diagnostic medical sonography, 126
Digital fluoroscopy, 88
Digital radiographs, 48
Disease(s)
    acute, 2
    chronic, 2
    defined, 2
    incidence of, 3
    monitoring trends of, 3
    prevalence, 3
    rate of incidence, 4-6
Disease classification
    congenital/hereditary disease, 6-7
    degenerative disease, 9
    inflammatory disease, 7-9
    metabolic disease, 9
    traumatic disease, 9
Dislocations, 280-282
    defined, 280
    hip, 281
    shoulder joint, 280-281
    subluxation, 280
Dissecting aneurysm, 213
Diverticula
    bladder, 150
    ureteral, 150
Diverticulitis, 113
Diverticulum, 111-113
Dohhoff tube, 90

Doppler sonography, cardiac, 196-198
Down syndrome, 6
Ductus arteriosus, 203
    patent, 204
Duodenum
    atresia of, 92-93
    ulcer, 95
Dysphagia, 84

E

Echocardiography
    stress, 196
    transesophageal, 197
Ectopic kidney, 148
Ectopic pregnancy, 180
Edema, pulmonary, 68
Edlich tube, 88
Elbow fat pad sign, 278
Electrolyte balances, 9
Electron beam CT, 203
Embolization, 200-201
Embolus, 210
Embryonal carcinomas, testicular, 184-187
Emergency medical system, 256-257
Emphysema, 67-68
    mediastinal, 56-57
    subcutaneous, 57
Empyemas, 71
Encephalitis, 239-240
Endocardium, 192
Endochondroma, 36
Endocrine disorder, 9
Endometriosis, 173
Endometrium, adenocarcinoma, 175-176
Endoscopic retrograde cholangiopancreatogram,
    125
Endoscopy, 84, 88-89
Endotracheal tube, 57-58
Enteral tube, 90
Ependymoma, 246
Epicardium, 192
Epidemiologic, defined, 3
Epididymo-orchitis, 184
Epidural hematoma, 263-264
Epiphrenic diverticulum, 111-112
Erythrocytes, 218
Esophagus, 81
    achalasia, 110
    atresia of, 91-92
    diverticula, 111-112

Esophagus—cont'd
    imaging consideration, 84
    strictures of, 94-95
    tumors of, 114-115
    varices of, 102-103
Etiology, defined, 2
Ewald tube, 88
Ewing's sarcoma, 41-42
Exostosis, 36
Extracorporeal shock wave lithotripsy, 142-143

F

Fallopian tubes, 168
Fatigue fractures, 273
Female reproductive system
    anatomy and physiology review, 167-169
    congenital abnormalities, 171-172
    disorders during pregnancy, 179-182
        amniotic fluid, 179-180
        ectopic pregnancy, 180
        hydatiform mole, 181-182
        placenta disorders, 180-181
    imaging considerations for, 169-171
        hysterosalpingogram, 169
        mammography, 171
        pelvimetry, 170
        ultrasound, 170-171
        xeromammography, 171
    inflammatory disease
        mastitis, 173
        pelvic inflammatory disease, 172-173
    neoplastic disease
        adenocarcinoma of endometrium, 175-176
        breast carcinoma, 178-179
        breast masses, 176-179
        carcinoma of cervix, 175
        cystadenocarcinoma, 174-175
        fibroadenoma, 176
        fibrocystic breasts, 176-178
        leiomyomas, 175
        ovarian cystic masses, 173-174
        uterine masses, 175-176
Fibroadenoma, 176
Fibrocaseous tuberculosis, 66
Fibrocystic breasts, 176-178
Fibrous joints, 16
Fluoroscopy
    cardiac, 196
    digital, 88
    of gastrointestinal system, 84-88

Foley catheter, 90-91, 146
Follicular ovarian cysts, 173
Foot, malformations, 19-20
Foramen ovale, 203
Fracture(s), 266-280
    avulsion, 271-272
    blow-out, 279-280
    Boxer's, 275
    butterfly, 270
    chip, 272
    classification of, 268
    closed, 268
    Colles', 275
    comminuted, 268-270
    complete, 270-271
    delayed union, 267-268
    fatigue, 273
    greenstick, 272
    growth plate, 272-273
    imaging considerations, 266-267
    impacted, 268
    incomplete, 272
    insufficiency, 273
    Maisonneuve, 276-277
    malunion, 268
    mandibular, 279
    maxillary, 279
    Monteggia's, 276
    nasal bone, 280
    noncomminuted, 270-271
    nonunion, 268
    oblique, 270
    occult, 274
    pathologic, 270
    penetrating, 272
    Pott's, 276
    simple, 268
    spiral, 270
    stress, 273
    stretch, 273
    torus, 272-273
    transverse, 270-271
    tripod, 280
    of vertebral body
        compression, 258-259
        Hangman's, 259
    visceral cranial, 278-280
    zygomatic arch fracture, 278
Fungal diseases, of respiratory system, 70-71
Fusiform, 213

G
Gallbladder. *See also* Hepatobiliary system
    anatomy and physiology review, 122-123
    cancer of, 135-136
    cholecystitis, 131
    cholelithiasis, 130
    diagnostic medical sonography, 126
Gallstone, 130-131, 158-159
Gallstone ileus, 108, 132
Ganglion, 28
Gastric tubes, 88-90
Gastric ulcers, 95
Gastroenteritis, 97-98
Gastrointestinal system. *See also* Abdomen
    abdominal tubes and catheters, 88-91
    anatomy and physiology review, 79-82
    bowel obstructions, 107-110
    congenital/hereditary anomalies
        atresia, 91-93
        hypertrophic pyloric stenosis, 93-94
        imperforate anus, 94
        malrotation, 94
    degenerative diseases, herniation, 104-107
    diverticular diseases
        colonic diverticula, 113
        esophageal diverticula, 111-112
    esophageal varices, 102-103
    imaging consideration, 84-88
        computed tomography, 87
        digital fluoroscopy, 88
        endoscopy, 88-89
        esophagus, 84
        other studies, 87-88
        small bowel, 85
        stomach, 84-85
    inflammatory diseases, 94-102
        appendicitis, 101
        esophageal strictures, 94-95
        gastroenteritis, 97-98
        malabsorption syndrome, 98-99
        peptic ulcer, 95-97
        regional enteritis, 99-100
        ulcerative colitis, 101-102
    neoplastic diseases
        colon cancer, 117-118
        colonic polyps, 116-117
        small-bowel neoplasms, 116
        tumors of esophagus, 114-115
        tumors of stomach, 115-116
    neurogenic disease

Gastrointestinal system—cont'd
  neurogenic disease—cont'd
    achalasia, 110
    Hirschsprung's disease, 111
Gated cardiac blood pool scans, 199
Giant cell tumor, 39
Giantism, 248
Gilomas, 243-246
Glioblastoma multiforme, 246
Glomerulonephritis, acute, 154
Gouty arthritis, 30-31
Granulomatous colitis, 99-100
Greenfield filters, 202-203
Greenstick fracture, 272
Growth plate fractures, 272-273

H

Hand, malformations, 19-20
Hangman's fracture, 259
Harris tube, 90
Health care, costs of, 3, 6
Heart
  anatomy and physiology review, 190-192
  murmur, 204
Hemangloma, 133-134
Hematocrit, 218
Hematoma
  brain, 263-266
  epidural, 263-264
  intracerebral, 264-266
  subarachnoid, 264-265
  subdural, 264-265
Hemocytoblasts, 218-219
Hemophilia, 6
Hemopoietic system
  acquired immune deficiency syndrome,
    222-223
  anatomy and physiology review of, 218-220
  imaging considerations, 220-222
    lymphadenograms, 230-231
    magnetic resonance imaging, 221
  neoplastic disease
    Hodgkin's disease, 225
    leukemia, 224-225
    multiple myeloma, 223-224
Hemorrhagic stroke, 210-213
Hemothorax, 72
Hepatitis
  type A, 130
  type B, 130

Hepatitis—cont'd
  type C, 130
  viral, 129-130
Hepatobiliary scans, 126-127
Hepatobiliary system
  anatomy and physiology review of, 121-123
  imaging considerations
    computed tomography, 126
    diagnostic medical sonography, 126
    endoscopic retrograde
      cholangiopancreatogram, 125
    hepatobiliary scans, 126-127
    operative cholangiography, 125
    oral cholecystogram, 124
    percutaneous transhepatic
      cholangiography, 124-125
    plain films, 123
    T-tube cholangiography, 125-126
  inflammatory disease
    cholelithiasis, 130-132
    cirrhosis, 128-129
    pancreatitis, 132-133
    viral hepatitis, 129-130
  metabolic disease, 133
    jaundice, 133
  neoplastic diseases
    carcinoma of gallbladder, 135-136
    hemangloma, 133-134
    hepatoma, 134-135
Hepatoma, 134-135
Hepatomegaly, 130
Hereditary diseases, 6-7
  defined, 2
  of respiratory system, 60-61
  of skeletal system, 17-22
Hernia, 104-107
  hiatal, 104-107
  incarcerated, 104
  inguinal, 104
  paraesophageal, 107
  strangulated, 104
Hiatal hernia, 104-107
Hickman catheter, 59-60
Hip
  congenital dislocation of, 20, 281
  traumatic dislocation of, 281
Hirschsprung's disease, 111
Histoplasmosis, 3, 70-71
Hodgkin's disease, 225
Horseshoe kidney, 147-148

Human immunodeficiency virus, 222
Hyaline membrane disease, 61
Hydatiform mole, 181-182
Hydroceles, 184
Hydrocephalus, 236
Hydronephrosis, 158
Hyperostosis frontalis interna, 36
Hyperparathyroidism, 9
Hyperplasia, renal, 147
Hyperthyroidism, 32-33
Hypertrophic pyloric stenosis, 93-94
Hypoplasia, renal, 146-147
Hysterosalpingogram, 169

I

Iatrogenic reaction, defined, 2
Ileal atresia, 92
Ileostomies, 86-87
Imaging considerations
    abdomen, 82-83
    cardiovascular system, 193-203
    central nervous system, 231-235
    female reproductive system, 169-171
    fractures, 266-267
    hepatobiliary system, 123-127
    male reproductive system, 182-183
    respiratory system, 46-57
    for skeletal system, 16-17
    urinary system, 140-146
Impacted fracture, 268
Imperforate anus, 94
Incarcerated hernia, 104
Incomplete fracture, 272
Infants, sail sign, 56
Infarct, 209
Infection, defined, 8
Inflammatory diseases
    autoimmune disorders, 7
    central nervous system, 238-240
    chronic vs. acute, 7
    defined, 7
    female reproductive system, 172-173
    of gastrointestinal system, 94-102
    hepatobiliary system, 128-133
    of respiratory system, 61-74
    of skeletal system, 22-30
    tissue regeneration and, 7
    of urinary system, 152-155
Inguinal hernia, 104
Insufficiency fractures, 273

Intervertebral disk, 230, 231
Intra-aortic balloon pump, 60
Intracerebral hematoma, 264-266
Intrathoracic stomach, 107
Intravenous urogram
    nephrogram radiograph, 141
    preliminary film, 141
Intussusception, 109
Involucrum, 23
Ischemia, 209
Ischemic stroke, 210

J

Jaundice, 133
    medical, 133
    surgical, 133
Joints, 16

K

Kaposi's sarcoma, 223
Kidney(s), 139-140. *See also* Urinary system
    agenesis of, 146
    anomalies of
        fusion, 147-148
        number, 146
        position, 148-149
        size of, 146-147
    calculi, 141-142
    carcinoma, 161-163
    colic, 157
    crossed ectopy of, 147-148
    cysts, 159-161
    ectopic, 148
    horseshoe, 147-148
    hyperplasia, 147
    hypoplasia, 146-147
    malrotation of, 148
    medullary sponge, 151-152
    nephroptosis, 149
    polycystic, 150-151
    supernumerary, 146
KUB, 83

L

Lactose insufficiency, 99
Lacunar infarction, 210
Left-sided appendicitis, 113
Legg-Perthes disease, 282-283
Legionnaires' disease, 63-64
Leiomyoma, 114, 175

Lesion, 9
Leukemia, 224-225
Leukocytes, 219
Levacuator tube, 88-90
Level I medical center, 258
Level II medical centers, 258
Level III medical centers, 258
Levin tubes, 88
Linear fracture, 261
Liver. *See also* Hepatobiliary system
    anatomy and physiology review of, 121-122
    cirrhosis, 128-129
    diagnostic medical sonography, 126
    hemangloma, 133-134
    hepatoma, 134-135
    viral hepatitis, 129-130
Lungs, 46-47. *See also* Respiratory system
    abscess of, 71-72
    traumatic disease
        atelectasis, 285-287
        pneumothorax, 284-285
Lymph, 220
Lymphadenograms, 220
Lymphatic system, 220
Lymph nodes, 220
Lymphocytes, 220

M

Magnetic resonance imaging
    of abdomen, 87-88
    central nervous system, 233-234
    hemopoietic system, 221
    respiratory system, 52
    skeletal system, 16
Maisonneuve fracture, 276-277
Malabsorption syndrome, 98-99
Male reproductive system
    anatomy/physiology review, 182
    congenital anomalies, 183
    imaging considerations, 182-183
    neoplastic diseases, 183-187
        adenocarcinoma of prostate, 183-184
        prostatic hyperplasia, 183
        testicular masses, 184-187
Malignant neoplasm, 10
Malrotation, 94
    of kidneys, 148
Mammography, female reproductive system, 171
Mandibular fracture, 279
Mantoux test, 66

Marble bone, 18
Marie-Strumpell disease, 26-27
Mastitis, 173
Maxillary fracture, 279
Mechanical bowel obstruction, 108-109
Mediastinal emphysema, 56-57
Mediastinum, 46
    imaging considerations for, 56-57
Medical jaundice, 133
Medullary canal, 14
Medullary sponge kidneys, 151-152
Medulloblastoma, 246
Meningiomas, 252-253
Meningitis, 238-239
Meningloma, 246-248
Meningocele, 236
Meningomyelocele, 235-236
Metabolic disease, 9
    hepatobiliary system, 133
    of skeletal system, 30-34
Metabolism, defined, 9
Metastasis(es)
    in bone, 42-43
    to brain, 252
    defined, 10
    pulmonary, 75-76
Military tuberculosis, 66
Milk of calcium, 123
Miller-Abbott tube, 90
Mobile automatic exposure control, 48
Monteggia's fracture, 276
Morbidity rate, defined, 3
Mortality rate
    defined, 3
    infant, 3
    table of, 4-6
Multiple myeloma, 223-224
Multiple sclerosis, 242-243
Murmur, 204
Mycoplasma pneumonia, 64
Myelocele, 236
Myocardial infarction, 210
Myocardial perfusion scan, 198-199
Myocardium, 192

N

Nasoenteric decompression tubes, 90
Neoplasm
    benign, 10
    malignant, 10

Neoplastic disease(s), 9-10
    central nervous system, 243-253
    of female reproductive system, 173-175
    of gastrointestinal system and abdomen, 114-118
    hemopoietic system, 223-225
    hepatobiliary system, 133-137
    male reproductive system, 183-187
    of respiratory system, 74-76
    of skeletal system, 35-43
    urinary system, 159-163
Nephroblastoma, 162-163
Nephrocalcinosis, 155
Nephrogram, 141
Nephrons, 140
Nephroptosis, of kidney, 149
Nephrosclerosis, 155
Nephrostomy tube, 145
Nephrotomography, urinary system, 142
Neurofibromas, 252-253
Neurogenic bladder, 154
Neurogenic diseases, of gastrointestinal system,
    110-111
Noncomminuted fractures, 270-271
Nosocomial disease, defined, 2
Nuclear medicine
    for cardiac assessment, 198-203
    central nervous system, 234
    respiratory system, 53
    skeletal system, 17
Nucleus pulposus, 231

O

Oblique fracture, 270
Occult fracture, 274
Oligodendroglioma, 246
Oligohydramnios, 179
Open fracture, 268
Operative cholangiography, 125
Oral cholecystogram, 124
Osteitis deformans, 31-32
Osteoarthritis, 9, 27-28
Osteoblastoma, 37-38
Osteoblasts, 14
Osteochondroma, 36
Osteoclasts, 14
Osteogenesis imperfecta, 17
Osteogenic sarcoma, 32
Osteoid osteoma, 37-38
Osteoma, 36
Osteomalacia, 31

Osteomyelitis, 22-23
Osteopetrosis, 18-19
Osteophytes, 28
Osteoporosis, 9, 30-31
Osteosarcoma, 39-41
Osteoscleroses, 18
Ovaries
    cysts of, 173-174
    polycystic, 173-174

P

Paget's disease, 31-32
Pancreas. *See also* Hepatobiliary system
    anatomy and physiology review of, 123
    cancer of, 136-137
Paraesophageal hernia, 107
Patent ductus arteriosus, 204
Pathogenesis, defined, 2
Pathologic fracture, 270
Pectus excavatum, 195
Pelvic inflammatory disease, 172-173
Pelvimetry, 170
Penetrating fractures, 272
Peptic ulcer, 95-97
Percutaneous transhepatic cholangiography,
    124-125
Percutaneous transluminal angioplasty, 201-202
Periosteum, 15-16
Pessary, 168
PET scanning, central nervous system, 234
Phlebitis, 214
Pituitary adenoma, 248-249
Placental abruption, 180
Placental accreta, 180-181
Placenta previa, 180
Plain films, hepatobiliary system, 123
Platelets, 219-220
Pleural effusion, 72
Pleurisy, 72
Pneumococcal lobar pneumonia, 62
Pneumoconioses, 68-70
    anthracosis, 70
    asbestosis, 70
    silicosis, 69-70
Pneumocystis carinii pneumonia, 223
Pneumonia, 7, 61-64
    aspiration, 64
    Legionnaires' disease, 63-64
    mycoplasma, 64
    pneumococcal lobar, 62

Pneumonia—cont'd
  staphylococcal, 63
  streptococcal, 63
  viral, 64
Pneumoperitoneum, 288-289
Pneumothorax, 284-285
Polycystic kidney disease, 150-151
Polycystic ovaries, 173-174
Polydactyly, 19
Polyhydramnios, 179-180
Polyps
  colonic, 116-117
  epithelium, 116
  pedunculated, 116
  sessile, 116
Portable radiographs, 48
Pott's disease, 24
Pott's fracture, 276
Pregnancy
  disorders during, 179-182
  ectopic, 180
  hydatiform mole, 181-182
  placenta disorders, 180-181
Preliminary film, 141
Prognosis, defined, 3
Prostate
  carcinoma of, 183-184
  transurethral resection of prostate, 183
Prostate gland, 182
Prostatic hyperplasia, 183
Pseudocyst, 132
Pulmonary artery catheter, 59
Pulmonary edema, 68
Pulmonary metastases, 75-76
Pulmonary tuberculosis, 65
Pulsion diverticulum, 111
Pyelonephritis, 152-153
Pyogenic arthritis, 25
Pyuria, 152-153

R

Radiography
  chest, 194-196
  of gastrointestinal system, 84-88
Red bone marrow, 14
Reed-Sternberg cells, 225
Reflux esophagitis, 95
Regional enteritis, 99-100
Renal agenesis, 146-147
Renal angiography, 144

Renal pelvis, 149
Reproductive system, 166-187. *See also* Female reproductive system; Male reproductive system
Respiratory distress syndrome, 61
Respiratory system
  anatomy/physiology review of, 46
  chest tubes, vascular access lines and catheters for, 57-60
  congenital/hereditary diseases
    cystic fibrosis, 60-61
    hyaline membrane disease, 61
  imaging consideration
    bony structure of chest, 54-55
    for computed tomography, 51-52
    exposure factor conditions, 46, 48
    magnetic resonance imaging, 52
    for mediastinum, 56-57
    nuclear medicine, 53
    perfusion scan of, 53
    position and projection, 49
    soft tissue of chest, 54
    for standard chest radiograph, 49-50
    ventilation scan, 53
  inflammatory diseases, 61-74
    bronchiectasis, 64
    chronic obstructive pulmonary disease, 68-70
    fungal diseases, 70-71
    lung abscess, 71-72
    pleural effusion, 72
    pleurisy, 72
    pneumoconioses, 68-70
    pneumonias, 61-64
    sinusitis, 72-74
    tuberculosis, 64-67
  neoplastic diseases
    bronchial adenomas, 74
    bronchogenic carcinoma, 74-75
    metastases from other sites, 75-76
  traumatic disease
    atelectasis, 285-287
    pneumothorax, 284-285
Reticuloendothelial system, 219
Retrograde pyelograph, urinary system, 142
Rheumatic fever, 206
Rheumatoid arthritis, 7, 25-26
  juvenile, 26
Rh factor, 219
Rib notching, 204-205
Rickets, 31

S

Saccular aneurysm, 213
Sail sign, 56
Sarcoma
  chondrosarcoma, 42
  defined, 10
  Ewing's, 41-42
  osteogenic, 32, 39-41
Schatzki's ring, 104, 106
Schwannoma, 250-251
Scoliosis, 20-21
Scout, 141
Seminomas, testicular, 184-186
Septal defects, 204
Sequestrum, 23
Shoulder joint, dislocation of, 280-281
Sigmoidoscopy, 102
Sign, defined, 2
Silicosis, 69-70
Simple fracture, 268
Single-photon emission computed tomography
  central nervous system, 234-235
  liver and, 126-127
Sinoatrial node, 192
Sinuses, 46
Sinusitis, 72-74
Skeletal modeling, 18
Skeletal system. *See also* Bones
  anatomy/physiology review of, 13-16
  congenital/hereditary diseases, 17-22
    achondroplasia, 17-18
    congenital dislocation of hip, 20
    cranial anomalies, 21-22
    hand/foot malformations, 19-20
    osteogenesis imperfecta, 17
    osteopetrosis, 18-19
    vertebral anomalies, 20-21
  imaging considerations for
    computed tomography, 16-17
    magnetic resonance imaging, 16
    nuclear medicine, 17
    radiography, 16
  inflammatory disease, 22-30
    ankylosing spondylitis, 26-27
    arthritis, 24-26
    gouty arthritis, 29-30
    inflammation, 28-29
    osteomyelitis, 22-23
    tuberculosis, 24

Skeletal system—cont'd
  metabolic diseases
    acromegaly, 33-34
    hyperparathyroidism, 32-33
    osteomalacia, 31
    osteoporosis, 30-31
    Paget's disease, 31-32
  neoplastic disease, 35-43
    chondrosarcoma, 42
    endochondroma, 36-37
    Ewing's sarcoma, 41-42
    metastases from other sites, 42-43
    osteochondroma, 36
    osteoclastoma, 39
    osteoid osteoma/osteoblastoma, 37-38
    osteoma, 36
    osteosarcoma, 39-41
    simple bone cyst, 37
  traumatic disease
    Battered Child syndrome, 282
    dislocation, 280-282
    fractures, 266-280
    Legg-Perthes disease, 282-283
    vertebral column, 258-260
  vertebral column injuries, 34
    spondylolisthesis, 34
    spondylolysis, 34
Sonography. *See* Ultrasound
Spermatoceles, 184
Spina bifida, 21, 235
Spinal cord
  anatomy/physiology review, 228-231
  traumatic injuries to, 258-260
  tumors of, 252-253
Spiral fracture, 270
Spleen, 220
Spondylolisthesis, 34
Spondylolysis, 34
Staghorn calculus, 157
Staphylococcal pneumonia, 63
Stein-Leventhal syndrome, 173-174
Stomach, 81
  imaging consideration for, 84-85
Strangulated hernia, 104
Streptococcal pneumonia, 63
Stress echocardiography, 196
Stress fractures, 273
Stretch fractures, 273
Stroke, 210-213
  hemorrhagic, 210-213

Stroke—cont'd
    ischemic, 210
Subarachnoid hematoma, 264-265
Subcutaneous emphysema, 57
Subdural hematoma, 264-265
Subluxation, 280
Supernumerary kidney, 146
Surgical jaundice, 133
Swan-ganz catheter, 59
Sylvian triangle, 248-249
Symptom, defined, 2
Syndactyly, 19
Syndrome, defined, 2
Synovial joints, 16
Systole, 192

T

Tendinitis, 29
Tenosynovitis, 28
Teratomas, testicular, 184, 186-187
Testes
    carcinoma of, 184-187
    masses of, 184-187
Tetralogy of Fallot, 206
Thrombocytes, 219-220
Thrombolysis, 200
Thrombophlebitis, 214
Thrombus, 210
Thyroid gland, 57
TNM staging system, 10
Tomography, urinary system, 142
Torus fractures, 272-273
Toxic megacolon, 102
Trabeculae, 14
Traction diverticulum, 112
Transesophageal echocardiography, 197
Transient ischemic attack, 212
Transitional vertebra, 21
Transjugular intrahepatic portosystemic
        stent, 201
Transurethral resection of prostate, 183
Transverse fracture, 270-271
Traumatic disease, 9
    of abdomen, 287-289
    of chest and thorax, 283-287
    introduction to, 256-258
    level I, II and III trauma centers, 258
    of skeletal system, 34, 266-283
    vertebral column and head, 258-260
Traumatic spondylosis, 259

Treatment
    curative, 10
    palliative, 10
Tripod fracture, 280
T-tube cholangiography, 125-126
Tuberculosis, 24, 64-67
Tubes
    cantor, 90
    chest, 57-58
    Dohhoff, 90
    endotracheal, 57-58
    enteral, 90
    Ewald or Edlich, 88
    gastric, 88-90
    Harris, 90
    Levacuator, 88-90
    Levin, 88
    Miller Abbott, 90
    nasoenteric decompression, 90
    nephrostomy, 145
Tumor(s)
    of bone, 35-43
    brain, 243-250
    of central nerve sheath cells, 250-251
    of esophagus, 114-115
    gastric, 115-116
    giant cell, 39
    of liver, 133-134
    spinal, 252-253
    testicular, 184-187

U

Ulcer
    duodenal, 95
    gastric, 95
    peptic, 95-97
Ulcerative colitis, 101-102
Ultrafast CT, 203
Ultrasound
    central nervous system, 234
    Doppler sonography, 196-198
    echocardiography, 196-198
    female reproductive system, 170-171
    urinary system, 144
Unicornuate uterus, 172
Universal precautions, 221-222
Uremia, 156
Ureteral diverticula, 150
Ureteral stents, 145-146
Ureterocele, 149-150

Ureters, 139-140
Urethral valves, 150-151
Urinary system, 138-163. *See also* Kidneys
  anatomy and physiology review of, 139-140
  congenital/hereditary diseases
    lower tract, 149-150
    renal, 149
  degenerative/metabolic disease
    calcifications, 156-159
    nephrocalcinosis, 155
    nephrosclerosis, 155
    renal failure, 155-156
  imaging considerations
    computed tomography, 144
    cystogram, 144
    extracorporeal shock wave lithotripsy, 142-143
    intravenous urography, 140-142
    nephrotomography, 142
    renal angiography, 144
    retrograde pyelography, 142
    tomographs, 142
    ultrasound, 144
    urinary tubes and catheters, 145-146
  inflammatory diseases
    acute glomerulonephritis, 154
    cystitis, 154
    neurogenic bladder, 154
    pyelonephritis, 160-161
    urinary tract infection, 152
    vesicoureteral reflux, 154
  neoplastic diseases
    adenocarcinoma, 161-162
    bladder carcinoma, 163
    nephroblastoma, 162-163
    renal cysts, 159-161
Urokinase, 200

Uterine fibroids, 175
Uterine tubes, 168
Uterus, 167-168
  bicornuate, 171-172
  carcinoma, 175-176
  didelphys, 172
  unicornuate, 172

V

Valvular stenosis, 206-207
Veins, 192-193
Ventricles, right/left, 190-191
Ventricular pacing electrodes, 60
Ventricular septal defects, 204
Vertebra
  anomalies of, 20-21
  transitional, 21
  traumatic injuries to, 34, 258-260
Vesicoureteral reflux, 154
Viral hepatitis, 129-130
Viral pneumonia, 64
Virulence, defined, 8
Visceral cranial fractures, 278-280
Volvulus, 108-109

W

Whiplash, 34
Wilms' tumor, 162-163

X

Xeromammography, 171

Z

Zenker's diverticulum, 111-112
Zygomatic arch fracture, 278